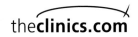

NEUROSURGERY CLINICS

OF NORTH AMERICA

Pediatric Spine Surgery (Part I):
Normal and Abnormal
Development of the Spine

GUEST EDITORS
Paul Klimo, Jr, MD, MPH, Maj, USAF
Jonathan R. Slotkin, MD
Douglas Brockmeyer, MD

CONSULTING EDITORS
Andrew T. Parsa, MD, PhD
Paul C. McCormick, MD, MPH

July 2007 • Volume 18 • Number 3

SAUNDERS

An Imprint of Elsevier, Inc.
PHILADELPHIA LONDON TORONTO MONTREAL SYDNEY TOKYO

W.B. SAUNDERS COMPANY
A Division of Elsevier Inc.

Elsevier Inc. • 1600 John F. Kennedy Blvd., Suite 1800 • Philadelphia, Pennsylvania 19103-2899

http://www.theclinics.com

NEUROSURGERY CLINICS OF NORTH AMERICA
July 2007
Editor: Joanne Husovski

Volume 18, Number 3
ISSN 1042-3680
ISBN-13: 978-1-4160-5095-7
ISBN-10: 1-4160-5095-7

Copyright © 2007 Elsevier Inc. All rights reserved. No part of this publication may be reproduced or transmitted in any form or by any means, electronic or mechanical, including photocopy, recording, or any information retrieval system, without written permission from the Publisher.

Single photocopies of single articles may be made for personal use as allowed by national copyright laws. Permission of the publisher and payment of a fee is required for all other photocopying, including multiple or systematic copying, copying for advertising or promotional purposes, resale, and all forms of document delivery. Special rates are available for educational institutions that wish to make photocopies for non-profit educational classroom use. Permission may be sought directly from Elsevier's Global Rights Department in Oxford, UK; phone: (+1) 215-239-3804 or +44 (0) 1865 843830, fax: +44 (0) 1865 853333, email healthpermissions@elsevier.com. Requests may also be completed online via the Elsevier homepage (http://www.elsevier.com/permissions). You may also contact Rights & Permissions directly through Elsevier's home page (http://www.elsevier.com), selecting first 'Customer Support', then 'General Information', then 'Permission Query Form'. In the USA, users may clear permissions and make payments through the Copyright Clearance Center, Inc., 222 Rosewood Drive, Danvers, MA 01923, USA; phone: (978) 750-8400; fax: (978) 750-4744, and in the UK through the Copyright Licensing Agency Rapid Clearance Service (CLARCS), 90 Tottenham Court Road, London WIP 0LP, UK; phone: (+44) 171 436 5931; fax: (+44) 171 436 3986. Other countries may have a local reprographic rights agency for payments.

The ideas and opinions expressed in *Neurosurgery Clinics of North America* do not necessarily reflect those of the Publisher. The Publisher does not assume any responsibility for any injury and/or damage to persons or property arising out of or related to any use of the material contained in this periodical. The reader is advised to check the appropriate medical literature and the product information currently provided by the manufacturer of each drug to be administered to verify the dosage, the method and duration of administration, or contraindications. It is the responsibility of the treating physician or other health care professional, relying on independent experience and knowledge of the patient, to determine drug dosages and the best treatment for the patient. Mention of any product in this issue should not be construed as endorsement by the contributors, editors, or the Publisher of the product or manufacturers' claims.

Neurosurgery Clinics of North America (ISSN 1042-3680) is published quarterly by Elsevier Inc., 360 Park Avenue South, New York, NY 10010-1710. Months of issue are January, April, July, and October. Business and Editorial Offices: 1600 John F. Kennedy Blvd., Suite 1800, Philadelphia, PA 19103-2899. Customer Service Office: 6277 Sea Harbor Drive, Orlando, FL 32887-4800. Periodicals postage paid at New York, NY, and additional mailing offices. Subscription prices are $231.00 per year (US individuals), $369.00 per year (US institutions), $253.00 per year (Canadian individuals), $440.00 per year (Canadian institutions), $303.00 per year (international individuals), $440.00 per year (international institutions), $116.00 per year (US students), and $149.00 per year (international students). International air speed delivery is included in all *Clinics* subscription prices. All prices are subject to change without notice. POSTMASTER: Send address changes to *Neurosurgery Clinics of North America*, Elsevier Periodicals Customer Service, 6277 Sea Harbor Drive, Orlando, FL 32887-4800. **Customer Service: 1-800-654-2452 (US). From outside of the US, call 1-407-345-4000.** E-mail: hhspcs@harcourt.com.

Neurosurgery Clinics of North America is covered in *Index Medicus*, *EMBASE/Excerpta Medica*, and *Current Contents/Clinical Medicine (CC/CM)*.

Printed in the United States of America.

CONSULTING EDITORS

ANDREW T. PARSA, MD, PhD, Assistant Professor, Department of Neurological Surgery, Neurospinal Research Center and The Brain Tumor Research Center, University of California San Francisco, San Francisco, California

PAUL C. McCORMICK, MD, MPH, Professor, Department of Clinical Neurosurgery, Columbia University College of Physicians and Surgeons, New York, New York

GUEST EDITORS

PAUL KLIMO, Jr, MD, MPH, Maj, USAF, Neurosurgeon, Medical Group, Wright-Patterson Air Force Base, Wright Patterson AFB, Ohio

JONATHAN R. SLOTKIN, MD, Chief Resident, Department of Neurosurgery, Brigham and Women's Hospital, The Children's Hospital, Harvard Medical School, Boston, Massachusetts

DOUGLAS BROCKMEYER, MD, Department of Neurosurgery, University of Utah; and Professor, Division of Pediatric Neurosurgery, Primary Children's Medical Center, Salt Lake City, Utah

CONTRIBUTORS

PANKAJ K. AGARWALLA, BS, Department of Neurosurgery, Children's Hospital of Boston, Boston, Massachusetts

RICHARD C.E. ANDERSON, MD, Department of Neurosurgery, Columbia University, College of Physicians and Surgeons, New York

DOUGLAS BROCKMEYER, MD, Professor, Department of Neurosurgery, University of Utah; and Division of Pediatric Neurosurgery, Primary Children's Medical Center, Salt Lake City, Utah

SHARON E. BYRD, MD, Professor of Radiology, Rush Medical College; and Attending Neuroradiologist, Section of Neuroradiology, Department of Diagnostic Radiology and Nuclear Medicine, Rush University Medical Center, Chicago, Illinois

MAURICIO A. CAMPOS, MD, Spine Surgery Fellow, Department of Orthopaedics and Rehabilitation, University of Iowa Hospitals and Clinics, Iowa City, Iowa; and Associated Instructor, Department of Orthopaedics, Pontificia Universidad Católica de Chile, Santiago, Chile

ELIZABETH M. COMISKEY, MD, Associate Professor of Radiology, Rush Medical College; and Attending Pediatric Radiologist, Section of Pediatric Radiology, Department of Diagnostic Radiology and Nuclear Medicine, Rush University Medical Center, Chicago, Illinois

MARK S. DIAS, MD, FAAP, Professor and Vice Chair for Clinical Neurosurgery, Department of Neurosurgery, Penn State Milton S. Hershey Medical Center, Penn State University College of Medicine, Hershey, Pennsylvania

IAN F. DUNN, MD, Department of Neurosurgery, Children's Hospital of Boston, Boston, Massachusetts

NEIL A. FELDSTEIN, MD, Department of Neurosurgery, Columbia University, College of Physicians and Surgeons, New York

TODD C. HANKINSON, MD, Department of Neurosurgery, Columbia University, College of Physicians and Surgeons, New York

PAUL KLIMO, Jr, MD, MPH, Maj, USAF, Neurosurgeon, Medical Group, Wright-Patterson Air Force Base, Wright Patterson AFB, Ohio

CORMAC O. MAHER, MD, Assistant Professor, Department of Neurosurgery, University of Michigan, Ann Arbor, Michigan

ROD J. OSKOUIAN, Jr, MD, Department of Neurological Surgery, University of Virginia, Charlottesville, Virginia

GANESH RAO, MD, Assistant Professor, University of Texas M.D. Anderson Cancer Center, Houston, Texas

CHARLES A. SANSUR, MD, Department of Neurological Surgery, University of Virginia, Charlottesville, Virginia

R. MICHAEL SCOTT, MD, Department of Neurosurgery, Children's Hospital of Boston, Boston, Massachusetts

CHRISTOPHER I. SHAFFREY, MD, Professor, Department of Neurological Surgery, University of Virginia, Charlottesville, Virginia

JONATHAN R. SLOTKIN, MD, Chief Resident, Department of Neurosurgery, Brigham and Women's Hospital, The Children's Hospital, Harvard Medical School, Boston, Massachusetts

EDWARD R. SMITH, MD, Department of Neurosurgery, Children's Hospital of Boston, Boston, Massachusetts

DEBBIE SONG, MD, Resident, Department of Neurosurgery, University of Michigan, Ann Arbor, Michigan

STUART L. WEINSTEIN, MD, Ignacio V. Ponseti Chair and Professor of Orthopaedic Surgery, Department of Orthopaedics and Rehabilitation, University of Iowa Hospitals and Clinics, Iowa City, Iowa

CONTENTS

Congenital malformations of the vertebrae are best understood in the context of our understanding of normal vertebral development. The author provides an in-depth discussion of normal vertebral development from gastrulation through vertebral ossification and provides multiple examples of how various disorders of vertebral development could lead to a variety of observed vertebral malformations.

Postnatal maturation of the spine is marked by the ossification process and by changes in the shape of the vertebrae, spinal curvature, spinal canal, discs, and bone marrow. Different aspects of the spine's maturation process are demonstrated on the three most common radiologic modalities used to evaluate the spine. Conventional plain spine imaging (plain spine radiography) provides a good initial evaluation of the bony spine. CT provides better bone detail and allows finer evaluation of subtle structures, the soft tissues of the spine (discs, ligaments), and the spinal cord. MRI provides excellent resolution of the bone marrow, ligaments, and discs of the spine, and can be used as an adjunct for evaluating the soft tissue of the spine and intraspinal contents.

There are numerous congenital anomalies of the cervical spine. They can be simple and clinically inconsequential to complex with serious neurologic and structural implications. They can occur in isolation or as one of several maldeveloped organs in the patients. Many are discovered incidentally. The more common anomalies seen by pediatric spine surgeons include defects of the anterior or posterior arches of C1, occipital assimilation of the atlas, basilar invagination or impression, os odontoideum, and Klippel-Feil syndrome. Management begins with a detailed history, physical examination, and imaging studies. In general, those lesions that are causing or have caused neurologic injury, chronic pain, or spinal deformity or place the patient at high risk for developing these require treatment.

FORTHCOMING ISSUES

RECENT ISSUES

THE CLINICS ARE NOW AVAILABLE ONLINE!

Access your subscription at
http://www.theclinics.com

ELSEVIER
SAUNDERS

Neurosurg Clin N Am 18 (2007) ix–x

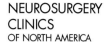
NEUROSURGERY
CLINICS
OF NORTH AMERICA

Preface

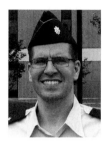 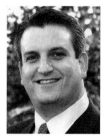 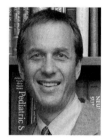

Paul Klimo, Jr, MD, MPH, Maj, USAF   Jonathan R. Slotkin, MD   Douglas Brockmeyer, MD
Guest Editors

In few areas of medicine is the old clinical axiom, "children are not just small adults" more true than in pediatric spinal disorders. The diseases that affect the pediatric spine are wholly different than those that occur in the adult spine. As such, knowledge of embryology, development, anatomy, biomechanics and pathophysiology are all necessary for any practioner caring for a child with a spinal disorder.

Management of these disorders has been strictly segregated to the domains of the neurosurgeon or the orthopedic surgeon, primarily on the basis of the type of disease. For example, deformity has been and continues to be primarily treated by orthopedic surgeons, whereas the tethered spinal cord is usually managed by neurosurgeons. However, this historically rigid model is showing signs of change as a growing number of neurosurgeons are taking an interest in all areas of pediatric spinal disease and there is a greater sense of interdepartmental cooperation to provide the best care for the children. Our goal in putting this project together was to present all of the major issues in pediatric spinal disorders in a comprehensive, up-to-date and easy to use format. Despite the seemingly inexorable move towards sub-specialization across all fields of medicine, we strongly believe that not only the pediatric neurosurgeon and the pediatric orthopedic surgeon, but others that help us on the "front line" in managing these disorders such as the generalist neurosurgeon and orthopedic surgeon, pediatrician, family physician, emergency room physician and radiologist need to have a firm grasp on the advancing concepts surrounding the pediatric spine. We originally set out to provide a broad yet complete single volume on the state of the art in the normal and abnormal pediatric spine. It quickly became apparent that this rapidly growing field would require more coverage than a single volume of *Neurosurgery Clinics of North America* would allow. The editor has kindly provided us with a wonderful opportunity to divide our coverage on The Pediatric Spine into two volumes, which should reach you, the reader, within a short time apart. This first volume that you hold will cover areas such as the normal development of the spine, congenital anomalies, postnatal maturation of the growing

1042-3680/07/$ - see front matter © 2007 Elsevier Inc. All rights reserved.
doi:10.1016/j.nec.2007.06.001

spine, skeletal dysplasias and other syndromes that affect the spine, an introduction to spinal deformity, the tethered cord, syringohydromyelia and the Chiari malformations.

We are quite pleased to have convened an outstanding group of authors to write these two volumes. All of our senior neurosurgical and orthopedic authors are true experts in the fields they cover for you within these pages. It is our hope that you get even a portion of the enjoyment and knowledge out of reading these outstanding contributions that we got out of assembling them.

Paul Klimo, Jr, MD, MPH, Maj, USAF
Wright-Patterson Air Force Base
4881 Sugar Maple Drive
Wright Patterson Air Force Base, OH 45433, USA

E-mail address: atomkpnk@yahoo.com

Jonathan R. Slotkin, MD
Department of Neurosurgery, University of Utah
Division of Pediatric Neurosurgery, Primary
Children's Medical Center
100 North Medical Drive
Salt Lake City, Utah 84113, USA

E-mail address:
jonathan.slotkin@childrens.harvard.edu

Douglas Brockmeyer, MD
Department of Neurosurgery
Brigham and Women's Hospital
The Children's Hospital
Harvard Medical School
300 Longwood Avenue, Bader 3
Boston, MA 02115, USA

E-mail address:
Douglas.brockmeyer@hsc.utah.edu

NEUROSURGERY
CLINICS
OF NORTH AMERICA

Neurosurg Clin N Am 18 (2007) 415–429

Normal and Abnormal Development of the Spine

Mark S. Dias, MD, FAAP

Department of Neurosurgery H110, Penn State Milton S. Hershey Medical Center,
Penn State University College of Medicine, 500 University Drive, Hershey, PA 17033, USA

Embryology of the spine

The development of the spine includes six separate but overlapping phases: (1) gastrulation and the formation of the somitic mesoderm and notochord, (2) condensation of the somitic mesoderm to form the somites, (3) reorganization of the somites to form dermomyotome and sclerotome, (4) the membranous phase of somitic development and resegmentation of the somites to form the definitive vertebrae, (5) vertebral chondrification, and (6) vertebral ossification.

Gastrulation and formation of somites and notochord

Within the first 2 weeks after fertilization, the embryo undergoes several cell divisions and cellular rearrangements to form a blastocyst—a two-layered embryo suspended between the amnionic and yolk sacs (Fig. 1). Cells on the dorsal surface of the embryo adjacent to the amnionic cavity comprise the epiblast, whereas cells on the ventral surface adjacent to the yolk sac comprise the hypoblast [1]. At this point, the embryo exhibits a craniocaudal orientation, with the prochordal plate visible as a cranial thickening.

During the second week, the embryo undergoes gastrulation. A midline primitive streak develops at the caudal end of the embryo and elongates cranially over 3 days (Fig. 2), occupying the midline in the caudal half of the embryo at its longest. The primitive streak subsequently becomes progressively shorter (regresses) and occupies a more caudal position in the embryo [1]. Throughout gastrulation, coordinated cell movements convert the embryo from two layers (epiblast and hypoblast) to three layers (ectoderm, mesoderm, and endoderm). Epiblast cells migrate toward the primitive streak and invaginate through the primitive groove within the primitive streak (see Fig. 2). During early gastrulation, while the primitive streak is still elongating, these invaginating cells form the endoderm [2–4]. Later, as the primitive streak regresses toward the caudal pole, the invaginating cells migrate between the epiblast and the newly formed endoderm to form the somitic mesoderm [3,5]. The remaining epiblast cells spread out to replace the cells that have invaginated through the primitive groove and form neuroectoderm and cutaneous ectoderm.

At the cranial end of the primitive streak is Hensen's node, within which is a cranial extension of the primitive groove called the primitive pit (Fig. 2B). As the primitive streak regresses, cells within Hensen's node invaginate through the primitive pit to form the midline notochord (see Fig. 2B) [3,5,6]. The notochord continues to elongate as the primitive streak regresses caudally and is flanked bilaterally by the newly developed somitic mesoderm; together, the notochord and somites form the axial skeleton. Both are laid down in a rostral-to-caudal direction. The caudal-most vertebrae are formed last from somitic cells derived from the caudal cell mass (the remnants of the primitive streak) and from caudal notochordal cells derived from the posterior notochordal center immediately cranial to the caudal cell mass.

Condensation of the somitic mesoderm to form the somites

The newly formed somitic mesoderm aggregates into discrete blocks of tissue, the somites (Fig. 3). The formation of somites is influenced by but does not require the adjacent notochord and

E-mail address: mdias@psu.edu

1042-3680/07/$ - see front matter © 2007 Elsevier Inc. All rights reserved.
doi:10.1016/j.nec.2007.05.003

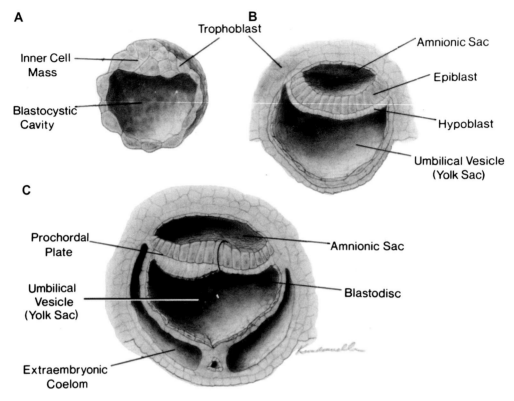

Fig. 1. Development of the blastocyst; midsagittal illustrations. (*A*) Continued proliferation of cells produces a sphere containing a blastocystic cavity surrounded by an eccentrically located inner cell mass and a surrounding ring of trophoblast cells. (*B*) Inner cell mass develops further into a two-layered structure, the blastodisc, containing the epiblast adjacent to the amnionic cavity and the hypoblast adjacent to the yolk sac. (*C*) With further development, the blastodisc thickens cranially to form the prochordal plate. (*From* McLone DG, Dias MS. Normal and abnormal early development of the nervous system. In: Cheek WR, editor. Pediatric Neurosurgery. Neurosurgery of the Developing Nervous System, 3rd edition. W.B. Saunders Co., Philadelphia, 1994; with permission.)

neural tube; somitic mesoderm cultured in isolation is still capable of forming segmented somites [7,8]. The first somites form early during the third week to form the cervical vertebrae [9].

Approximately five somites are present at the time the neural tube begins to close; succeeding somites thereafter form at the level of the closing neural tube in a rostral-to-caudal sequence.

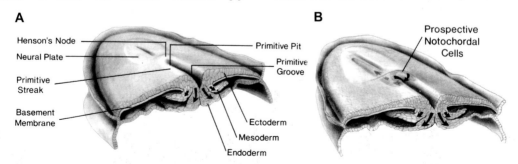

Fig. 2. Normal human gastrulation. (*A*) Prospective endodermal and mesodermal cells of the epiblast migrate toward the primitive streak and ingress (*arrows*) through the primitive groove to become the definitive endoderm and mesoderm. (*B*) Prospective notochordal cells in the cranial margin of Hensen's node ingress through the primitive pit during primitive streak regression to become the notochordal process. (*From* Dias MS, Walker ML. The embryogenesis of complex dysraphic malformations: a disorder of gastrulation? Pediatr Neurosurg 1992;18(5–6):229–53; with permission.)

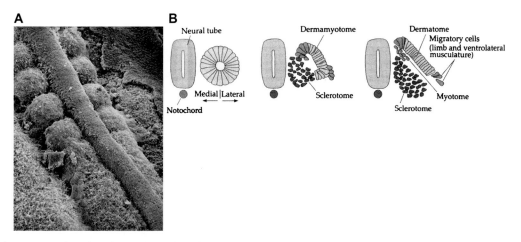

Fig. 3. Formation of somites. (*A*) Scanning electron micrograph of a chick embryo shows the somitic mesoderm forming as blocks of tissue from the unsegmented somitic mesoderm lying on either side of the midline neural tube. (*B*) Somite initially forms immediately lateral to the neural tube and notochord. Reorganization within the somite forms the dorsolateral demomyotome that gives rise to the skin and muscle, and the ventromedial sclerotome that gives rise to the vertebrae.

The patterning of the somites is determined by the interaction of various homeobox genes and their gene products. The specification of a vertebra along the craniocaudal axis is thought to be attributable to its Hox profile—the expression of various homeobox genes. Misexpression of one or another homeobox gene in mice can result in cranial or caudal transformation of various vertebrae. For example, the overexpression of Hoxa-7 results in a caudal translocation of the last occipital somites to form an aberrant proatlas rather than contributing to the occiput, whereas the true atlas, which normally would comprise only a ring, instead expresses a full vertebral body. In contrast, overexpression of Hox-6 results in a cranial translocation of the first lumbar somite pair to form a rib-bearing vertebra [10]. The misexpression of homeobox genes in human beings could similarly account for such malformations as the occipitalized atlas, cervical ribs, and lumbarized or sacralized lumbosacral vertebrae.

The maximum number of somites in the human embryo is generally given as 42 to 44, although no more than 38 or 39 are required for the formation of the axial skeleton [9]. Most of the "overage" is attributable to coccygeal somitic segments that disappear during subsequent growth, although a rearrangement or loss of the most cranial segments can occur as well [11]. The number and size of the somites seem to be species specific [12]. If somites are experimentally removed, the embryo is capable of compensating (regulating) to generate a normal number of somites of normal size [13,14]. Vertebral

malformations of the type seen in clinical practice are rare after experimental excision of somites, suggesting that such malformations may arise later in embryogenesis.

Formation of the sclerotome and dermomyotome

The developing somite becomes reorganized dorsoventrally into two parts: a ventral sclerotome forming the axial skeleton and a more dorsal dermomyotome forming the subcutaneous tissues and dorsal trunk musculature (see Fig. 3) [8]. The sclerotome and dermomyotome are distinguished by the expression of molecular markers, with the sclerotome expressing Pax-1 and Pax-9 and the dermomyotome expressing Pax-3, Pax-7, and Myo-D [15]. The formation of the sclerotome and dermomyotome is regulated by the notochord or neural tube floor plate (the ventral portion of the neural tube); the sclerotome can be obliterated by experimentally removing the notochord or duplicated by implanting an additional dorsal notochord [8].

The subsequent development of the somites can be divided into three phases: the membranous phase during the fifth week of embryogenesis, the chondrification phase beginning at the sixth embryonic week, and the ossification phase beginning at around the ninth embryonic week.

Formation of the membranous somite and resegmentation

The membranous phase begins during the fifth embryonic week, with sclerotomal cells from each somitic pair migrating ventrally to surround the notochord and dorsally to surround the neural tube. Ventral somitic cells form the vertebral centra. Each centrum develops a craniocaudal polarity during somitogenesis, with cranial and caudal portions having a unique histology and expressing a unique set of molecular markers [8,15]. The cranial portion of each sclerotome is more loosely organized, whereas the caudal portion contains more densely packed cells. Between the cranial and caudal portions lies a hypocellular cleft, the fissure of von Ebner. The craniocaudal organization of the sclerotome is critical to axonal outgrowth, because the outgrowth of spinal nerves at each level of the neuraxis is restricted to the more loosely organized cranial portion [7,15]. The dorsal vertebral arch seems to be exclusively derived from the caudal more densely packed half of the sclerotome.

There has been ongoing debate about whether each centrum is derived from a single sclerotome or from the fusion of the caudal and cranial halves of two adjacent sclerotomes with the hypocellular fissure of von Ebner contributing to the intervening intervertebral disc (a process called resegmentation, or *Neugliederung*). Resegmentation was originally proposed by Remak [16] in 1855 to account for the anatomic arrangement of the vertebral centra, dorsal vertebral arch, and spinal nerves. Because the spinal nerve passes through the cranial half-sclerotome at each sclerotomal level and the posterior vertebral arch is derived from the caudal half-sclerotome, one would predict that the spinal nerve would exit cranial to the corresponding pedicle. The

observation that each spinal nerve passes caudal to the corresponding pedicle could only be accounted for by resegmentation, such that the cranial loose-celled region of one sclerotome would join with the caudal dense-celled region of the next more cranial sclerotome to form a single vertebral unit (Fig. 4).

The concept of resegmentation was opposed by Verbout [17], Theiler [18], and others, who have suggested that each vertebra is derived exclusively from a single sclerotome. Experimental evidence favors the concept of resegmentation [19–21]. For example, labeling single somites by chick-quail chimeras (in which a single chick somite is replaced with a quail somite) or retrovirally mediated gene transfer (in which a somite is labeled with a recombinant retrovirus expressing a β-galactosidase marker) produces embryos containing label in two adjacent vertebral centra.

Chondrification phase

Chondrification centers appear within the sclerotomes during the sixth embryonic week. Three paired chondrification centers appear for each vertebra (Fig. 5A, B): one pair within the vertebral centrum, a second pair dorsolaterally within the posterior vertebral arches and spinous process, and a third pair between the first two and within the transverse process and costal arch. Chondrification begins in the cervicothoracic region and extends cranially and caudally thereafter; chondrification of the vertebral centra occurs before the dorsal arches. During the chondrification phase, physaliphorous cells of the notochord form the

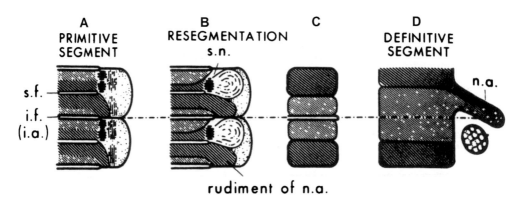

Fig. 4. (*A–D*) Resegmentation of the somites to form the definitive vertebrae. The densely hatched area is the dense-celled area, and the more lightly hatched area is the loose-celled area. For details, see text. i.a., intersegmental artery; i.f., intersegmental fissure; n.a., neural arch; s.f., segmental fissure (of von Ebner); s.n., spinal nerve. (*From* Tanaka T, Uhthoff HK. Significance of resegmentation in the pathogenesis of vertebral body malformation. Acta Orthop Scand 1981;52(3):337; with permission.)

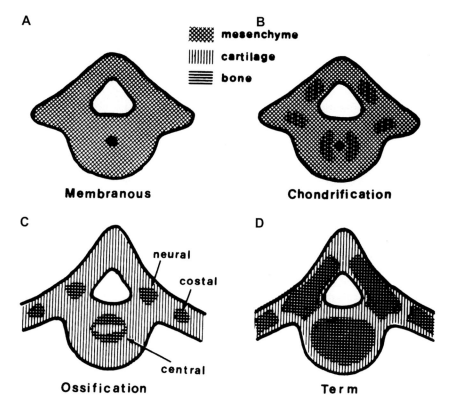

A Membranous
B Chondrification

mesenchyme
cartilage
bone

C Ossification
neural
costal
central

D Term

Fig. 5. (*A–D*) Chondrification and ossification of the vertebrae. For details, see text. (*From* Parke WW. Development of the spine. In: Herkowitz HN, Garfin SR, Balderston RA, et al, editors. Rothman-Simeone, the spine. 4th edition. Philadelphia: WB Saunders; 1999. p. 4; with permission.)

more centrally located nucleus pulposus and are surrounded by perinotochordal cells from the somites, which form the disc annulus [22]. The anterior and posterior longitudinal ligaments are formed during the chondrification phase from mesenchymal cells surrounding the cartilaginous vertebrae.

Ossification phase

Ossification of the vertebrae begins during the eighth embryonic week [23] and continues after birth (Fig. 5C). The number of ossification centers is still debated. Most authors describe three primary ossification centers—one for the vertebral centrum and one for each side of the dorsal vertebral arch. Within each side of the dorsal arch, the ossification centers form three independent ossification zones—one each for the pedicles, lamina, and transverse processes. Other authors have suggested two independent ossification centers within each vertebral centrum—one dorsal and one ventral—that fuse by the twentieth to twenty-fourth embryonic week. Still others have suggested that as many as six primary ossification centers may be present—two forming the vertebral centrum; two forming the pedicles, lateral masses, and transverse processes; and two forming the lamina and spinous process (reviewed by Ogden and colleagues [22]).

The centra first begin to ossify at the thoracolumbar junction (T10-L1) and spread quickly to T2 to L4 vertebrae. Thereafter, ossification proceeds in a bidirectional fashion to involve progressively more cranial and caudal vertebrae. In contrast, ossification of the dorsal arches begins simultaneously from C1 to L1 and proceeds craniocaudally thereafter. The centrum ossifies slightly before the dorsal arch [23,24]. All ossification centers are visible by 14 weeks of gestation [23,24]. The expanding dorsal and ventral ossification centers meet to form the neurocentral joint of Luschka. It is important to recognize that the neurocentral joint lies not at the junction of the vertebra and pedicle but within the vertebral body. The vertebral body is therefore derived from the centrum and dorsal ossification centers, and the terms *centrum* and *vertebral body* are therefore not strictly synonymous. Secondary ossification centers develop later in embryogenesis and are located in the ring apophysis and the tips of the spinous and transverse processes. The primary and secondary ossification centers fuse by the age of 15 to 16 years.

Cartilaginous end plates arise cranial and caudal to the ventral ossification centers. The ring apophysis develops at the periphery of the cartilaginous end plates between the developing intervertebral disc and the expanding ossification center of the vertebral centrum and is the analogue of the secondary ossification centers of long bones. The ring apophysis has a horseshoe shape, with a relative deficiency dorsally. At between 11 and 14 years of age, progressive ossification within the ring apophysis forms a radiographic "ring" [22] that eventually fuses with the vertebral centrum during middle to late adolescence. During childhood, fractures of the ring apophysis with displaced fracture fragments into the vertebral canal can simulate a herniated intervertebral disc clinically and radiographically.

The notochord proper contributes cells only to the intervertebral discs. During the embryonic period, the notochord develops craniocaudal segmented "undulations" with a more vacuolated appearance within the discs and a "mucoid streak" in the intervening centra. The mucoid streak largely regresses as the ossification centers appear within the centra; the remaining notochordal cells contribute only to the nucleus pulposus, although microscopic rests may sometimes be found within the vertebral bodies. The proliferation of physaliphorous cells largely ceases by the age of 5 years, and no viable cells usually remain in the disc; persistent notochordal rests likely give rise to chordomas [11].

Embryology of the craniovertebral junction

The embryology of the craniovertebral junction (CVJ) is unique and complex and produces malformations that are seen only in this region. The CVJ develops from the four occipital sclerotomes (formed from somite pairs 1–4) and the first and second cervical sclerotomes (formed from somites 5 and 6) (Fig. 6). The occipital bone, clivus, and occipital condyles are derived from the four occipital sclerotomes (somites 1–4), with sclerotome 4 forming the condyles, paracondylar processes, and the

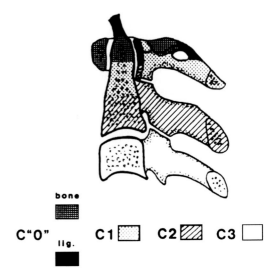

bone

C"O"   lig.   C1   C2   C3

Fig. 6. Development of the CVJ from the fourth occipital and first three cervical somites. For details, see text. lig., ligament. (*From* Parke WW. Development of the spine. In: Herkowitz HN, Garfin SR, Balderston RA, et al, editors. Rothman-Simeone, the spine. 4th edition. Philadelphia: WB Saunders; 1999. p. 9; with permission.)

bones surrounding the foramen magnum. The anterior arch of the atlas is derived from a dense band of tissue, the hypochordal bow, which is derived from the fourth occipital sclerotome (somite 4). The posterior arch of the atlas is derived from contributions from the fourth occipital sclerotome (somite 4) as well as the first cervical sclerotome (somite 5). The apical, cruciate, and alar ligaments are also derived from the fourth occipital sclerotome. The atlas ossifies from a single ventral and paired dorsal ossification centers. The anterior arch of the atlas is nonossified in 80% of newborns and usually ossifies between 6 and 24 months after birth [22].

The axis is derived from the fourth occipital sclerotome (somite 4) and the first and second cervical sclerotomes (somites 5 and 6). Rather than forming the centrum of the atlas, the ventral portion of the first cervical sclerotome (somite 5) instead forms most of the odontoid process. Notochordal remnants within the odontoid process confirm its origin from the centrum [11]. The odontoid process separates from the atlas between the sixth and seventh weeks of gestation. The cranial tip of the odontoid (the phylogenetic equivalent of the proatlas in reptile and avian species) is formed from the fourth occipital sclerotome (somite 4). The axis body and dorsal vertebral arch are derived from the second cervical sclerotome (somite 6).

Chondrification of the CVJ begins at 45 days of gestation, and chondrification of the C1 anterior arch begins at approximately 50 to 53 days of gestation [25]. O'Rahilly and colleagues [26] have described three parts to the cartilaginous axis in human embryos at 8 weeks of gestation, labeled X, Y, and Z. Parts X and Y form the future odontoid process, and part Z forms the axis body. The junction of parts X and Y can occasionally be seen as a lobulation in the midportion of the odontoid on lateral radiographs in infancy or early childhood.

Axis ossification involves six ossification centers. The odontoid contains bilateral ossification centers that may not fuse until 3 months after birth [22]; the odontoid tip (derived from the fourth occipital sclerotome) contains an additional ossification center. The axis body contains three ossification centers: a single ventral ossification center forming the centrum and bilaterally paired dorsal ossification centers forming the dorsal arch. Fusion of the odontoid and axis body at the dentocentral synchondrosis begins at approximately 4 years of age and is completed by 8 years of age; fusion of the apex of the odontoid to the odontoid proper occurs at around 12 years.

Development of the sacrum

The sacral and coccygeal vertebrae are the last to develop at 31 days of gestation. Chondrification is similar to chondrification at other levels, but the first three sacral elements contain an additional pair of ossification centers. Fusion of the sacral vertebrae begins during early puberty and is complete by the middle part of the third decade. The coccyx is formed from rudimentary segments. Ossification of the first segment begins between 1 and 4 years of age, with remaining coccygeal segments ossifying craniocaudally from 5 through 20 years of age. The coccyx is usually segmented, although fusion occasionally occurs.

Spinal malformations

Several classification schemes for spinal malformations have been proposed. The most recent and comprehensive classification by Tsou and colleagues [27] (Fig. 7) is based on alleged embryogenetic mechanisms, with modifications in response to more recent embryonic data obtained by Tanaka and Uhthoff [28]. These schemes propose that most vertebral malformations arise during the membranous (resegmentation) or early chondrification phase of vertebral formation, although certain malformations may arise during the ossification phase [27,28]. Vertebral malformations can be divided into at least seven categories according to reputed embryogenetic mechanism(s), although more than one mechanism may account for each malformation: (1) abnormalities of gastrulation (vertebral anomalies associated with split cord and other complex dysraphic spinal cord malformations), (2) disordered alignment of sclerotomal rests giving rise to hemimetameric shifts (hemivertebrae), (3) disordered formation of whole vertebrae (single or multiple) or of vertebral elements from sclerotomal precursors (vertebral wedging, hemivertebrae, or caudal agenesis), (4) disordered segmentation of vertebrae with or without associated vertebral formation defects (block vertebrae or Klippel-Feil syndrome [KFS]), (5) disordered alignment of vertebrae (congenital vertebral dislocation), (6) disordered assimilation of sclerotomal cells across the midline (butterfly vertebrae), and (7) disordered ossification and fetal growth (isolated defects of vertebral centra or dysplastic spondylolysis). Although this list is not intended to be comprehensive, the author gives concrete examples to illustrate the various vertebral malformations and attempts to place them into the context of disordered embryogenesis. Neither the cellular nor the molecular mechanisms underlying these malformations are understood.

Disordered gastrulation

Several vertebral malformations are associated with spinal dysraphism, particularly with split cord malformations. Dias and Walker [29] proposed that malformations of the neuraxis and axial skeleton involving tissues derived from all three primary germ cell layers, including split cord and other "complex dysraphic malformations," represent disorders of gastrulation. According to this theory, disordered midline axial integration during the period of primitive streak regression could result in paired notochordal processes and neural tubes (Fig. 8) as well as disruption of the adjacent somitic mesoderm. Subsequent embryonic repair of this initial disturbance could result in a variety of malformations that share a common embryonic mechanism, although they are phenotypically

CONGENITAL VERTEBRAL ANOMALIES

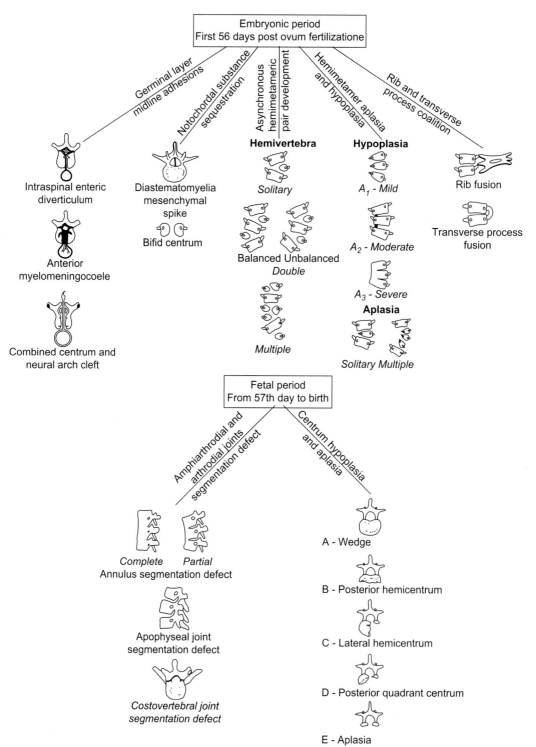

Fig. 7. Proposed schematic of vertebral malformations. For details, see text. (*From* Tsou PM, Yau A, Hodgson AR. Embryogenesis and prenatal development of congenital vertebral anomalies and their classification. Clin Orthop 1980;(152):214; with permission.)

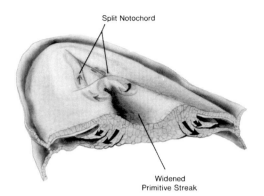

Split Notochord

Widened
Primitive Streak

Fig. 8. Proposed embryogenesis of split cord malforma-tions and other "complex dysraphic malformations." Abnormal gastrulation results in failure of midline axial integration. The primitive streak is abnormally wide; prospective notochordal cells therefore begin ingressing more laterally than normal. As a result, two notochordal processes are formed. The caudal neuroepithelium flank-ing the primitive streak also fails to become integrated to form a single neuroepithelial sheet and instead forms two "hemineural plates." The displaced somites (not yet formed) form abnormal vertebrae. (*From* Dias MS, Walker ML. The embryogenesis of complex dysraphic malformations: a disorder of gastrulation? Pediatr Neu-rosurg 1992;18(5–6):241; with permission.)

different. Hemivertebrae; sagittally clefted (butter-fly) vertebrae; fused (block) vertebrae; midline os-seous or fibrocartilaginous spurs or bands; and some types of the Klippel-Feil anomaly, inience-phaly, and sacral agenesis have all been described in association with these neural tube defects (re-viewed by Dias and Walker [29]). The association with elements of the split cord malformation and its sequelae is the key to identifying this embryopathy.

Malalignment of somitic columns: hemimetameric shift

Lehman-Facius [30] first suggested in 1925 that hemivertebrae may arise as a result of a "hemime-tameric shift" of the somitic column on one side of the embryo relative to the contralateral side. Tsou and colleagues [27] argued that whereas nor-mal vertebral centra arise from the midline inte-gration of paired somites at the same stage of development, tardy development of a somite on one side might lead to a caudal metameric (seg-mental) shift of one somitic column with respect to the other, an unpaired sclerotome, and a resul-tant hemivertebra (Fig. 9). The key characteristic

of this malformation is a hemivertebra having a rounded medial border that does not cross the midline. The contralateral portion of the centrum and the corresponding dorsal vertebral arch are congenitally absent [27]. The ipsilateral posterior arch is present but often incorporated into the ver-tebral arch above or below the hemivertebra and is difficult to see. The malformation may be uni- or multisegmental. This type of hemivertebra accounted for 58 (92%) of 63 cases in one series [27].

Disordered vertebral formation

Disruption or injury to the somitic mesoderm during gastrulation, to the somites during seg-mentation, or to the sclerotomal precursors dur-ing the membranous phase could unilaterally decrease the ability of the sclerotome to contrib-ute cells to the formation of the vertebra, resulting in unilateral vertebral hypoplasia or agenesis. Although disordered ossification was originally proposed by Junghanns [31], the presence of these malformations in embryos at 7 to 11.5 weeks of gestation [28,32] suggests that ossification is likely affected only secondarily. Examples of partially disordered vertebral formation are wedge verte-brae and less than 10% of hemivertebrae.

Tsou and colleagues [27] have applied the term *hemimetameric hypoplasia or aplasia* to these mal-formations and identify three types related to the severity of the deficiency. A key component is the involvement of the vertebral centrum and the pos-terior vertebral arch. In the mildest form, the quantity of cells from the ventral sclerotome is re-duced; decreased centrum height produces a wedge vertebra (see Fig. 9). In the moderate form, the posterior vertebral arch is deficient and the hypo-plastic posterior segments of adjacent vertebrae fuse to form a dorsolateral unsegmented bar, with additional rib malformations if the thoracic region is involved (see Fig. 9). In the most severe form, involvement of the centrum and dorsal arch leads to another type of hemivertebra. In contrast to the hemivertebra formed by hemime-tameric shift, contributions from the hypoplastic ipsilateral sclerotome produce a hemivertebra that is irregular and crosses the midline to a vari-able degree; a rudimentary rib may mark the site of the ipsilateral sclerotome. In the extreme, mul-tisegmental failure can occur and the hemiverte-bral elements are replaced at multiple levels with poorly differentiated fibrocartilaginous tissue [27].

424 DIAS

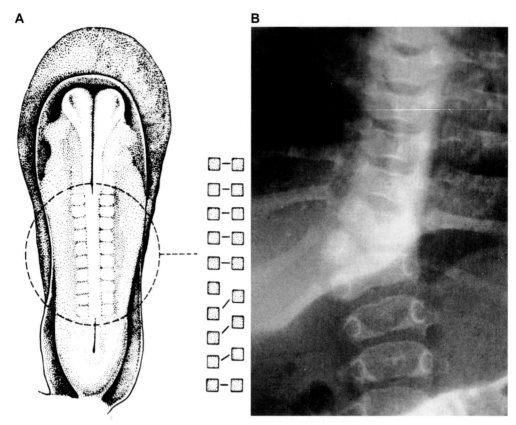

Fig. 9. Hemivertebra. (*A*) Schematic illustration of hemimetameric somitic shift producing a hemivertebra. If paired somites are not at the same stage of maturation at the time of somitic midline fusion, the tardy side shifts one segment caudad, producing an isolated hemisomite that develops into a solitary hemivertebra. (*From* Tsou PM, Yau A, Hodgson AR. Embryogenesis and prenatal development of congenital vertebral anomalies and their classification. Clin Orthop 1980;(152):218; with permission.) (*B*) Anterior-posterior radiograph of a hemivertebra.

Hemivertebrae of this type have been associated with dysraphic malformations, most commonly split cord and related malformations. The combination of a single hemivertebra with a contralateral congenital dorsolateral unsegmented bar is the malformation most frequently (50% of cases) associated with an underlying spinal cord malformation [33]. Associated renal malformations are also common with lower thoracic and lumbar lesions and are predicted embryologically by the close physical and temporal proximity of embryonic intermediate mesoderm during development, lying lateral to the somitic mesoderm and giving rise to the mesonephros. When renal malformations coexist with hemivertebrae, they are always ipsilateral to the side of the missing half-vertebra [34]. The underlying cause of the disruption is unknown, although a vascular

disruption of the intersegmental arteries during the membranous phase has been proposed by Tanaka and Uhthoff [32]. Those associated with dysraphic malformations may arise before neural tube closure and involve a disorder of gastrulation as discussed previously [29].

Disordered vertebral segmentation

Several malformations could be ascribed to disordered somitic segmentation. The simplest example of isolated failure of vertebral segmentation would be the block vertebra (fusion of two adjacent vertebrae). These may be ventral (affecting only the vertebral body), dorsal (affecting only the dorsal vertebral arch), or both. An example of more restricted dorsolateral failure would be the unsegmented bar (discussed previously). Multilevel vertebral fusions constitute the KFS.

The simplest mechanistic explanation would be failure within the prospective somitic mesoderm to segment properly into discrete somites, perhaps because of disordered expression of homeobox genes, cell adhesion molecules, or other molecular species. Keynes and colleagues [7] have described "segmentation-class" gene mutations in mice that display a variety of vertebral fusions, deletions, and malformations. For example, in the mouse mutant pudgy, only rudimentary segmentation takes place, resulting in multiple segmentation anomalies and irregular misshapen vertebrae [10]. Homologs of the *Drosophila* genes Delta and Notch seem to be particularly important in somite segmentation [8]; mouse mutants lacking in Notch expression exhibit severe defects of somitic segmentation and polarity, and microinjections of a dominant negative form of X-Delta-2 into Xenopus embryos cause multiple disorders of segmentation.

Alternatively, Tsou and colleagues [27] suggested that osseous metaplasia of the annulus ventrally or of the apophyseal or costovertebral joint dorsally during the ossification phase could account for vertebral fusions. Descriptions of block vertebrae at 5 to 7.5 weeks in human embryos suggest that these malformations occur much earlier, however, during or before the membranous phase [28,32]. Cervical vertebral fusions seen in KFS may reflect a disruption in subclavian or vertebral artery blood supply to the involved structures during or shortly before the sixth embryonic week, yielding not only cervical vertebral fusions but a Sprengel's deformity of the scapula, hypoplastic pectoralis muscles, and breast as well as terminal limb defects that are sometimes associated with KFS [35,36].Vascular mechanisms fail to explain the rare associated thoracolumbar or lumbar fusions (KFS type III) and sacral agenesis (KFS type IV), however [37]. Finally, the reported association of KFS with split cord malformations [29,38] raises the possibility that some cases may arise through disordered gastrulation.

Disordered vertebral alignment

Congenital vertebral dislocation is a rare condition that may represent disordered vertebral alignment during early development. Congenital vertebral dislocation (Fig. 10) results in a complete vertebral spondyloptosis at a single vertebral level (most commonly at or near the thoracolumbar junction) as if the entire vertebral column has been translocated. The spinal canal at the involved level is widened; the pedicles of the more superior vertebra are peculiarly elongated (see Fig. 10), and the dorsal vertebral arch is often dysraphic. The spinal cord is intact across the lesion but is almost always low lying (suggesting spinal cord tethering). Despite the severe disruption of the vertebral canal, these patients often have few or no neurologic deficits. Reported instances of tracheoesophageal fistula and unilateral renal agenesis suggest an early embryonic insult. Dias and colleagues [39] have proposed that these malformations could arise from simple mechanical buckling of the embryo between the fourth and sixth embryonic weeks, after neurulation but before chondrification has been completed.

Failed fusion of sclerotome, chondrification, or ossification centers

Various vertebral malformations may be attributable to disordered assimilation, or "fusion," of the various chondrification or ossification

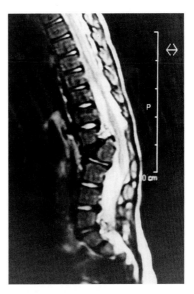

Fig. 10. Congenital vertebral dislocation. T2-weighted sagittal MRI scan demonstrates a complete and abrupt spondyloptosis of T11 on T12. Note the alignment of the T12 body with the more caudal vertebral column. (*From* Dias MS, Li V, Landi M, et al. The embryogenesis of congenital vertebral dislocation: early embryonic buckling? Pediatr Neurosurg 1998;29(6):284; with permission.)

centers. For example, sagittally clefted or butterfly vertebra could arise from disordered integration of sclerodermal pairs around the notochord, perhaps because of an abnormal perinotochordal sheath [40]. Butterfly vertebrae are experimentally produced in rabbits by maternal oxygen deprivation at stages corresponding to postconception days 23 to 27 in the human embryo and have been described in Danforth's short-tail mice (reviewed by Muller and colleagues [41]); notochordal abnormalities have been described in both. Experimental models and observations of human fetal malformations [41] suggest that these defects arise during the initial formation of the somites. Alternatively, a failure of bilateral (left and right) chondrification centers to become properly integrated could occur as late as the sixth embryonic week [41].

Localized failure of fusion of the ventral and dorsal ossification centers could result in malformations of the pedicles or facets, such as dysplastic spondylolysis. Similarly, failure to fuse the paired dorsal chondrification or ossification centers could result in spina bifida occulta, with a missing or malformed spinous process. A homeobox gene, Msx-2 (formerly known as Hox-8), is expressed in the spinous process and seems to be involved in the development of the dorsal vertebral arch during early embryogenesis. Mutations of the Msx-2 gene produce mouse embryos that lack a spinous process [10].

Isolated failure of ossification and growth

Isolated hypoplasia or aplasia of the vertebral centrum, without corresponding alterations in the dorsal vertebral arch, likely reflects a failure of centrum growth during later fetal stages [27]. All or part of the centrum is reduced or absent, but the pedicles and posterior body up to the neurocentral synchondrosis are intact. In the absence of corresponding dorsal arch anomalies, a primary sclerotomal disorder is unlikely; a disruption of the vascular supply has been proposed as a possible cause [27]. The posterior (dorsal) hemivertebra with isolated absence or wedging of the ventral portion of the centrum may also occur during later vertebral development, because the growth of the centrum is most rapid ventrally and would therefore be at greatest risk for vascular compromise. Conversely, if there are indeed ventral and dorsal ossification centers within the centrum, as some have described, an isolated failure of the ventral

ossification center could also produce such a malformation.

Malformations of the craniovertebral junction

Several malformations are unique to the CVJ and reflect the unique embryology of this region. These malformations include the following:

1. Dysplastic or aplastic occipital condyles
2. Atlas assimilation
3. Congenital absence of the anterior C1 arch
4. Absence or hypoplasia of the posterior atlas arch
5. Absence or hypoplasia of the odontoid tip
6. Absence or hypoplasia of the odontoid proper
7. Occipitalized odontoid tip
8. Failure of fusion of the odontoid tip to the odontoid body (os avis or ossiculum terminale)
9. Failure of fusion of the odontoid proper to the axis body (os odontoideum [OO])

Mechanistically, these anomalies can also be assigned to various reputed embryopathologic processes. For example, hypoplasia or aplasia involving any of the first six somites could result in isolated absence or hypoplasia of portions of the CVJ: an absent anterior atlas arch (inadequate development of the hypochordal bow), a hypoplastic or absent posterior atlas arch or absent odontoid tip (inadequate development of the fourth occipital sclerotome [somite 4]), or a hypoplastic or absent odontoid proper (inadequate development of the first cervical sclerotome [somite 5]). Unilateral failures have also been described and could be attributed to unilateral somitic aplasia: absence of one side of the anterior atlas arch (unilateral failure of the hypochordal bow) or posterior arch (unilateral aplasia of the first cervical sclerotome [somite 4]). Dubousset [42] described three types of atlas hypoplasia: type I involves an isolated hemiatlas, type II represents a hemiatlas with congenital cervical vertebral fusions, and type III is a partial or complete atlanto-occipital fusion with uni- or bilateral atlas aplasia. Type I represents isolated atlas aplasia, and types II and III represent a combination of aplasia and segmentation anomalies. Familial cervical dysplasia, an autosomal dominant condition, involves multiple malformations of the atlas and axis, most commonly posterior arch hypoplasia or aplasia [43]. Occipital condylar hypoplasia or aplasia has also been described and may represent another form of occipital somite maldevelopment [44].

Segmentation failures of the first six somites may account for other malformations of the CVJ. Atlas assimilation likely arises from failure of segmentation of the fourth occipital sclerotome from the first cervical sclerotome. Taitz [45] has described four types of incomplete atlas assimilation: the paracondylar process, epitransverse process, hypocondylar arch, and third occipital condyle. The first two represent bony projections between the transverse process of the atlas and the occipital condyle (paracondylar process) or jugular process of the occipital bone (epitransverse process), usually with a pseudoarthrosis [45]. The hypocondylar arch represents persistence of the hypochordal bow forming a rim of bone within the anterior rim of the foramen magnum between the two occipital condyles. The third condyle represents a rudiment of the hypocondylar arch as a small ventral "condyle" situated in the ventral midline of the foramen magnum [45].

A segmentation failure also likely accounts for congenital fusion of the odontoid tip to the anterior clivus (failure of the hypochordal bow to separate from the fourth occipital sclerotome), isolated or occurring in combination with other vertebral malformations. Recent attention has focused on the Hox genes, particularly the Hox gene Cdx1 in mice. This gene is expressed in the caudal primitive streak during gastrulation and extends as far rostrally as the caudal hindbrain. Inactivation of Cdx1 results in anterior homeotic transformation of the vertebrae—the anterior arch of the atlas is fused with the occiput, the posterior arch is hypoplastic, the second and third vertebrae are malformed, and scattered malformations are found as far caudal as the ninth thoracic vertebra. Disruption of Hoxb-4 leads to homeotic transformation of the atlas to the axis, whereas disruption of Hoxd-3 leads to cranial homeotic transformations of C1 and C2. These experiments suggest an important role of Hox genes and their gene products in the proper specification and segmentation of the CVJ [46].

Incomplete chondrification or ossification may give rise to several malformations. For example, incomplete atlantal chondrification or ossification may produce hypoplasia or aplasia of one or both posterior atlas arches. Failure of fusion of the posterior atlas arch generally is thought to represent a failure of chondrification, because the midline defect is filled with connective tissue rather than cartilage [47].

Abnormal fusion of adjacent ossification centers at the CVJ may produce several well-known malformations. Within the atlas or axis, failure of anterior and posterior ossification centers to fuse properly produces characteristic defects involving the predictable sites of normal fusion—anterolaterally and at the posterior midline. Failure of midline fusion between the paired odontoid ossification centers results in a bifid odontoid process. In an analogous manner, failure of fusion between the odontoid tip (fourth cervical sclerotome) and the odontoid process (first cervical sclerotome) results in ossiculum terminale (or os avis); in some cases, the odontoid tip fuses instead with the distal clivus.

The genesis of OO is a particularly fascinating study in the embryology of the CVJ. Traumatic and congenital forms have been proposed. Several illustrative cases in which OO developed months or years after trauma, with previously documented radiographs showing a normal odontoid, support the view that at least some forms of OO represent posttraumatic pseudoarthroses [48]. Others seem more clearly to be congenital in origin. The original embryogenetic theory to explain OO proposed a failure of fusion between the first and second cervical sclerotomes (somites 5 and 6). In a more recent study, however, Currarino and colleagues [49] suggest an alternative mechanism. A close inspection of radiographs in 10 patients with OO revealed that all had defects in the midportion of the odontoid (ie, within the odontoid proper) rather than at the synchondrosis between the odontoid and axis base. Six of these patients had various forms of skeletal dysplasia (diastrophic dysplasia, spondyloepiphyseal dysplasia, pseudoachondroplasia, and Larsen syndrome). Because no transverse segmentation exists in the midportion of the normal odontoid at any time during embryonic life, these findings led Currarino and colleagues [49] to conclude that OO represents an abnormal complete or partial embryonic segmentation within the odontoid itself. They proposed that OO arises because of an embryologically abnormal segmentation (complete or partial) of the midportion of the odontoid between chondrification segments X and Y.

Summary

It has been the author's intention in this article to prepare the reader to identify and organize the various congenital vertebral malformations that one sees clinically, the clinical aspects and surgical management of which are described in other articles in this issue. The developmental origin(s) of many of these malformations cannot be known with certainty, and it is likely that some, and perhaps even all, of the current models may eventually be proven wrong. Attempts to attribute these malformations simplistically to one embryogenetic mechanism (eg, failure of segmentation) are likely to be supplanted by more sophisticated models that involve the interplay of various genes (eg, Hox genes) in a complicated "developmental dance." Despite the limitations of our current models, however, the classification of various congenital vertebral malformations according to their reputed embryonic mechanism(s) at least provides a framework on which to base a better understanding of their anatomy and biomechanics. The next contributions to our understanding of this complex subject are anxiously awaited.

References

[1] O'Rahilly R, Mèuller F, Streeter GL. Developmental stages in human embryos: including a revision of Streeter's "Horizons" and a survey of the Carnegie collection. Washington, DC: Carnegie Institution of Washington; 1987.

[2] Vakaet L. Some new data concerning the formation of the definitive endoblast in the chick embryo. J Embryol Exp Morphol 1962;10:38–57.

[3] Rosenquist GC. A radioautographic study of labeled grafts in the chick blastoderm. Development from primitive streak stages to stage 12. Contrib Embryol 1966;38(262):73–110.

[4] Modak SP. [Experimental analysis of the origin of the embryonic endoblast in birds]. Rev Suisse Zool 1966;73(4):877–908.

[5] Nicolet G. Analyse autoradiographique de la localisation des différentes ébauches présomptives dans la ligne primitive de l'embryon de poulet [French]. J Embryol Exp Morphol 1970;23:79–108.

[6] Nicolet G. Avian gastrulation [French]. Adv Morphog 1971;9:231–62.

[7] Keynes RJ, Stern CD. Mechanisms of vertebrate segmentation [French]. Development 1988;103(3): 413–29.

[8] Gossler A, Hrabe de Angelis M. Somitogenesis. Curr Top Dev Biol 1998;38:225–87.

[9] Muller F, O'Rahilly R. Somitic-vertebral correlation and vertebral levels in the human embryo. Am J Anat 1986;177(1):3–19.

[10] Dietrich S, Kessel M. The vertebral column. In: Thorogood P, editor. Embryos, genes, and birth defects. Chichester (UK): John Wiley and Sons; 1997. p. 281–302.

[11] Parke WW, et al. Development of the spine. In: Herkowitz HN, Garfin SR, Balderston RA, editors.

Rothman-Simeone, the spine. 4th edition. Philadelphia: W.B. Saunders; 1999. p. 3–27.

[12] Flint OP, Ede DA, Wilby OK, et al. Control of somite number in normal and amputated mutant mouse embryos: an experimental and a theoretical analysis. J Embryol Exp Morphol 1978;45: 189–202.

[13] Smithells RW, et al. Apparent prevention of neural tube defects by periconceptional vitamin supplementation. Arch Dis Childh 1981;65:911–8.

[14] Bagnall KM, Sanders EJ, Higgins SJ, et al. The effects of somite removal on vertebral formation in the chick. Anat Embryol (Berl) 1988;178(2):183–90.

[15] Christ B, Schmidt C, Huang R, et al. Segmentation of the vertebrate body. Anat Embryol (Berl) 1998; 197(1):1–8.

[16] Remak R. Untersuchungen über die Entwicklung der Wirbelthiere. Berlin: Reimer; 1855.

[17] Verbout AJ. A critical review of the 'neugliederung' concept in relation to the development of the vertebral column. Acta Biotheor 1976;25(4):219–58.

[18] Theiler K. Vertebral malformations. Adv Anat Embryol Cell Biol 1988;112:1–99.

[19] Ewan KB, Everett AW. Evidence for resegmentation in the formation of the vertebral column using the novel approach of retroviral-mediated gene transfer. Exp Cell Res 1992;198(2):315–20.

[20] Bagnall KM. The migration and distribution of somite cells after labelling with the carbocyanine dye, Dil: the relationship of this distribution to segmentation in the vertebrate body. Anat Embryol (Berl) 1992;185(4):317–24.

[21] Bagnall KM, Higgins SJ, Sanders EJ. The contribution made by cells from a single somite to tissues within a body segment and assessment of their integration with similar cells from adjacent segments. Development 1989;107(4):931–43.

[22] Ogden JA, Ganey TM, Sasse J, et al. Development and maturation of the axial skeleton. In: Weinstein SL, editor. The pediatric spine: principles and practice. New York: Raven Press, Ltd.; 1994. p. 3–69.

[23] Bareggi R, Grill V, Sandrucci MA, et al. Developmental pathways of vertebral centra and neural arches in human embryos and fetuses. Anat Embryol (Berl) 1993;187(2):139–44.

[24] Bareggi R, Grill V, Zweyer M, et al. A quantitative study on the spatial and temporal ossification patterns of vertebral centra and neural arches and their relationship to the fetal age. Anat Anz 1994;176(4): 311–7.

[25] David K, McLachlan J, Aiton J, et al. Cartilaginous development of the human craniovertebral junction as visualised by a new three-dimensional computer reconstruction technique. J Anat 1998;192(Pt 2): 269–77.

[26] O'Rahilly R, Muller F, Meyer DB. The human vertebral column at the end of the embryonic period proper. 1. The column as a whole. J Anat 1980; 131(3):565–75.

[27] Tsou PM, Yau A, Hodgson AR. Embryogenesis and prenatal development of congenital vertebral anomalies and their classification. Clin Orthop 1980;(152): 211–31.

[28] Tanaka T, Uhthoff HK. The pathogenesis of congenital vertebral malformations. A study based on observations made in 11 human embryos and fetuses. Acta Orthop Scand 1981;52(4):413–25.

[29] Dias MS, Walker ML. The embryogenesis of complex dysraphic malformations: a disorder of gastrulation? Pediatr Neurosurg 1992;18(5-6):229–53.

[30] Lehman-Facius H. Die Keilwirbelbildung bei der Kongenitalen Skoliose [German]. Frankf Z Pathol 1925;31:389.

[31] Junghanns H. Die Fehlbildungen der Wirbelkörper [German]. Arch Orthop Unfallchir 1937;38:1–24.

[32] Tanaka T, Uhthoff HK. Significance of resegmentation in the pathogenesis of vertebral body malformation. Acta Orthop Scand 1981;52(3):331–8.

[33] McMaster MJ. Congenital scoliosis. In: Weinstein SL, editor. The pediatric spine: principles and practice. New York: Raven Press, Ltd.; 1994. p. 227–44.

[34] Tori JA, Dickson JH. Association of congenital anomalies of the spine and kidneys. Clin Orthop 1980;(148):259–62.

[35] Bavinck JN, Weaver DD. Subclavian artery supply disruption sequence: hypothesis of a vascular etiology for Poland, Klippel-Feil, and Mobius anomalies. Am J Med Genet 1986;23(4):903–18.

[36] Brill CB, Peyster RG, Keller MS, et al. Isolation of the right subclavian artery with subclavian steal in a child with Klippel-Feil anomaly: an example of the subclavian artery supply disruption sequence. Am J Med Genet 1987;26(4):933–40.

[37] Raas-Rothschild A, Goodman RM, Grunbaum M, et al. Klippel-Feil anomaly with sacral agenesis: an additional subtype, type IV. J Craniofac Genet Dev Biol 1988;8(4):297–301.

[38] David KM, Copp AJ, Stevens JM, et al. Split cervical spinal cord with Klippel-Feil syndrome: seven cases. Brain 1996;119(Pt 6):1859–72.

[39] Dias MS, Li V, Landi M, et al. The embryogenesis of congenital vertebral dislocation: early embryonic buckling? Pediatr Neurosurg 1998;29(6):281–9.

[40] Ehrenhaft JL. Development of the vertebral column as related to certain congenital and pathological changes. Surg Gynecol Obstet 1943;76:282–92.

[41] Muller F, O'Rahilly R, Benson DR. The early origin of vertebral anomalies, as illustrated by a 'butterfly vertebra'. J Anat 1986;149:157–69.

[42] Dubousset J. Torticollis in children caused by congenital anomalies of the atlas. J Bone Joint Surg Am 1986;68(2):178–88.

[43] Saltzman CL, Hensinger RN, Blane CE, et al. Familial cervical dysplasia. J Bone Joint Surg Am 1991;73(2):163–71.

[44] Nicholson JT, Sherk HH. Anomalies of the occipitocervical articulation. J Bone Joint Surg Am 1968; 50(2):295–304.

[45] Taitz C. Bony observations of some morphological variations and anomalies of the craniovertebral region. Clin Anat 2000;13(5):354–60.

[46] Subramanian V, Meyer BI, Gruss P. Disruption of the murine homeobox gene Cdx1 affects axial skeletal identities by altering the mesodermal expression domains of Hox genes. Cell 1995;83(4):641–53.

[47] Hierholzer J, Isalberti M, Hosten N, et al. A rare, complex developmental anomaly of the atlas: embryological and radiological considerations. Neuroradiology 1999;41(12):901–3.

[48] Ryken T, Menezes A. Cervicomedullary compression in achondroplasia. J Neurosurg 1994;81(1): 43–8.

[49] Currarino G, Rollins N, Diehl JT. Congenital defects of the posterior arch of the atlas: a report of seven cases including an affected mother and son. AJNR Am J Neuroradiol 1994;15(2):249–54.

Neurosurg Clin N Am 18 (2007) 431–461

Postnatal Maturation and Radiology of the Growing Spine

Sharon E. Byrd, MD[a,b,*], Elizabeth M. Comiskey, MD[a,c]

[a]Rush Medical College, 1653 West Congress Parkway, Chicago, IL 60612, USA
[b]Section of Neuroradiology, Department of Diagnostic Radiology and Nuclear Medicine,
Rush University Medical Center, 1653 West Congress Parkway, Chicago, IL 60612, USA
[c]Section of Pediatric Radiology, Department of Diagnostic Radiology and Nuclear Medicine,
Rush University Medical Center, 1653 West Congress Parkway, Chicago, IL 60612, USA

The spine is part of the supporting framework of the body and is composed of vertebrae, discs, and ligaments. It continues to mature postnatally, with marked changes occurring predominantly in the vertebrae during infancy, childhood, and early adolescence. Maturation of the spine is not only manifested by the ossification process but by changes in the shape of the vertebrae, spinal curvature, spinal canal, discs, and bone marrow. The parts of the spine and the maturation process can be evaluated by various imaging modalities such as conventional plain spine imaging (CPSI [plain spine radiography]), CT, and MRI. CPSI is historically one of the best modalities for imaging the bony spine. CT provides better bone detail and allows finer evaluation of subtle structures, the soft tissue of the spine (discs, ligaments), and the spinal cord. MRI is not the modality of choice to demonstrate bone detail but it provides excellent resolution of the bone marrow, ligaments, and discs of the spine. MRI can be used as an adjunct for visualization of the soft tissue of the spine and intraspinal contents (Fig. 1) [1–4].

* Corresponding author. Section of Neuroradiology, Department of Diagnostic Radiology and Nuclear Medicine, Rush University Medical Center, 1653 West Congress Parkway, Chicago, IL 60612.

E-mail address: sebyrd7730@sbcglobal.net (S.E. Byrd).

Anatomy

The spine consists of osseous and soft tissue components that provide support and mobility for the body and a protective covering for the central nervous system. The vertebral column is composed of 7 cervical, 12 thoracic, and 5 lumbar vertebrae; the sacrum (composed of 5 fused vertebrae that become progressively smaller); and the coccyx (3 to 5 rudimentary vertebrae). A typical vertebra consists of a body and neural arch. The neural arch is composed of bilateral pedicles, laminae, superior and inferior articulating facets, transverse processes, and a unilateral spinous process. The vertebral body is composed of an outer rim of cortical bone and an inner matrix of cancellous bone, marrow, and fat (see Fig. 1). Some minor differences exist at segmental levels of the bony spine. The cervical vertebrae (from C1 to C6) have a foramen in each of their transverse processes called the foramen transversarium (for the vertebral arteries) (Fig. 2). The first and second cervical vertebrae are unique and differ considerably from the other cervical vertebrae. The first cervical vertebra (atlas) has the shape of a ring. It consists of anterior and posterior arches with paired lateral masses. The arches form in the midline. Each lateral mass consists of a transverse process with a foramen transversarium and superior (condylar fossa) and inferior articular facets (Fig. 3). The second cervical vertebra (axis) consists of the odontoid process (dens), body, lateral masses, laminae, and a spinous process. Each paired lateral mass consists

1042-3680/07/$ - see front matter © 2007 Elsevier Inc. All rights reserved.
doi:10.1016/j.nec.2007.05.002

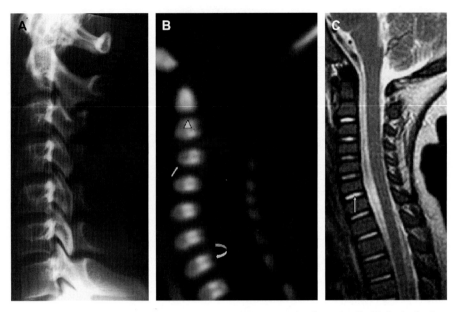

Fig. 1. Normal spine images. (*A*) Lateral CPSI in a 5-year-old demonstrating bone detail. (*B*) Sagittal reformatted CT (multiplanar reconstruction) of a 2-day-old demonstrating bone detail with oval-shaped ossification centers of vertebrae (*arrow*) with posterior channel for basivertebral vein (*curved arrow*) and subdental synchondrosis of C2 (*arrowhead*). (*C*) Sagittal MRI T2-W fast spin-echo in a 1-year-old showing bone marrow, hyperintense discs (*arrow*), and spinal cord.

of a pedicle, a foramen transversarium, and superior and inferior articular facets. The odontoid process consists of a tip (os terminale) and a body, which is connected to the main body of the axis at the subdental synchondrosis (Fig. 4). The thoracic vertebrae have costal facets for the rib attachments (see Fig. 2) [1–6].

Twenty-three intervertebral discs (IVDs) extend from the C2-3 to the L5-S1 intervertebral levels. No IVDs exist between the cranium and C1, between C1 and C2, in the sacrum, or in the coccyx. The IVD is composed of an outer fibrous tissue or fibrocartilage (the annulus fibrosus) and a central semiliquid gelatinous substance (the nucleus pulposus). The IVD is connected to the adjacent end plates of each vertebral body by its annulus fibrosus and is considered an amphiarthrosis, or half joint. The IVD becomes avascular after 4 to 5 years of age (Fig. 5) [1–15].

The other joints of the spine consist of the facet joints, the joints of Luschka, and the sacroiliac joints. The facets (apophyseal or zygapophyseal) are true synovial joints extending bilaterally from each vertebral level from C3 to S1, consisting of hyaline cartilage on the articular surfaces of the inferior articular facet of the superior vertebra to the superior articular facet of the inferior vertebra (Fig. 6) [1–15].

The joints of Luschka are not true synovial joints. They are bilateral articulation from C3 to C7 between the uncinate process of the superolateral margins of the vertebral body and the inferolateral margin of the above adjacent vertebral body. The joints of Luschka do not form until after 10 years of age when loose fibrous tissue in this area is reabsorbed, leaving a cleft that appears similar to an articulation. The sacroiliac joints are complex multiplanar articulations between the sacrum and pelvis. The costovertebral and costotransverse articulations are true synovial articulations between the ribs and vertebral bodies (costovertebral), and between the ribs and transverse processes. The craniocervical articulations are a complex set of synovial articulations that allow flexion, extension, and rotary motion of the head on the neck (see Fig. 6) [1–15].

The main ligaments of the spine are the anterior and posterior longitudinal ligaments running along the anterior and posterior surfaces of the vertebral bodies. The ligamentum flava join contiguous borders of adjacent laminae. The supraspinous and interspinous ligaments join adjacent spinous processes. The intertransverse ligaments join adjacent transverse processes (see Fig. 5) [1–15].

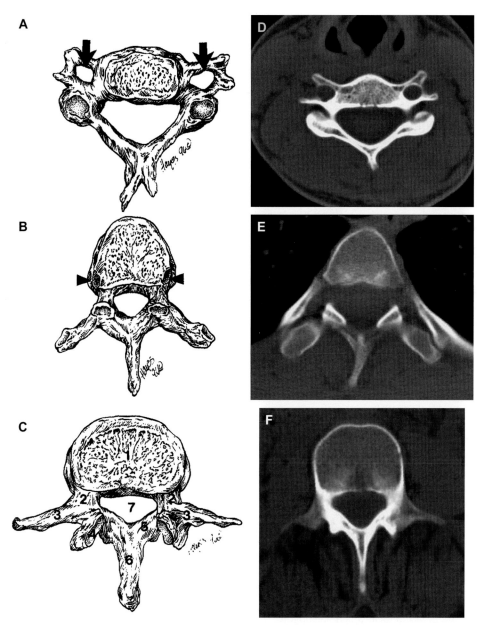

Fig. 2. Diagrams and CT scans of typical vertebra at each level. (*A* and *D*) Cervical vertebra diagram and CT axial with bilateral transverse foramina (*arrows in A*). (*B* and *E*) Thoracic vertebra diagram and CT axial with bilateral costal facets (*arrowheads in B*). (*C* and *F*) Lumbar vertebra diagram and CT axial; diagram shows body (*1*), pedicle (*2*), transverse process (*3*), superior articulating facet (*4*), lamina (*5*), spinal process (*6*), and spinal canal (*7*). (*From* McLone DG. Pediatric neurosurgery. 4th edition. Philadelphia: Saunders; 2001. p. 113; with permission [Fig. 2A–C].)

The major ligamentous attachments at the base of the skull, C1 and C2, consist of the anterior longitudinal ligament; the apical ligament (which extends from the tip of the dens to the tip of the clivus); the cruciform ligament (the transverse portion, which lies behind the tip of the dens between the inner aspect of the lateral masses of C1, and the vertical portion, which connects the body of the dens to the occiput); the posterior longitudinal ligament; the tectorial membrane (the

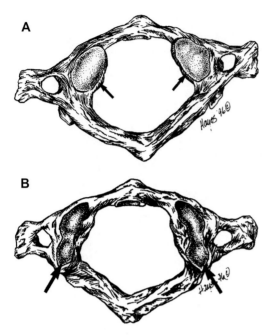

Fig. 3. C1 (atlas) vertebra: typical appearance. Superior surface (*A*) with condylar fossa (*short arrows*) for articulations with occipital condyles, and inferior surface (*B*) with inferior articulating facets (*long arrows*) for articulations with axis (C2). (*From* McLone DG. Pediatric neurosurgery. 4th edition. Philadelphia: Saunders; 2001. p. 113; with permission.)

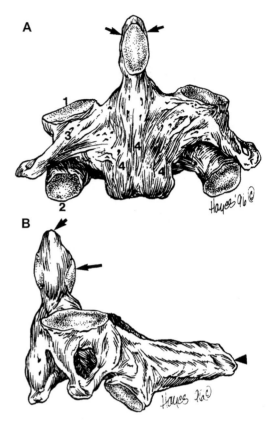

Fig. 4. C2 (axis) vertebra anterior view (*A*) with odontoid process (dens) (*short arrows*), superior (*1*) and inferior (*2*) articulating facets, transverse processes (*3*), and body of axis (*4*). Oblique lateral view (*B*) with tip (*small arrow*) and body (*large arrow*) of odontoid process and spinous process (*arrowhead*). (*From* McLone DG. Pediatric neurosurgery. 4th edition. Philadelphia: Saunders; 2001. p. 114; with permission.)

continuation of the posterior longitudinal ligament along the posterior border of the dens to the clivus); the atlantoaxial ligaments (which attach the body of C2 to the lateral masses of C1); the alar ligaments (which extend from the tip of the dens to the inferomedial aspects of the occipital condyles); the anterior atlantooccipital ligament (which is continuous with the anterior longitudinal ligament and extends from the anterior arch of C1 to the anterior portion of the foramen magnum ligamentum flavum at C1-C2); and the posterior atlantooccipital ligament analogous to the ligamentum flavum of the spine (which extends from the posterior arch of C1 to the posterior portion of the foramen magnum) (Fig. 7) [1–15].

The spinal canal is a bony tube lined with ligaments that contains primarily the spinal cord, spinal nerve roots, and cerebrospinal fluid. Its borders are anteriorly, the posterior aspect of the vertebral bodies, IVDs, and posterior longitudinal ligament; posteriorly, by the bony neural arch and ligamentum flavum; and laterally, by the pedicles and facet joints (see Fig. 5). It is round to oval in

shape in the cervical, thoracic, and upper lumbar regions. It becomes triangular in appearance in the mid- and lower lumbar and sacral regions. In the young adult, the sagittal diameter of the spinal canal measures 15 to 27 mm in the lumbar, 17 to 22 mm in the thoracic, and 15 to 27 mm in the cervical region of the spine [1–15].

The intervertebral foramina are bilateral bony openings extending the length of the spine, containing the spinal nerve roots, vessels, and fat. They are oval in shape and increase in size as they extend inferiorly down the spine. They are bounded anteriorly by the vertebral bodies and IVD, above and below by the pedicles, and posteriorly by the superior and inferior articular facets and ligamentum flavum [1–15].

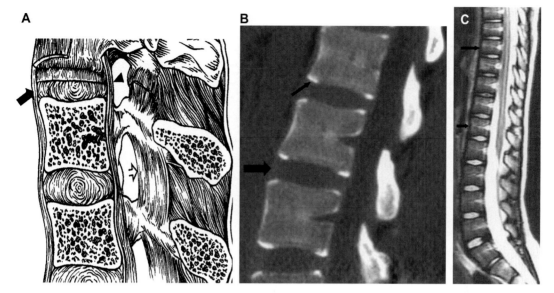

Fig. 5. IVDs and ligaments of the spine. (*A*) Lateral diagram of a segment of the upper lumbar spine with IVDs and ligamentous attachments: anterior (*closed arrow*) and posterior (*arrowhead*) longitudinal ligaments, ligamentum flavum (*open arrow*), and interspinous ligaments. (*From* McLone DG. Pediatric neurosurgery. 4th edition. Philadelphia: Saunders; 2001. p. 14; with permission.) (*B*) Sagittal multiplanar reconstruction CT of a 17-year-old upper lumbar spine. Vertebral body with ring apophysis increased density at end plates (*small arrow*) and isodense IVDs (*large arrow*). (*C*) Sagittal MRI T2-weighted image of an 11-year-old thoracolumbar spine with hypointense anterior longitudinal ligament (*arrows*).

Imaging modalities

Conventional plain spine imaging (plain spine radiography)

Various imaging modalities are available to evaluate the pediatric spine. CPSI is the initial modality of choice, with CT and MRI as adjuncts to define better the bone, soft tissue, or intraspinal contents. CPSI and CT use x-rays to create an image and thus are a form of radiation to the pediatric patient. Because CPSI uses ionizing radiation, care and experience are extremely important in obtaining adequate views. Initially, anterior-posterior (AP) and lateral views are obtained. Additional views, such as the lateral swimmers' view (to evaluate cervicothoracic junction), flexion and extension lateral views (to evaluate movement), oblique views, or views through the mouth AP (to evaluate atlas and axis) are obtained only depending on the history, the physical examination, or findings on the initial images (Fig. 8). Practices have changed and CT is now often used to evaluate the spine further, instead of obtaining some of these additional views (see Fig. 8).

The radiologic evaluation of CPSI consists of analyzing the soft tissues, alignment, vertebral bodies, posterior elements, spinal canal, and intervertebral (neural) foramina. All of the spine at each level should be visualized. For example, in evaluating the cervical spine, the craniocervical junction, C1 to C7, and the upper border of T1, should be seen. The prevertebral and paravertebral soft tissue symmetry, size, and delineation of normal planes are assessed. The prevertebral soft tissue of the cervical spine is best seen on the lateral view. The retropharyngeal space (between the posterior pharyngeal wall and the anterior-inferior margin of C2) should not be greater than 7 mm, with an average of 3.5 mm in children. The soft tissue space between the posterior tracheal wall and the anterior-inferior aspect of C6 should be less than 14 mm, with an average of 7 to 8 mm in children. Occasionally, a prevertebral fat stripe may be seen on the lateral view in children. This stripe is a thin radiolucent line adjacent to the anterior surface of the vertebrae, lying parallel to the anterior longitudinal ligament. These soft tissues planes can be seen not only on CPSI but also on CT and MRI (see Fig. 8). In the thoracic and lumbar spine, the paravertebral soft tissue is seen on the AP views. The soft tissue should be symmetric, with sharp planes [1–6,15].

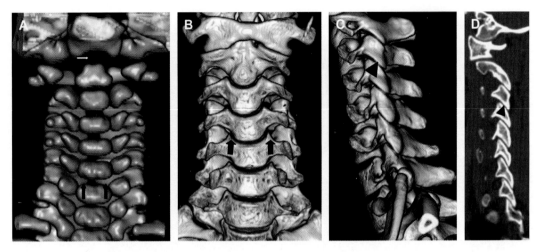

Fig. 6. (*A*) Three-dimensional volume rendering technique of anterior posterior view of cervical spine in a 2-day-old child; normally, the joints of Luschka (*black arrows*) and os terminale (*white arrow*) of C2 vertebra are not developed at this age. (*B*) Three-dimensional volume rendering technique of anterior posterior view of cervical spine in a 17-year-old with joints of Luschka (*large arrows*). (*C*) Three-dimensional volume rendering technique lateral view and (*D*) multiplanar reconstruction CT sagittal view of facet joints (*arrowheads*) of cervical spine in a 17-year-old.

The vertebrae should have normal alignment on all views. The spine should be straight on the AP view (Fig. 9). The normal lordotic curvature of the cervical and lumbar spine and the normal kyphosis of the thoracic and sacrococcygeal spine are seen on the neutral lateral view. Alignment of the spine is maintained by the ligaments, joints, vertebrae, discs, and adjacent musculature.

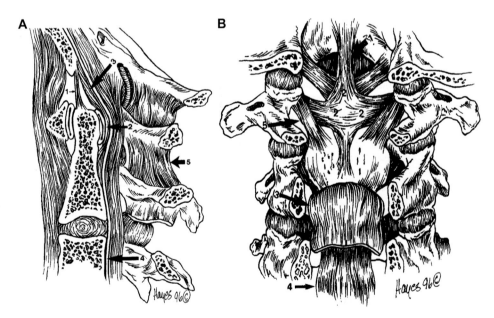

Fig. 7. (*A*) Lateral diagram of craniocervical junction with ligamentous attachments: apical (*1*), cruciate (*2*), tectorial membrane (*3*), posterior longitudinal (*4*), and spinous (*5*) ligaments. (*B*) Posterior-anterior diagram of ligaments at craniocervical junction with apical (*1*), vertical and transverse bands of cruciate (*2*), tectorial membrane (*3*), posterior longitudinal (*4*), and alar (*5*) ligaments. (*From* McLone DG. Pediatric neurosurgery. 4th edition. Philadelphia: Saunders; 2001. p. 115; with permission.)

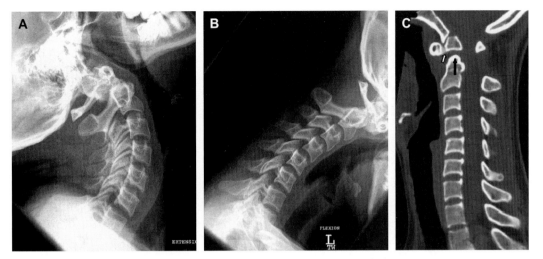

Fig. 8. CPSI lateral views in (*A*) extension and (*B*) flexion, and (*C*) multiplanar reconstruction CT sagittal in a 17-year-old with abnormal ununited os terminale of odontoid of C2 (os odontoideum) (*black arrow*) and fusion to body of C1 (*white arrow*).

Lordosis, kyphosis, and anterior and posterior subluxation are evaluated on the lateral views. Flexion and extension views may be necessary to evaluate abnormal movement of the spine. The degree of scoliosis, torticollis, and lateral subluxation is evaluated on AP views. The vertebra should align with those above and below. Imaginary lines can be seen, or lines drawn, on the CPSI images to connect parts of the spine to evaluate alignment. The most common lines are demonstrated on lateral views. The three lines are the anterior and posterior vertebral lines, and the laminar line connecting the laminae. These lines flow in gentle curves following the normal curvature of each specific level of the spine (Fig. 10). Straightening of the spine (loss of the normal curvature) on the lateral view is abnormal; some of the common causes are muscle spasm, trauma, infection, and poor posture [1–6,15].

Normal areas of pseudosubluxation can be seen on the lateral view. The most common locations of normal pseudosubluxation are in the cervical spine at C2-C3 and C3-C4 in young children and C4-5 or C5-6 in older children (Fig. 11). The C1-dens distance (atlantoaxial relationship between the posterior margin of the arch of C1 and the anterior margin of the odontoid process) should measure no more than 5 mm in children. This distance is usually between 3 and 5 mm in infants and young children, and can normally increase 1 to 2 mm on the flexion lateral view. Pseudospread of the lateral masses of C1 is a normal variant in infants, and could simulate a Jefferson fracture on AP views [1–6,15,16].

The vertebra (bodies and posterior elements), spinal canal, and neural foramina vary in appearance and size during the postnatal development of the spine. In general, in the older child, the vertebral bodies are rectangular in appearance. Unique vertebrae (C1, C2, sacrum, and coccyx) differ considerably in appearance from most vertebrae.

CT

CT is the next modality for evaluating the pediatric spine. CT is a computer-based non-invasive imaging modality that uses x-rays (ionizing radiation) to produce radiologic images in the axial, coronal, sagittal, or oblique planes. It provides the best bone detail, with some detail of the discs, paraspinal musculature, spinal cord, and nerve roots. State-of-the-art CT scanners can produce a submillimeter slice thickness image in less than a second. CT technology is based on a x-rays beam and detector system [17–21].

Introduced 30 years ago, CT has undergone breakthrough technology within the last 10 years, with the emergence of multislice CT (MSCT) scanners. One of the major advantages of MSCT is in postprocessing. MSCT, in comparison to single-slice CT, took a fundamental step from a cross-sectional view to a truly three-dimensional (3D) imaging modality that allows arbitrary cut

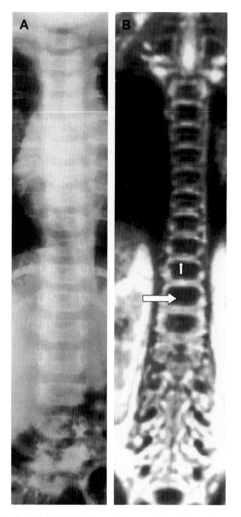

Fig. 9. (*A*) CPSI AP view with normal straight spine and paraspinal soft tissue planes in a 3-month-old child. (*From* McLone DG. Pediatric neurosurgery. 4th edition. Philadelphia: Saunders; 2001. p. 116; with permission.) (*B*) MRI T1-weighted coronal view with normal straight spine, hypointense bone marrow of the vertebral bodies (*large arrow*), and hyperintense cartilaginous end plates (*small arrow*) in a newborn.

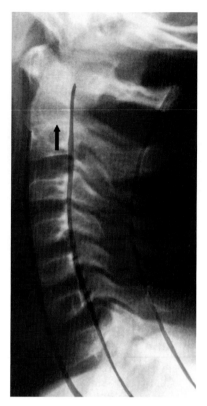

Fig. 10. Lateral cervical CPSI in a 3-year-old normal cervical spine with partial fusion (closing) of subdental synchondrosis (*arrow*), normal kyphosis curvature, and the three alignment lines (anterior, middle, and posterior).

planes and superb display of data sets. The newer generation of MSCT scanners allows near-isotropic voxel acquisitions, which is a prerequisite for delineation of highly detailed two-dimensional multiplanar reconstructions (MPR) and 3D reconstructed images (see Figs. 6 and 8). MSCT provides spine sections in the same image quality as the source. Any plane can be reformatted from the acquired volume. Three-dimensional postprocessing has different 3D rendering software packages. The two most common are the surface shaded display (SSD) and the volume rendering technique (VRT) (Figs. 12–14). SSD is capable of demonstrating gross 3D relationships but fails to display lesions hidden beneath the bone surface. The 3D VRT conveys more information than SSD and can show multiple internal and overlying features, such as the IVDs and ligaments and the bony vertebrae. One of the major disadvantages of MSCT is the increased radiation dose compared with conventional single-slice CT scanners; however, the radiation dose to the child can be significantly reduced by tailoring the image protocol (parameters) to the clinical question [17–21].

The spine is routinely scanned in the direct axial plane with the child supine. The x-ray beam is perpendicular to the long axis of the spine. With special software packages, the axial images can be postprocessed into coronal, sagittal, or oblique images with MPR, or into 3D images. The images are viewed with bone settings (high window and level settings) to evaluate bony detail and with soft

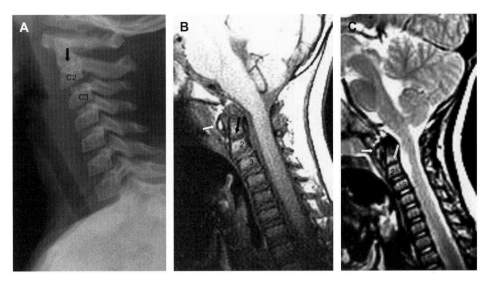

Fig. 11. (*A*) Lateral CPSI in a 2-year-old with normal pseudosubluxation C2-C3 and incompletely ossified subdental synchondrosis of C2 (*black arrow in A and B and large white arrow in C*). (*B*) MRI T1-weighted and (*C*) fast spin-echo T2-W in a 5-year-old with normal pseudosubluxation at C2-C3 and cartilaginous body of C1 (*small white arrow*).

tissue settings to evaluate discs, ligaments, spinal cord, nerve roots, and paraspinal muscles. In the infant and very young child, the discs and other soft tissue components are not well demonstrated (see Figs. 12–14). CT studies are routinely performed without intravenous iodinated contrast material. To evaluate the dura or soft tissue abnormalities of the spine, contrast may be required [17–21].

The anatomy demonstrated on the CT study of the spine is the routine spine anatomy, with bone anatomy and pathology being well demonstrated. Although soft tissue components such as bone marrow, discs, ligaments, spinal cord, nerve roots,

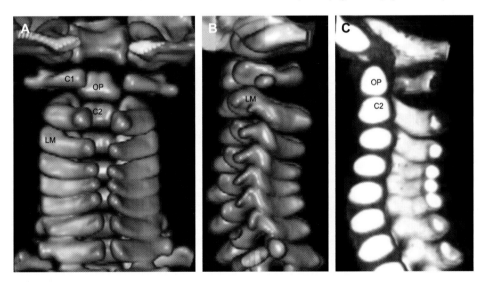

Fig. 12. 3D VRT images of 2-day-old cervical spine. (*A*) Posterior-anterior view with nonossified os terminale of odontoid process (*OP*), body of C2, lateral masses of vertebrae (*LM*) and nonossified laminae/spinous processes. (*B*) 3D VRT lateral view. (*C*) Midline section of the lateral view of 3D VRT with non visualization of body of C1 due to ossification centers not developed at this age, odontoid process (OP) and body of C2 ossification centers, cervical vertebral bodies demonstrate oval shaped ossification centers, as well as, ossification centers demonstrated in posterior elements of these cervical vertebrae.

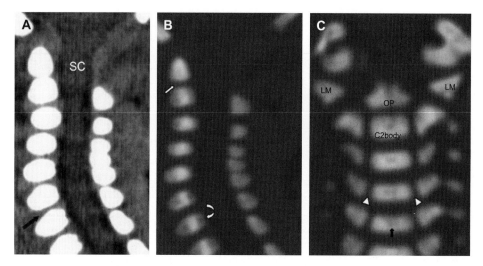

Fig. 13. CT of a 2-day-old newborn. (*A*) MPR sagittal soft tissue settings with spinal cord (*SC*), discs (*arrow*). (*B*) MPR sagittal bone settings with dense ossification centers of bodies and posterior elements of vertebrae, nonossified subdental synchondrosis of C2 (*small white arrow*), and posterior channel for basivertebral vein (*curved arrow*). (*C*) MPR coronal bone settings. No os terminale, not ossified, nonossified neurocentral synchondrosis at junction of bodies with lateral masses of vertebrae (*arrowheads*), C2 (body) and odontoid process (*OP*), channel for basivertebral vein (*black arrow*), C1 lateral masses (*LM*).

and paraspinal muscles are demonstrated on CT, these structures are better defined on MRI.

MRI

MRI is a computer-based imaging method that uses radio waves and a strong magnetic field to generate an image of the tissues and organs of the body. The contraindications to an MRI examination consist of various pacemakers, some aneurysmal clips, and any metal in the eye. MRI is the modality of choice in evaluating intraspinal pathology. It can be used as an adjunct in further evaluating bony abnormalities in children to

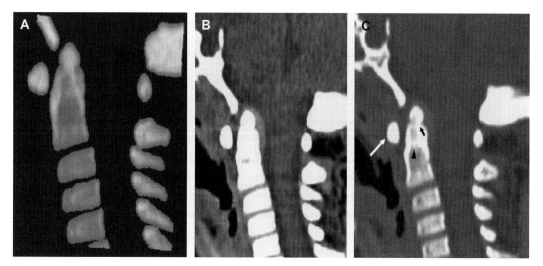

Fig. 14. CT of a 4-year-old cervical spine (sagittal views). (*A*) SSD bone settings. (*B*) MPR soft tissue settings. (*C*) Bone settings with body of C1 (*white arrow*), ossification of subdental synchondrosis (*arrowhead*), ossification of os terminale, and partial fusion with body of odontoid process of C2 (*black arrow*).

determine any compression or extension into the spinal canal. However, MRI's greatest role is in the evaluation of abnormalities affecting the soft tissues of the pediatric spine [7–10,18,22–24].

MRI is highly dependent on various factors that affect resolution (signal-to-noise ratio). These factors include the field strength of the MRI scanner and which technical parameters to use on the MR scanners, and the problems of physiologic and voluntary patient motion. Spin-echo T1- and gradient echo (GE) T2-weighted (W) or fast spin-echo (FSE) T2-W acquisitions are routinely used to evaluate the pediatric spine (Fig. 15). FSE T2-W pulse sequences scan times are shorter, and the resolution of the bone detail is better, than GE T2-W sequences. However, FSE T2-W pulse sequences do not suppress cere-brospinal fluid motion as well as GE T2-W sequences, and flow (motion) artifacts are more pronounced on the images of the spinal canal in infants and young children and may obscure intraspinal pathology. Therefore, flow compensation parameters should be used. The FSE T2-W pulse sequences do not effectively suppress fat, so if fat suppression is desired, a GE or FSE (with fat suppression) T2-W pulse sequence should be used [7–9,18,23–26].

It is important to obtain at least two MRI projections of the spine in children. The sagittal and axial projections are the most commonly obtained. However, in some children with severe scoliosis, some forms of spinal dysraphism, or paravertebral masses with spinal canal extension, the coronal projection may also have to be obtained.

Prenatal development of the spine

The development of the vertebral column occurs in three stages: membranous, cartilaginous, and osseous (Fig. 16 and 17). The notochord acts as a framework for the developing spine. Lack of development, or an arrest in the development, of the vertebra during the stages of chondrification or ossification can result in various anomalies in the pediatric spine. These anomalies range from sagittal and coronal clefting to an absent or hypoplastic body (Fig. 18) [1,6,10,27,28]. The prenatal development of the spine is discussed in detail in an article elsewhere in this issue.

Postnatal development of the spine

The spine continues to grow and develop postnatally, with major changes occurring in the curvature, vertebrae, ossification process, spinal canal, discs, ligaments, and bone marrow. These

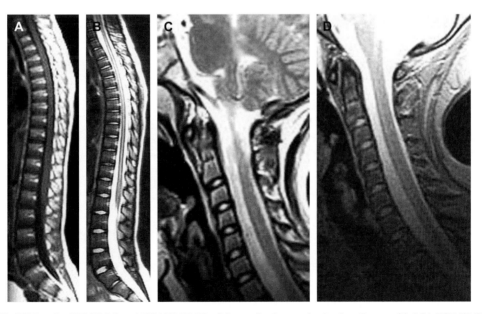

Fig. 15. MRI sagittal T1-W (*A*) and FSE T2-W (*B*) of thoracolumbosacral spine in a 7-year–old child. FSE T2-W (*C*) and GE T2-W (*D*) of cervical spine in an 11-year-old.

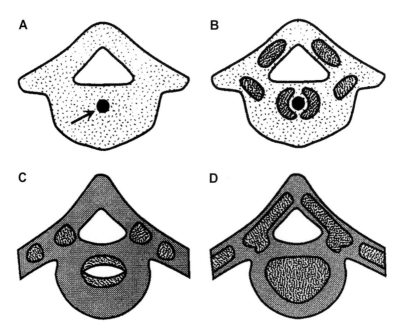

Fig. 16. Axial/transverse images of a thoracic vertebra demonstrating the three stages of development of the vertebral column: (*A*) membranous with notochord (*arrow*); (*B*) cartilaginous with chondrification centers; and (*C*) osseous with ossification centers. (*D*) The appearance of the vertebra at birth, with areas of ossification (centers) seen at birth on the imaging studies. (*From* McLone DG. Pediatric neurosurgery. 4th edition. Philadelphia: Saunders; 2001. p. 123; with permission.)

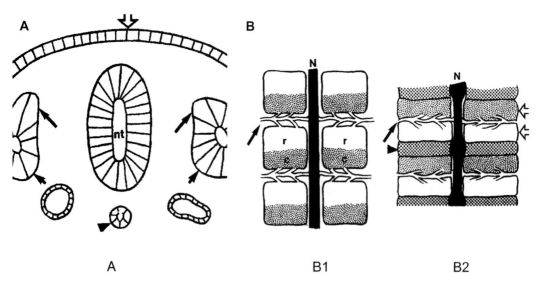

Fig. 17. (*A*) Differentiation of somites into sclerotomes anteriorly (*large arrows*) and demomyotomes posteriorly (*small arrows*) flanked by the neural tube (*nt*) and notochord (*arrowhead*), with all structures surrounded by ectoderm (*large open arrow*). (*B*) Development of sclerotomes into the vertebral column with division of sclerotomes into rostral (*r*) and caudal (*c*) halves (*B1*) and formation of vertebral bodies (*open arrows*) from the fusion of the caudal half of one sclerotome and the rostral half of the adjacent sclerotome; the IVD (*arrowhead*) forms from the caudal half of the somite (*B2*). (*From* McLone DG. Pediatric neurosurgery. 4th edition. Philadelphia: Saunders; 2001. p. 112–4; with permission.)

changes can be seen on the various imaging modalities used to evaluate the pediatric spine [1–6,29–40].

Curvature

At birth, the neonate has a very mild posterior convex curve seen on the lateral view. This gentle kyphosis is the primary curvature of the spine and is seen over its entire length. A totally straight spine is abnormal, even in the newborn. At 3 months, with development of head control, a secondary convex anterior cervical curve develops. This development is the beginning of the normal lordosis of the cervical spine. At 12 months, when the infant begins to crawl and walk, another secondary anterior convex curve develops in the lumbar spine. This development is the beginning of the normal lordosis of the lumbar spine. As the child continues to grow, movement is improved and the paraspinal muscles, ligaments, vertebrae, and discs develop further. The spinal curvature continues to develop into its adult configuration, with its primary curves of kyphosis at the thoracic and sacrococcygeal levels and secondary curves of lordosis at the cervical and lumbar levels (Fig. 19) [1–6].

Vertebrae

The shape of the vertebral bodies in the neonate is usually oval with slightly rounded anterior margins. This shape extends throughout the entire spine, although occasionally it may be more prominent at the lumbar level and the thoracic level may have a slightly squared appearance. The height of a vertebral body is about equal to, or slightly smaller than, the height of the IVD space as seen on lateral CPSI. This simulation of a smaller-sized vertebral body in the neonate is not a true finding. On the CPSI, only the ossified portion of the vertebral bodies is visualized, and the body and the IVD are not visualized, simulating a disc larger than it actually is. Two central indentations or clefts exist within the anterior and posterior walls of the midportion

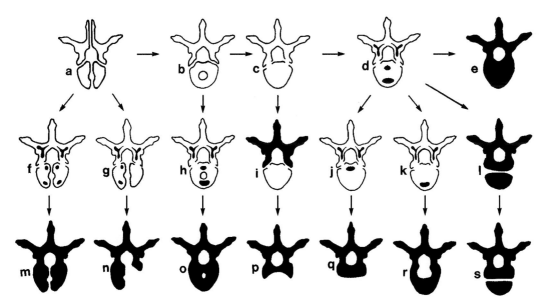

Fig. 18. Axial view of the normal and abnormal development of the vertebrae, with osseous formation in black and cartilaginous formation in white. (*a–e*) Normal formation of a vertebra. (*f–l*) Abnormal formation. (*m–s*) End-stage abnormality. The abnormalities are (*m*) vertebral body sagittal cleft due to nonfusion of the cartilaginous centers, (*n*) hemivertebra due to nonfusion of the cartilaginous centers with unilateral nondevelopment of an ossification center, (*o*) remnant of a notochord, (*p*) agenesis of a vertebral body due to nondevelopment of the ossification centers, (*q*) anterior hypoplasia of a vertebral body due to nondevelopment of the anterior ossification center, (*r*) posterior hypoplasia of a vertebral body due to nondevelopment of the posterior ossification center, and (*s*) vertebral body coronal cleft due to failure of the anterior and posterior ossification centers. (*Modified from* Harwood-Nash DC, Fitz CR. Neuroradiology in infants and children. St. Louis (MO): CV Mosby; 1976. p. 1055; with permission.)

of the vertebral bodies. These anterior and poste-rior indentations represent vascular channels. The anterior channel consists of nutrient artery and a sinusoidal channel that disappears by the end of the first year of life. However, the anterior channel may be sharply visible up to 3 to 6 years of age and may persist as a slitlike channel with sclerotic margins. The posterior channel consists of a drain-ing vein (the basivertebral vein) and a nutrient artery. The posterior channel does not disappear but persists throughout childhood into adulthood (see Figs. 13, 19) [1–6,29,31,32,34–36].

In the neonate, a normal variation in appear-ance of the vertebral body of "bone within bone" can be seen on CPSI. This appearance of a lucent area within the outer aspect of the ossified vertebral body is more common in premature infants but can be seen in some series in as many as 50% of full-term normal infants. This appear-ance is related to the normal ossification process of the vertebral body. It is primarily seen before 6 weeks of age and disappears by 2 to 3 months of age (see Fig. 19) [6,40,41].

The coronal cleft in the vertebral body can be a normal variation or a pathologic process. The coronal cleft is an incidental finding that usually involves the lower lumbar vertebrae (L3-L5), with L4 being the most common. It can be seen occasionally at the thoracic level. It is usually single (38%) but it can involve two (18%), three (18%), or multiple (25%) vertebral bodies. It is seen on the lateral CPSI in the midhalf of the ver-tebral body. The coronal cleft is seen within the first few months of life and disappears by age 6 to 12 months, although it can persist for up to 2 to 3 years. The cleft is believed to be a result of slow or delayed fusion of the anterior and poste-rior ossification centers of the vertebral body. Per-sistence of a coronal cleft is not necessarily significant, although persistent coronal clefts are associated with other segmentation anomalies of the vertebral bodies and spinal dysraphic condi-tions [1–6].

On the lateral CPSI, the ossified vertebral body does not appear connected to the ossified neural arch (see Fig. 19; Fig. 20). The lucent area at this junction on the lateral CPSI is nonossified neuro-central synchondrosis. The neurocentral syn-chondroses are paired and connect both sides of the neural arch to the vertebral body. The paired

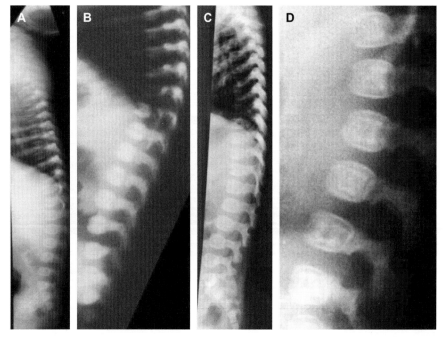

Fig. 19. Lateral CPSI normal spines. (*A*) Relatively straight thoracolumbosacreal spine of a newborn. (*B*) Relatively straight lower thoracic lumbosacreal spine of a 1-month-old with anterior notches for vessels and neurocentral syn-chondrosis. (*C*) Thoracolumbosacral spine of a 1-year-old with beginning of formation of curvatures. (*D*) Thoracolum-bar spine in 5-week-old demonstrating "bone with bone" appearance and anterior notch in vertebral body for anterior vascular channel.

neurocentral synchondroses are seen on AP CPSI along the lateral aspect of each side of the spine. The primary ossification centers of the posterior elements of the vertebrae are present, although the laminae are not fused [1–6,37].

Ossification is present within parts of all of the vertebrae from C1 to sacrum and can be seen on CPSI at birth. C1 and C2 ossify slightly differently than the other vertebrae, and certain important parts (such as the body of C1 and part of the odontoid process) are not seen on the CPSI at birth. The coccyx is not ossified at birth and is not demonstrated on CPSI [38,39].

With further development of the vertebrae at age 2 to 3, the vertebral bodies assume a more rectangular shape, which continues throughout life. The AP diameter of the vertebral body is greater than its vertical height, and its vertical height is greater than the IVD height. The vertebrae continue to ossify, with an increase in density (ossification) occurring within the neurocentral synchondroses by age 3 to 6 [1–6].

By age 5 to 8, superior and inferior steplike recesses appear on the anterior surface of the vertebral bodies, producing an anterior beaking on lateral CPSI (Fig. 21). This finding is caused by an annular rim of cartilage that develops at this time called the ring apophyses. This rim forms over the superior and inferior surfaces of the vertebral bodies. It extends more into the upper and lower anterior borders of the body. This cartilage rim develops outside of the cartilaginous end plates and does not take part in the growth of the vertebral body. This annular ring apophysis begins to ossify and small calcific foci are usually seen at the superior and inferior anterior borders of the vertebral body, most often at the lumbar and thoracic levels and less commonly at the cervical level (Fig. 22). The calcification of the ring apophysis begins to coalesce and ossify to form a complete ring by puberty and to fuse with the remainder of the vertebral body by age 18 to 25. The beaking of the vertebral bodies disappears by puberty (age 10 to 13) but the calcification and later ossification at the superior and inferior rims may persist until 18 to 25 years of age. This normal beaking of the vertebral bodies is never as severe as seen in pathologic conditions such as Morquio's syndrome [1–6].

The last important process that changes the shape and size of the vertebrae is the development of the secondary ossification centers. These centers occur at the tips of the transverse processes, superior and inferior articulating facets, spinous process, and ring apophysis by puberty, with complete ossification by age 18 to 25. These secondary ossification centers can be seen as small lucent areas just proximal to the tips of these processes on CPSI (Fig. 23) (Table 1) [1–6].

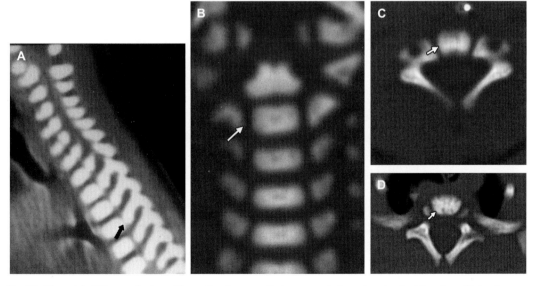

Fig. 20. Neonate's CT scan of spine with nonfused, nonossified neurocentral synchondrosis at junction of lateral masses with the bodies of the vertebrae (*arrows*). (*A*) MPR sagittal off-midline, slightly rotated cervicothoracic spine. (*B*) MPR coronal. (*C*) Axial of C4. (*D*) Axial of T1.

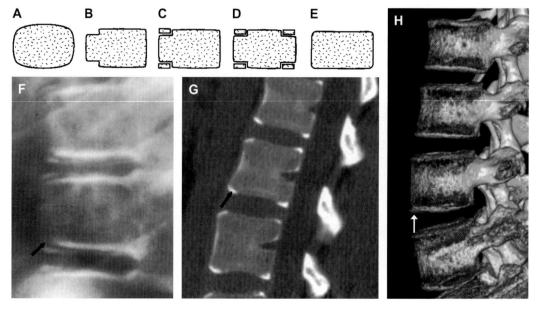

Fig. 21. (*A–E*) Lateral views of the postnatal development of the vertebral body. (*A*) Newborn with oval shape. (*From* McLone DG. Pediatric neurosurgery. 4th edition. Philadelphia: Saunders; 2001. p. 129; with permission.) (*B*) Age 5 to 8, with the beginning of development of the ring apophyses (with superior and inferior steplike indentations). (*C*) Beginning of calcification of the ring apophyses. (*D*) Vertebra with calcification in the anterior and posterior ring apophyses. (*E*) Ossified ring apophyses with a rectangular-shaped vertebral body in a teenager. (*F*) CPSI lateral view of upper lumbar vertebrae, (*G*) CT MPR sagittal of upper lumbar vertebrae, and (*H*) 3D VRT lateral view of lumbar vertebrae, with ossification of portions of the ring apophyses (*arrows*).

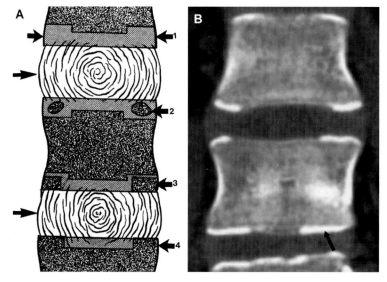

Fig. 22. (*A*) Sagittal view of the lumbar spine showing the relationship of IVDs (*large arrows*) to ossification of the ring apophysis with cartilaginous ring (*1*), appearance of ossification centers (*2*), further enlargement of ossification centers (*3*), and fusion of ossification of the ring to the vertebral body (*4*). (*Modified from* Silverman FN, Kuhn JP. Caffey's pediatric x-ray diagnosis: an integrated imaging approach. St. Louis (MO): CV Mosby; 1993. p. 134; with permission.) (*B*) CT MPR coronal view of upper lumbar spine with ossification in ring apophysis area of increased density (*arrow*). (*From* McLone DG. Pediatric neurosurgery. 4th edition. Philadelphia: Saunders; 2001. p. 112–4; with permission.)

Table 1
Maturation of the spine

Vertebrae	Primary ossification centers	Age at presentation	Age at closure	
			Neurocentral synchondrosis	Laminae
C3-L5	1 middle (body)	At birth	3–6 y	1–3 y
	2 lateral (1 in each half of neural arch)	At birth		
C1	Middle (body)	20% at birth; 80% 6–12 mo	5–7 y (average 6 y)	3–4 y
C2	1 body of C2	At birth	3–6 y	3–6 y
	2 lateral (1 in each half of neural arch)	At birth		
	1 body of dens (rarely, 2)	At birth		
	1 tip of dens (os terminale)	2–6 y fuses with body of dens (10–12 y)		

Vertebrae	Secondary ossification centers	Age at presentation	Ossification completed
C3-L5	Superior articulating facets	Puberty (10–13 y)	18–25 y
	Inferior articulating facets	10–13 y	18–25 y
	Transverses processes	10–13 y	18–25 y
	Spinous process	10–13 y	18–25 y
C3-L5	Ring apophyses	Puberty (10–13 y)	18–25 y

From McLone DG. Pediatric neurosurgery. 4th edition. Philadelphia: Saunders; 2001. p. 125; with permission.

Ossification process

The ossification process within the vertebrae is an ongoing process from fetal development until early adulthood. Most primary ossification centers develop with the vertebral bodies and neural arches during the ossification stage of development of the bony spine, beginning at the eighth week of gestation. At birth, these primary ossification centers can be seen as three bony centers within each vertebra from C3 to L5. Each of these vertebrae has one center in the centrum (the vertebral body) and one in each half of the neural arch (Fig. 24). These ossification centers can be seen at birth as areas of increased density (ossification) within the vertebral body and neural arch. Cartilaginous attachments called

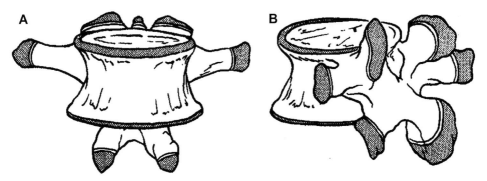

Fig. 23. Vertebra. Anteroposterior (*A*) and oblique lateral (*B*) views of development of secondary ossification centers at the tips of the superior and inferior articulating facets, transverse processes, spinous process, and ring apophysis at the superior and inferior surfaces of the vertebral body. (*From* McLone DG. Pediatric neurosurgery. 4th edition. Philadelphia: Saunders; 2001. p. 129; with permission.)

neurocental synchondroses are on each side of the neural arch to the vertebral body. These synchondroses appear lucent on CPSI but they ossify and become dense on CPSI by age 3 to 6. This ossification proceeds in an orderly fashion from cephalad to caudal, with ossification occurring first in the cervical vertebrae at age 2 to 3 and progressing inferiorly, with completion by age 6 to 7 in the lumbar region. When the ossification process is complete in the neurocentral synchondroses, the vertebral body is fused to the neural arch. The laminae fuse posteriorly in the midline by age 1 to 3. This process continues in an orderly fashion from inferior to superior, with the laminae fusing in the lumbar area beginning at the end of the first year of life and progressing superiorly, with fusion of the cervical laminae by 3 years of age (Fig. 25) [1–6].

The primary ossification centers of C1, C2, sacrum, and coccyx appear at slightly different times when compared with the rest of the vertebrae (C3-L5). The atlas (C1) commonly has two primary ossification centers at birth, one in each half of the neural arch. The primary ossification center in the body of C1 is only present 20% of the time at birth. It usually appears between the sixth to the twelfth month of life. The neurocentral synchondroses of C1 usually fuse by age 5 to 7 (about 6) and the laminae fuse by age 3 to 4, although nonfusion of the laminae is a common malformation seen at C1 (Figs. 26 and 27) [1–6,38,42].

The axis (C2) has four primary ossification centers at birth, one within the half of each neural arch, one in the body of C2, and one in the body of the dens of C2. The body of the dens (odontoid process) initially has two ossification centers (one on each side) during fetal development. These two ossification centers usually fuse before birth, with one center appearing at birth on CPSI. At times, the two ossification centers may not fuse until 3 months, or up to 1 to 2 years after birth. When this occurs, the odontoid process (body of the dens) has a bifid appearance on AP CPSI. The primary ossification center at the tip of the dens, called the os terminale, usually does not develop until age 5 to 6, although it may be seen as early as the first or second year of life. It appears as a small triangle or round area of density at the tip of the dens (atop the body of the dens). The os terminale fuses with the body of the dens by age 10 to 12, although, rarely, it may not fuse and may persist as a small ossicle. The body of the dens joins the body of C2 at the subdental synchondrosis, which appears as a lucent line slightly below the plane of

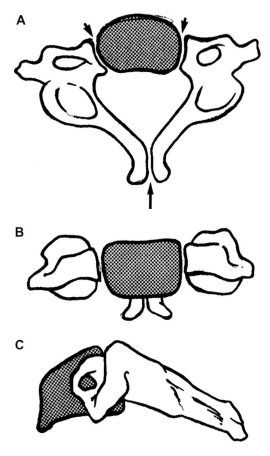

Fig. 24. (*A–C*) Vertebra from C3-7, which is representative of the vertebra from C3-L5, demonstrating the three ossification centers for the body and each of the neural arches. The neurocentral synchondroses (*small arrows*) and ununited laminae (*large arrow*) are present. (*From* Malone DG. Pediatric neurosurgery. 4th edition. Philadelphia: Saunders; 2001. p. 130; with permission.)

the superior border of the body of C2. This line disappears (ossifies) by age 4 to 6, although it may persist as a small lucent line up to age 10. Complete ossification of the subdental synchondrosis fuses the body of the dens to the body of C2. The neurocentral synchondroses of C2 ossify by age 3 to 6 and the laminae fuse posteriorly by age 3 to 4 (Figs. 28 and 29) [1–6,39,42].

An ossification center is seen in each of the bodies of the sacrum at birth and within each side of the neural arch (see Fig. 19A, C). Ossification may vary and may not be complete in the sacrum until age 18 to 20. During infancy, the sacral vertebrae are separated from each other by intervertebral fibrocartilage. The two lower vertebrae fuse around the 18th year of life, and fusion proceeds gradually

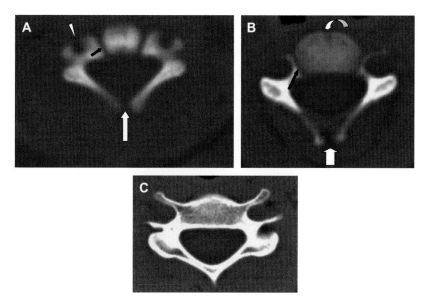

Fig. 25. CT axial (bone settings) of representative cervical vertebrae of C3-7. (*A*) A 3-day-old child with ossification in the body (centrum) and each half of the neural arch, with neurocentral synchondrosis (*black arrow*), transverse foramina (*white arrowhead*), and ununited laminae (*large white arrow*). (*B*) A 4-day-old child with incomplete ossification of the neurocentral synchondrosis (*small arrow*) and laminae (*large arrow*), and persistent anterior channel (*curved arrow*). (*C*) A 16-year-old with complete ossification of vertebra. (*From* McLone DG. Pediatric neurosurgery. 4th edition. Philadelphia: Saunders; 2001. p. 112–4; with permission.)

in a cranial direction until the entire sacrum is united. The vertebral arches unite with the bodies of the lower sacral vertebrae at approximately age 2, and the upper segments unite at approximately age 6. This development occurs by fusion (ossification) of the neurocentral synchondrosis.

The coccyx is not ossified at birth. Each coccygeal segment ossifies from a single center. The ossification center for the first coccygeal vertebra appears approximately at age 4, the second between ages 5 and 10, the third between ages 10 and 15, and the fourth between ages 14 and 20. At times, the segments may undergo bony fusion, but generally, they are united with one another by fibrocartilage.

Secondary ossification centers appear in the vertebrae from C3 to L5 at around puberty (age 10 to 13) and completely ossify by age 18 to 25. These secondary ossification centers appear at the tips of the transverse processes, superior and inferior articulating processes, spinous process, and ring apophyses [1–6].

Simple spina bifida, ununited laminae posteriorly at one or two spinal levels, can occur without any significance or it can be associated with certain forms of spinal dysraphism, especially if multiple segments are involved. Simple spina bifida can be seen in 9% to 22% of children and 1% to 9% of adults in certain series based on

CPSI. The overall occurrence of simple spina bifida is seen more commonly at L5-S1, C1, C7-T1, and the lower thoracic level, in decreasing order of frequency. Transitional vertebrae exist in the vertebral column at the cervicothoracic, thoracolumbar, and lumbosacral levels. Variations that are not malformations, including those involving the cervical ribs, hypoplastic or absent twelfth ribs, lumbarization of the first sacral segment or first lumbar ribs, and sacralization of the fifth lumbar segment, occur at these levels [6,42].

Other anatomic variations consist of occipitalization of the C1 vertebral body, third condyle (spur attached to the inferior edge of the anterior border of the foramen magnum); absence of the posterior arch of C1 (usually a fibrous ring is seen); anterior cleft in the anterior ring of C1, secondary to failure of the central ossification center to develop; bifurcation or duplication of the odontoid, os terminale; absence of pedicles: and thinning of pedicles at the thoracolumbar junction (commonly T11-L2) [6,42].

Pseudosubluxations

During the postnatal maturation of the spine, certain spine measurements and pseudodisplacements in children differ in comparison with adults. The

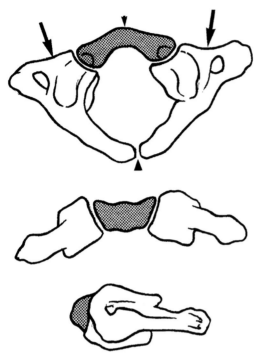

Fig. 26. C1 in an infant with the body of C1 (*small arrow*), lateral masses (*large arrows*), and ununited laminae (*arrowhead*). (*From* McLone DG. Pediatric neurosurgery. 4th edition. Philadelphia: Saunders; 2001. p. 132; with permission.)

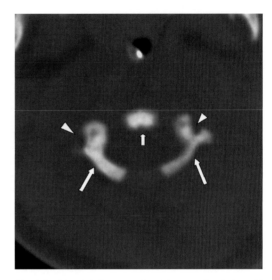

Fig. 27. CT axial (bone settings) image of a 2-day-old neonate with ossification center in each lateral mass of C1 (*large arrows*), transverse foramen (*arrowheads*), and ossification center of odontoid process of C2 (*small arrow*). The ossification center in the body of C1, which lies anterior to odontoid process, is not seen. It is commonly not present on CT or CPSI until the 6th to 12th month of life.

atlantoaxial relationship between the posterior margin of the arch of C1 and the anterior margin of the odontoid process (C1-dens) usually measures 2 to 4 mm but may be as great as 5 mm in children or young adults. This distance can normally increase 1 to 2 mm on the flexion lateral view but the overall measurement should not exceed 5 mm. The variance in this distance is felt to be a combination of laxity of surrounding ligaments and incomplete ossification of the dens.

Pseudosubluxations (anterior displacements) of the body of C2 and C3 or C3 onto C4 are 3 to 4 mm but can vary from 1 to 5 mm when the spine is flexed from the neutral position on lateral CPSI. These pseudosubluxations occur during infancy and childhood, up to 10 years of age (usually seen between ages 1 and 7) (see Fig. 11). After age 10, pseudosubluxations can be seen at C4-5 or C5-6. Differentiation of these pseudosubluxations from true subluxations depends on the maintenance of the normal alignment of the spinolaminar line. Normally, the alignment of the posterior arches (spinolaminar junction lines) is maintained in these pseudosubluxations. These

areas of pseudosubluxations occur at the principle cervical motion, which in the infant and young child occurs at the C2-3 or C3-4 level. The principle cervical motion changes to the C4-5 or C5-6 level at approximately 10 years of age [1–6,42–45].

Intervertebral disc

Changes also occur in the maturation of the IVD. The disc is ovoid in appearance on CPSI and blends into the nonossified vertebral end plates in the neonate and infant. With ossification and development of the vertebral bodies, the disc appears rectangular in shape on CPSI by age 2 to 3. However, the true shape of the disc in the neonate is best seen on the T2-W sagittal view as a hyperintense ovoid or rectangular structure separate from the cartilaginous end plates of the vertebral body. It is approximately one third to one fourth the size of the body, depending on the age of the child. The disc is larger in the newborn and infant [1–6,23,33–35,46].

The disc is a vascular structure at birth. It receives its vascularity from the adjacent vertebrae. The arterial supply is primarily from nutrient arteries of the body extending to the

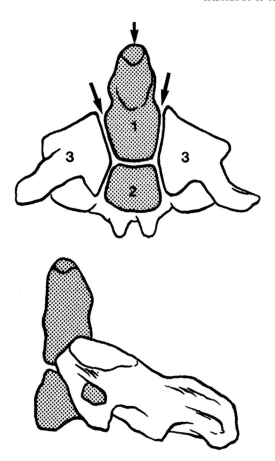

Fig. 28. Ossification centers of C2 with os terminale (at tip of dens) (*small arrow*), body of dens (*1*), body of C2 (*2*), lateral masses (*3*), and neurocentral synchondroses (*large arrows*). (*From* McLone DG. Pediatric neurosurgery. 4th edition. Philadelphia: Saunders; 2001. p. 133; with permission.)

cartilaginous end plates and adjacent discs. This vascularity gradually decreases throughout infancy and early childhood until about age 4, when the disc becomes an avascular structure. The disc is composed of a central nucleus pulposus and an outer ring, the annulus fibrosus. The nucleus pulposus develops from notochordal and perichordal mesenchyme. It consists of a mucoid substance, oncotic proteoglycan (product of notochordal degeneration), water (88% at birth), and a few fibrocartilaginous strands. The annulus fibrosus develops only from perichordal mesenchyme and consists of fibrocartilage and water (78% at birth). As the disc matures through childhood and into early adulthood, it loses water. By age 25 to 30, the water content of the nucleus pulposus has decreased to 76%, and that of the

annulus fibrosus to 70%. The normal disc is not visualized on CPSI but it can be seen on CT (see Figs. 1, 5, 12, 13, and 21). It is best imaged on MRI because of its high water content (see Figs. 1, 5, 12, 13 and 22) [1–10,23,27].

The ligamentous attachments of the spine are not seen on CPSI. Some of the ligaments can be demonstrated on the soft tissue settings on CT but they are not well delineated. The ligaments are best seen on MRI on T2-W images. The spine has two types of joints. The IVDs form amphiarthroses and the facets form diarthrodeses joints, which are demonstrated on CT and MRI.

Spinal canal and intervertebral foramina

The bony spine grows by enchondral and membranous ossification. The vertebral body grows in height by enchondral ossification at its cartilaginous end plates and in width by membranous ossification. The posterior elements grow by membranous ossification. At birth, the average length of the spine without the sacrum is 20 cm, during first 2 years of life it is 45 cm, at puberty it is 50 cm, and in the adult it averages 60 to 75 cm. The maximum length is attained at age 22 to 24. The parts of the spine grow at different rates. At birth, the cervical spine is 25%, the thoracic spine is 50%, and the lumbar spine is 25% of the total length of the spine without the sacrococcygeal region. In the adult, the cervical is 17%, the thoracic 50%, and the lumbar 33% of the total length of the spine [4,47].

The spinal canal grows by enchondral and membranous ossification of the vertebrae and by enchondral ossification of the neurocentral synchondroses. The spinal canal grows as the vertebrae grow, but once the neurocentral synchondroses and the midline posterior arch ossify and close, the spinal canal can no longer grow. The spinal canal diameter reaches adult size by age 6 to 8, after which very little diametric canal growth occurs. In the newborn and during infancy, the spinal canal is oval in shape and its transverse diameter is larger than its sagittal diameter. By late childhood, it assumes a more round-to-oval configuration in the cervical, thoracic, and upper lumbar regions, and is round to triangular in the lumbar and sacral regions [1–6].

At birth to age 3 months, the sagittal diameter of the spinal canal is 1.0 cm in the cervical region and 1 to 1.3 cm in the lumbar region. At the end of the first decade of life, the spinal canal should approach adult size, whereby the sagittal diameter is 15 to 27 mm in the cervical, 17 to 22 in the thoracic, and 15 to 27 mm in the lumbar spine. The transverse diameters are larger than the sagittal diameters. The interpedicular (transverse) measurements of the spinal canal have been used and delineated more succinctly in the literature; Elsberg and Dyke in adults, French and Peyton in infants and children, Simril and Thurston in children, Landdmesser and Heublein in children from 1 to 15, and Hinck, Clark and Hopkins in children and adults [48–57].

Vascularity and vascular structures

The vascularity to the bony spine is provided by arteries and draining venous plexuses and veins. The arterial trunks to the spine are virtually complete by the seventh month of gestation. The cervical region is supplied by arterial vessels from the vertebral, ascending cervical, cervical, and occipital arteries. The thoracic spine receives arteries from the dorsal branches of the intercostal arteries. The lumbar spine is supplied by the posterior branches of the lumbar arteries. These arteries eventually supply the bony spine by nutrient arterial branches. In the newborn, arterial vessels can be seen extending anteriorly into the middle of the vertebral body. The main vessel is a nutrient artery and it forms an anterior channel and anterior notch seen at birth and during infancy in the middle of the vertebral body on CPSI and CT. This anterior channel usually disappears by age 1; however, it may persist and be sharply visible for up to age 3 to 6, or even in older children, as a slitlike notch with sclerotic margins. On MRI, this anterior nutrient artery can be seen on sagittal T1-W images in the neonate and young infant (Fig. 30) [1–10,24,58,59].

The venous drainage of the spine is by way of venous plexuses and veins that drain into vertebral veins. Epidural veins posterior to the posterior border of the vertebral body within the anterior epidural space can be seen as soft tissue densities running as bilateral parallel bundles along the anterolateral aspect of the spinal canal. These bundles are best appreciated in the epidural fat on the axial CT scans filmed with soft tissue settings and as vascular bundles with signal void or mixed signal on axial MRI scans. These venous bundles represent a combination of the retrovertebral plexus of veins and paired anterior internal vertebral veins. The basivertebral vein is part of the venous drainage of the vertebral body. It is at the midpoint of the vertebral body, best seen on

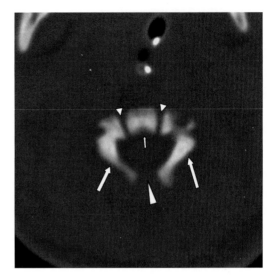

Fig. 29. CT axial (bone settings) image of C2 in a 2-day-old child with ossification in the body (*small arrow*), lateral masses (*large arrows*), neurocentral synchondroses (*small arrowheads*), and ununited laminae (*large arrowhead*).

axial CT scan as a Y or V lucent structure draining posteriorly into the retrovertebral plexus at the midline, as a single venous channel, or as two channels separated by a bony septum. On the lateral CPSI, sagittal MPR CT, and sagittal T1-W and T2-W MRI, the basivertebral vein can be seen as a posterior channel and notch in the middle of the vertebral body. It is present at birth and persists throughout life. These venous channels will enhance with contrast [1–10,18,23,24].

Bone marrow

The marrow spaces in the spine are predominantly within the vertebral bodies. At birth, the vertebral body consists of cartilaginous end plates, an outer shell of cortical bone, and an inner matrix composed of cancellous (trabeculae) bone and cellular (bone) marrow. Bone marrow is composed of hematopoietic cells, fat cells, and reticulum cells. Marrow can be categorized as red (hematopoietically active) or yellow (hematopoietically inactive). Red marrow is a rich vascular network made up of water (40%), protein (20%), and fat (40%). Yellow marrow consists of a sparse vascular network of water (15%), protein (5%), and fat (80%) [7–10,23,27].

During fetal development, all bone marrow is red. At birth, the marrow is almost totally red. Over the next 10 years, the red marrow begins its progressive conversion to yellow marrow. By age

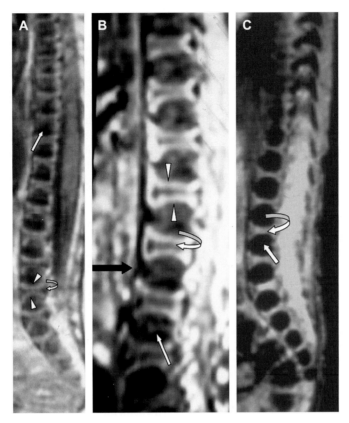

Fig. 30. MRI of newborn spine lower thoracolumbosacral. (*A*) Sagittal T1-W, with marked hypointense vertebral bodies' ossification center (*white arrow*), marked hyperintense cartilaginous end plates (*white arrowheads*), iso/hypointense discs (*curved arrow*). (*B*) Sagittal T1-W of thoracolumbar area with nutrient artery extending into anterior channel of the vertebral bodies (*back arrow*). (*C*) Sagittal GE T2-W of thoracolumbosacral spine with marked hypointense vertebral bodies' ossification center (*arrow*), marked hyperintense cartilaginous end plates, and hyperintense discs (*curved arrow*).

10, only 58% of the bone marrow is red, with 42% being yellow. The conversion to the dominant pattern of yellow marrow (adult pattern) is completed by early adulthood, around age 25. Red marrow is still present, but most of the marrow is yellow. MRI is the best modality to evaluate the changes in bone marrow [7–10,23,27,46,60–63].

MRI of the normal pediatric spine

The MRI appearance of the pediatric spine is related to signal from the vertebrae and IVDs. The signal intensity of the vertebrae is caused by its outer cortical shell and inner matrix of bone marrow. The signal intensity of the disc is primarily from the water content of the nucleus pulposus. The pediatric spine demonstrates changes related to the development of the vertebrae during the first

2 years of life. The changes in the development of the vertebrae are related to the cartilaginous end plates and the ossification centers, consisting of mainly red (hematopoietic) marrow. The vertebral bodies/ossification centers and the cartilaginous end plates are considered one unit. The cartilage is hyaline, which forms the endochondral growth layer around the ossification centers at the end plates. These changes are more pronounced on MRI during the first 24 months of life and more readily demonstrated in the vertebral bodies on the different pulse sequences. The GE T2-W pulse sequence suppresses fat and the red bone marrow appears more hypointense on these images, compared with the FSE T2-W pulse sequence at all ages. Changes also occur with the shape of the vertebral column and the IVDs [7,8,24,46,63]. The MRI signal changes outlined in the following discussion of the postnatal maturation of the spine

are based on a high field strength 1.5 Tesla MRI scanner (Table 2).

From birth to 1 month of life (neonatal period), the spine is relatively straight because weight-bearing forces are inconsequential at this time. The vertebral body (ossification center) is oval in shape and demonstrates marked hypointensity on T1-W, marked hypointensity on GE T2-W, and moderate hypointensity on FSE T2-W images because of the almost totally red marrow content of the ossification center. The cartilaginous end plates are markedly hyperintense on T1-W and GE T2-W images, with mild hyperintensity on T2-W images. The cartilaginous end plates comprise about 25% to 50% of the vertebral body height. The IVD is a thin band that is iso- or hypointense on T1-W images and hyperintense on T2-W images, and is about 20% to 30% of the height of the vertebral body. The

posterior elements with their ossification centers follow the same signal as the vertebral bodies. The neural foramina are round (see Fig. 30; Figs. 31 and 32) [24,46,63,64].

By age 1 month to 6 months, the spine is still relatively straight. During this stage, a thin black rim/cortex surrounding the ossification center becomes visible on some of the pulse sequences. The vertebral body (ossification center) is oval in shape and demonstrates the beginning of mild, slight hyperintensity to its superior or inferior aspects, with a larger central area of hypointensity on T1-W and FSE T2-W images and continued hypointensity on the GE T2-W images. The cartilaginous end plates are iso- to moderately hyperintense on T1-W images, iso- to mildly hyperintense on T2-W images, and mild to moderately hyperintense on GE T2-W images, and comprise 20% to 30% of the vertebral body

Table 2
MRI changes in the normal pediatric spine from birth to age 3

Vertebral body	T1-W	GE T2-W	FSE T2-W
Birth to 1 month of age			
Ossification center	Marked hypointensity	Marked hypointensity	Moderate hypointensity
Cartilaginous End plates	Marked Hyperintensity	Marked Hyperintensity	Mild Hyperintensity
Intervertebral disc	Iso- or hypointensity	Hyperintensity	Hyperintensity
1 to 6 months of age			
Ossification center	Slight hyperintensity; superior or inferior aspect with larger central area of hypointensity	Hypointensity	Slight hyperintensity; superior or inferior aspect with larger central area of hypointensity
Cartilaginous End plates	Iso- to moderate Hyperintensity	Mild to moderate Hyperintensity	Iso- to mild Hyperintensity
Intervertebral disc	Iso- or hypointensity	Hyperintensity	Hyperintensity
6 to 12 months of age			
Ossification center	Iso- or slight hyperintensity	Slight hypointensity	Iso- or slight hyperintensity
Cartilaginous End plates	Not well seen Iso- to hypointensity	Not well seen Iso- to hypointensity	Not well seen Iso- to mild hyperintensity
Intervertebral disc	Iso- to hypointensity	Hyperintensity	Hyperintensity
1 to 2 years of age			
Ossification center	Mild to moderate hyperintensity	Slight hypointensity	Iso- to slight hyperintensity
Cartilaginous End plates	Not well seen Hypointensity	Not well seen Hypointensity	Not well seen Hypointensity
Intervertebral disc	Hypointensity	Hyperintensity	Hyperintensity
2 to 3 years of age			
Ossification center	Slight hyperintensity	Slight hypointensity	Slight hyperintensity
Cartilaginous End plates	Not well seen Cortical rim surrounding body	Not well seen Cortical hypointense rim surrounding body	Not well seen Cortical hypointense rim surrounding body
Intervertebral disc	Hypointensity	Hyperintensity	Hyperintensity

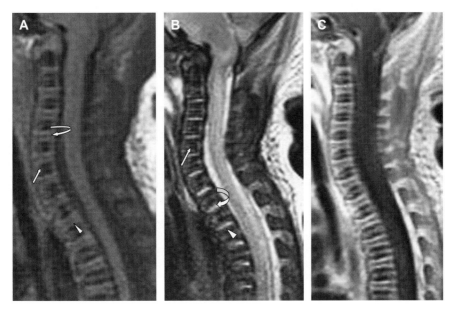

Fig. 31. Cervical spine of newborn sagittal MRI. (*A*) T1-W hypointense vertebral bodies' ossification centers (*white arrow*), hyperintense cartilaginous end plates (*arrowhead*), and isointense discs (*curved arrow*). (*B*) FSE T2-W with hypointense vertebral bodies' ossification centers (*white arrow*), mild hyperintense cartilaginous end plates (*arrowhead*), and isointense discs (*curved arrows*). (*C*) T1-W postgadolinium contrast demonstrating some enhancement of the vertebrae and cartilaginous end plates.

height. During this stage, the signal intensity of the ossification center/vertebral body becomes equal to that of the cartilaginous end plates. The IVD is band shaped, iso- or hypointensive on T1-W images and hyperintense on T2-W images, and 20% to 30% of the height of the vertebral body. The posterior elements follow the same signal as the vertebral body. The neural foramina are round (Fig. 33) [24,46,63,64].

By age 6 to 12 months, the cartilaginous end plates are not as well seen. They blend into the signal of the adjacent disc. The ossification within the cortical rim is more apparent and demonstrates no signal. The cortical rim appears as black on all of the pulse sequences. The spine starts to develop a mild cervical and lumbar lordosis. The normal cervical lordosis develops when the infant begins to have head control. The thoracic kyphosis and lumbar lordosis begin to develop when the child starts to bear weight (crawling and walking). The vertebral body (ossification center) is ovoid to slightly rectangular in shape and demonstrates

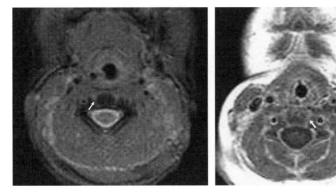

Fig. 32. MRI newborn cervical spine axial images. (*A*) GE T2-W hyperintense neurocentral synchondrosis (*arrow*). (*B*) T1-W postgadolinium contrast image with some enhancement of the neurocentral synchondrosis (*arrow*).

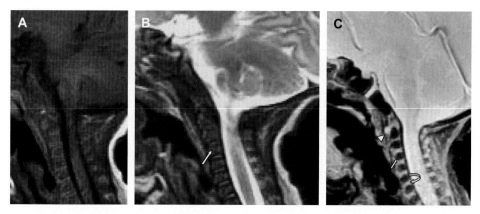

Fig. 33. MRI sagittal of a 3-month-old cervical spine. (*A*) T1-W slight hyperintense peripheral aspect of vertebral bodies' ossification centers with larger central area of hypointensity and a midlinear area of slight hyperintensity related to the basivertebral vein, hyperintense cartilaginous end plates. (*B*) FSE T2 iso- to slight hyperintense ossification centers of the vertebrae (*arrow*). (*C*) GE T2-W hypointense ossification centers (*arrow*), cartilaginous hyperintense body of C1 (*arrowhead*), and hyperintense cartilaginous end plates and discs (*curved arrow*).

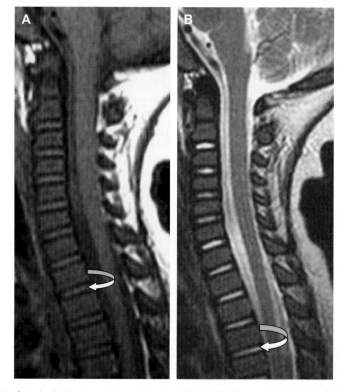

Fig. 34. Sagittal MRI of cervical spine in an 11-month-old child. (*A*) T1-W iso- to slightly hyperintense ossification centers of the vertebrae, isointense discs (*curved arrow*), and iso- to hypointense cartilaginous end plates that are not well seen, hypointense cortical rim. (*B*) GE T2-W iso- to slightly hypointense ossification centers, hyperintense discs (*curved arrow*) and iso- to hypointense cartilaginous end plates that are not well seen, hypointense cortical rim.

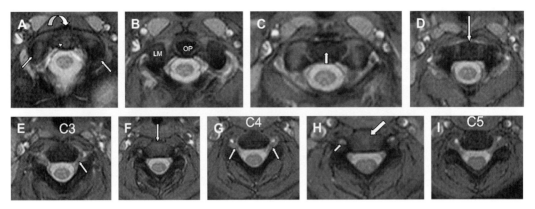

Fig. 35. MRI GE T2-W axial of cervical spine in an 11-month-old child. (*A*) anterior arch (body of C1) (*curved arrow*), cartilaginous tip of the odontoid process (*arrowhead*), superior articulating facets of lateral masses of C1 (*short white arrows*). (*B*) Inferior articulating facets of lateral masses of C1 (*LM*) and odontoid process (*OP*) of C2. (*C*) Junction of odontoid process with body of C2 (*arrow*). (*D*) Body (*arrow*) and lateral masses of C2. (*E*) C3 vertebra with nerve root (*arrow*) in intervertebral foramen. (*F*) C3-4 disc (*arrow*). (*G*) C4 intervertebral neural foramen (*arrows*). (*H*) C4-5 disc (*large arrow*) and transverse foramen (*small arrow*). (*I*) C5 vertebra.

either iso- or slight hyperintensity on T1-W images and FSE T2-W images, or slightly greater superior or inferior areas of mild hyperintensity, with a central area of hypointensity on T1-W images, and slight hyperintensity of the vertebral body on T2-W images. The cartilaginous end plates are not well seen and are mainly iso- to hypointense on T1-W images and iso- to mildly hyperintense on T2-W images, and comprise 20% to 30% of the vertebral body height. The IVD is rectangular shaped, iso- to hypointense on T1-W images, hyperintense on T2-W images, and 20% to 30% of the height of the vertebral body. The posterior elements/spinous processes are iso- to slightly hyperintense on T1- and T2-W images. The neural foramina are round to oval in shape (Figs. 34 and 35) [24,46,63,64].

From 1 to 2 years of age, the spinal curvature has a mild cervical and lumbar lordosis and mild thoracic kyphosis. The vertebral body is more rectangular in shape and demonstrates mild to moderate hyperintensity on T1-W images, iso- to slight hyperintensity on FSE T2-W images, and slight hypointensity on GE T2-W images. By age 2, the cartilaginous end plates and ossification center have reversed their relationship with

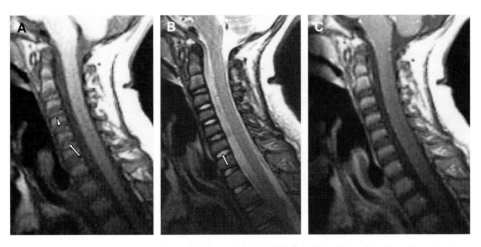

Fig. 36. MRI of cervical spine in 3-year-old sagittal images. (*A*) T1-W slight hyperintensity of vertebrae, isointense discs (*arrow*) and thin cortical hypointense rim (*arrow head*). (*B*) FSE T2-W slight hyperintense vertebrae and more marked hyperintense discs (*arrow*). (*C*) T1-W post gadolinium contrast with no enhancement of the vertebrae.

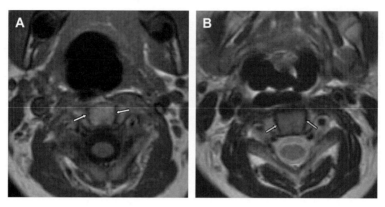

Fig. 37. MRI of 2 and one half year old cervical C4 vertebra axial. (*A*) T1-W and (*B*) FSE T2-W hypointense neuro-central synchondroses (*arrows*).

respect to signal. The cartilage is hypointense, becoming thinner and more difficult to visualize, and comprises 10% to 15% of the vertebral body height. The IVD is rectangular shaped, hypointense on T1-W images and hyperintense on T2-W images, and 20% to 25% of the height of the vertebral body. The posterior elements/spinous processes are the same signal as the vertebral bodies. The neural foramina are ovoid in shape [24,46,63,64].

The spine of a 2- to 3-year-old child can be used as the norm for the pediatric patient. By this time, the normal spinal curvature has developed.

The lack of signal from the ossified cortex of the vertebral bodies is seen on all pulse sequences, with some very mild changing in the marrow of the vertebrae producing a slightly high signal on T1-W and FSE T2-W images. The developing slight hyperintensity seen in the vertebrae on the T1-W and FSE T2-W images in infants and young children is felt to be related to some lipid infiltration of the marrow early in life. However, true conversion to fatty marrow appears to be a different process because 80% to 90% of the marrow in young children is red and not yellow (fat) (Figs. 36–38). The neurocentral

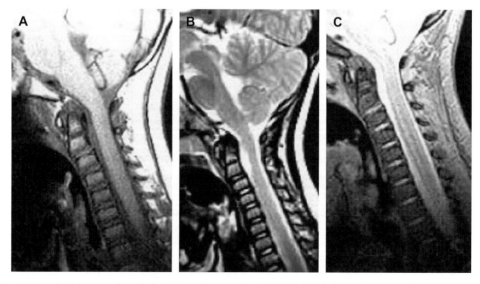

Fig. 38. MRI sagittal images of cervical spine in a 6-year-old. (*A*) T1-W slightly hyperintense vertebrae. (*B*) FSE T2-W slightly hyperintense vertebrae. (*C*) GE T2-W slightly hypointense vertebrae.

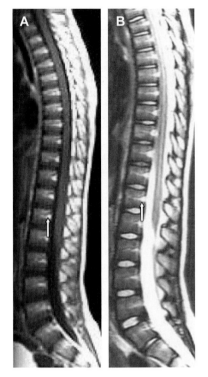

Fig. 39. MRI sagittal images of thoracolumbosacral spine in a 7-year-old. (*A*) T1-W slightly hyperintense vertebrae. (*B*) FSE T2-W slight hyperintense vertebrae. The posterior channel in the midportion of the vertebral body for the basivertebral vein demonstrates hyperintensity (*arrows*).

synchondroses are hypointense on T1-W and FSE T2-W images, and hyperintense on GE T2-W images (see Fig. 32 and 37). The disc is hypointense on T1-W images and markedly hyperintense on T2-W images. The parts of the disc, the annulus fibrosus (outer part) and nucleus pulposus (inner part), may begin to be differentiated by age 5. The anterior artery of the vertebral body can be seen in the newborn and young infant (see Fig. 30). However, the posterior channel with the basivertebral vein can be seen throughout life on some of the different pulse sequences (Fig. 39) [24,46,63,64].

The spinal ligaments demonstrate no signal on either the T1- or T2-W images in all age groups. The T2-W images better demonstrate the ligaments, with easy differentiation of the anterior and posterior spinal ligaments. The ligamentous attachments at the base of the skull with C1 and C2 and the ligamentous attachments of the posterior elements, although demonstrated on MRI, cannot be separated into individual attachments (see Fig. 39; Fig. 40) [7–9,64].

During infancy and childhood, enhancement on MRI using a routine intravenous dose of gadolinium 0.1 mmol/kg or 0.2 mL/kg can be seen in certain structures such as vertebrae and their cartilaginous end plates. In the newborn to children age 2, marked to mild homogeneous enhancement can be seen in the vertebrae (body and posterior elements) (see Figs. 31 and 32). Mild homogeneous enhancement can be seen in

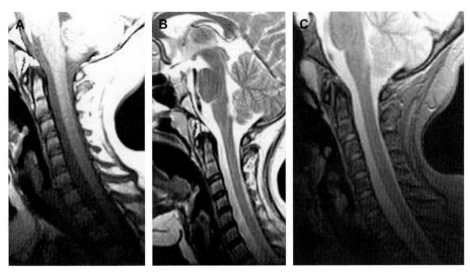

Fig. 40. MRI sagittal images of cervical spine in an 11-year-old. (*A*) T1-W slightly hyperintense vertebrae. (*B*) FSE T2-W slightly hyperintense vertebrae. (*C*) GE T2-W slightly hypointense vertebrae.

the vertebrae from 2 to 7 years of age. No enhancement in the vertebrae should be seen after 7 years of age (Figs. 39 and 40). Enhancement of the hyaline cartilaginous end plates of the vertebral bodies can be seen in the newborn to age 18 months. Enhancement of the basivertebral venous plexus can be seen in all pediatric patients but it is most pronounced in newborns, infants, and young children. The normal IVDs and spinal cord should not demonstrate enhancement on MRI. Enhancement of the vertebrae and cartilaginous end plates are related to their rich vascular supply, the permeability of the endothelium of their capillaries, and their extensive extravascular spaces [65].

References

[1] Weinstein SL, editor. The pediatric spine: principles and practice. 2nd edition. Philadelphia: Lippincott Williams & Wilkins; 2001.

[2] Kirks DR, editor. Practical pediatric imaging: diagnostic radiology of infants and children. 3rd edition. Philadelphia: Lippincott Williams & Wilkins; 1998.

[3] Swischuk LE, editor. Imaging of the newborn, infant, and young child. 5th edition. Philadelphia: Lippincott Williams & Wilkins; 2003.

[4] Kuhn JP, Slouis T, Haller J. Caffey's pediatric imaging. 10th edition. Philadelphia: Elsevier; 2004.

[5] Epstein B, editor. The spine: a radiologic text and atlas. 4th edition. Philadelphia: Lea & Febiger; 1976.

[6] Harwood-Nash DC, Fitz CR. Neuroradiology in infants and children. St. Louis (MO): Mosby; 1976.

[7] Ball WS Jr. Pediatric neuroradiology. Philadelphia: Lippincott-Raven Press; 1997.

[8] Barkovich AJ. Pediatric neuroimaging. 4th edition. Philadelphia: Lippincott Williams & Wilkins; 2005.

[9] Atlas SW. Magnetic resonance imaging of the brain and spine. 3rd edition. Philadelphia: Lippincott Williams & Wilkins; 2002.

[10] Tortori-Donati P, Rossi A. Pediatric neuroradiology brain, head, neck and spine. Berlin: Springer-Verlag; 2005.

[11] Pick TP, Howden R, editors. Gray's anatomy: the anatomical basis of medicine and surgery. 39th edition. Philadelphia: Elsevier Churchill Livingstone; 2005.

[12] Clemente C. Anatomy: a regional atlas of the human body. 5th edition. Philadelphia: Lippincott Williams & Wilkins; 2006.

[13] Sinnatamby CSS, Last RJ. Last's anatomy: regional and applied. 10th edition. Philadelphia: Elsevier; 2000.

[14] Pansky B. Review of Gross Anatomy. 6th edition. New York: McGraw-Hill; 1995.

[15] Byrd SE, Darling CF. Chapter 7: Postnatal maturation of the spine. In: McLone DG, editor. Pediatric

[16] neurosurgery surgery of the developing nervous system. 4th edition. Philadelphia: W.B. Saunders Co.; 2001.

[16] Swischuk LE. Emergency imaging of the acutely ill or injured child. 4th edition. Philadelphia: Lippincott Williams & Wilkins; 2000.

[17] Kricun R. Computed tomography. In: Kricun ME, editor. Imaging modalities in spinal disorders. Philadelphia: Harcourt Brace Jovanovich, Inc.; 1988. p. 376–467.

[18] Zimmerman RA, Gibby WA, Carmody RF. Neuroimaging: clinical and physical principles. 1st edition. New York: Springer-Verlag; 2000.

[19] Knollmann F, Coakley FV. Multislice CT principles and protocols. 1st edition. Philadelphia: Saunders-Elsevier; 2006.

[20] Lipson SA. MDCT and 3D workstations: a practical guide and teaching file. New York: Springer; 2006.

[21] Rydberg J, Buckwalter KA, Caldemeyer KS, et al. Multislice CT: scanning techniques and clinical applications. Radiographics 2000;20:1787–806.

[22] Carty H, Brunelle F, Stringer DA, et al. Imaging children. 2nd edition. Philadelphia: Elsevier; 2005.

[23] St. Amour TE, Hodges SC, Laakman RW, et al. MRI of the spine. New York: Raven Press; 1994.

[24] Khanna AJ, Wasserman BA, Sponseller PD. Magnetic resonance imaging of the pediatric spine. J Am Acad Orthop Surg 2003;4(4):797–833.

[25] Byrd SE, Darling CF, McLone DG, et al. MR imaging of the pediatric spine. Magn Reson Imaging Clin N Am 1996;4(4):797–833.

[26] Byrd SE, Fitz CR. Chapter 3: The brain and spine. In: Silverman FN, Kuhn JP, editors. Caffey's pediatric x-ray diagnosis. 9th edition. St. Louis (MO): Mosby. p. 201–343.

[27] McLone DG. Pediatric neurosurgery: surgery of the developing nervous system. 4th edition. Philadelphia: W.B. Saunders; 2001.

[28] Verbout AJ. The development of the vertebral column. Adv Anat Embryol Cell Biol 1998;90:1–122.

[29] Keim H. The adolescent spine. New York: Grune & Stratton; 1976.

[30] Bailey DK. The normal cervical spine in infants and children. Radiology 1952;59:712–9.

[31] O'Rahilly R, Benson DR. The development of the vertebral column. In: Bradford DS, Hensinger RM, editors. The pediatric spine. New York: Thieme; 1985.

[32] Gadow HF. The evolution of the vertebral column. Cambridge University Press; 1933.

[33] Bradner ME. Normal values of the vertebral body and intervertebral disk index during growth. AJR Am J Roentgenol 1970;110:618–27.

[34] Gooding CA, Neuhauser EBD. Growth and development of the normal vertebral body in the presence and the absence of stress. AJR Am J Roentgenol 1965;93:388–94.

[35] Taylor JR. Growth of human intervertebral discs, vertebral bodies. J Anat 1975;120:49–68.

[36] Knutsson F. Growth and differentiation of the postnatal vertebrae. Acta Radiol 1961;55:401–8.

[37] Ford DM, McFadden KD, Bagnall KM. Sequence of ossification in human vertebral neural arch centers. Anat Rec 1982;203:175–8.

[38] Ogden JA. Radiology of postnatal skeletal development: XI. The first cervical vertebra. Skeletal Radiol 1984;12:12–20.

[39] Ogden JA. Radiology of postnatal skeletal development: XII. The second cervical vertebra. Skeletal Radiol 1984;12:169–77.

[40] Brill PW, Baker DH, Ewing ML. "Bone-within-bone" in the neonatal spine: stress change or normal development? Radiology 1973;108:363–6.

[41] Ebel KD, Blickman H, Willich E, et al. Differential diagnosis in pediatric radiology. New York: Thieme; 1999.

[42] Lustrin ES, Karakas SP, Ortiz AO, et al. Pediatric cervical spine: normal anatomy, variants, and trauma. Radiographics 2003;23:539–60.

[43] Overton LM, Grossman JW. Anatomical variations in the articulation between the second and third cervical vertebrae. J Bone Joint Surg [Am] 1952;34:155–61.

[44] Catell HS, Filtzer DL. Pseudosubluxation and other normal variations in the cervical spine in children. A study of one hundred sixty children. J Bone Joint Surg [Am] 1965;47:1295–309.

[45] Jacobson G, Leecker HH. Pseudosubluxation of the axis in children. AJR Am J Roentgenol 1959;82:472–81.

[46] Sze G, Baierl P, Bravo S. Evolution of the infant spinal column: evaluation with MR imaging. Radiology 1991;181:819–27.

[47] Silverman FN, Kuhn JP. Introduction to the spine. In: Caffey's pediatric x-ray diagnosis: an integrated imaging approach. St. Louis (MO): Mosby; 1993. p. 116–25.

[48] Simril WA, Thurston D. Normal intrepediculate space in the spines of infants and children. Radiology 1955;64:340–7.

[49] Markuske H. Sagittal diameter measurements of the bony cervical spinal cord in children. Pediatr Radiol 1977;6:129–31.

[50] Hinck VC, Clark WM Jr, Hopkins CE. Normal interpediculate distances (minimum and maximum) in children and adults. AJR Am J Roentgenol 1966;97:141–53.

[51] Hinck VC, Hopkins CE, Savara BS. Sagittal diameter of the cervical spinal canal in children. Radiology 1962;79:97–108.

[52] Hinck VC, Hopkins CE, Clark WM. Sagittal diameter of the lumbar spinal cord in children and adults. Radiology 1966;85:929–37.

[53] Yousefzadeh DK, El-Khoury GY, Smith WL. Normal sagittal diameter and variation in the pediatric cervical spine. Radiology 1982;144:319–25.

[54] Naik DR. Cervical spinal canal in normal infants. Clin Radiol 1970;21:323–6.

[55] Schwarz GS. Width of spinal canal in growing vertebra with special reference to sacrum; maximum interpediculate distance in adults and children. AJR Am J Roentgenol 1956;76:476–86.

[56] Elsberg CA, Dyke CG. Diagnosis and localization of tumors of spinal cord by means of measurements made on x-ray films of vertebrae and the correlation of clinical and x-ray findings. Bull Neurol Inst New York 1936;3:359–69.

[57] Landmesser WE, Heublein GW. Measurement of the normal interpedicular space in the child. Conn Med 1953;17:310–3.

[58] Brookes M. The blood supply of bone: an approach to bone biology. New York: Appleton; 1971.

[59] Crock HV, Yoshizawa H. The blood supply of the vertebral column and spinal cord in man. New York: Springer-Verlag; 1977.

[60] Dooms GC, Fisher MR, Hricak H, et al. Bone marrow imaging: magnetic resonance studies related to age and sex. Radiology 1985;155:429–32.

[61] Vogler JB III, Murphy WA. Bone marrow imaging. Radiology 1988;168:679–93.

[62] Ricci C, Cova M, Kang YS, et al. Normal age-related patterns of cellular and fatty bone marrow distribution in the axial skeleton: MR imaging study. Radiology 1990;177:83–8.

[63] Sebag GH, Dubois J, Tabet M, et al. Pediatric spinal bone marrow assessment of normal age-related changes in the MRI appearance. Pediatr Radiol 1993;23(7):515–8.

[64] Walker HS, Dietrich RB, Flannigan BD, et al. Magnetic resonance imaging of the pediatric spine. Radiographics 7(6):L1129–52.

[65] Sze G, Bravo S, Baierl P, et al. Developing spinal column: gadolinium-enhanced MR imaging. Radiology 1991;180(2):497–502.

ELSEVIER
SAUNDERS

Neurosurg Clin N Am 18 (2007) 463–478

NEUROSURGERY
CLINICS
OF NORTH AMERICA

Congenital Anomalies of the Cervical Spine

Paul Klimo, Jr, MD, MPH, Maj, USAF[a],*, Ganesh Rao, MD[b],
Douglas Brockmeyer, MD[c]

[a]88th SGOS/SGCXN, 4881 Sugar Maple Drive, Wright-Patterson Air Force Base, OH 454333, USA
[b]University of Texas M.D. Anderson Cancer Center, 1515 Holcombe Boulevard, Houston, TX 77030, USA
[c]Division of Pediatric Neurosurgery, Primary Children's Medical Center,
100 North Medical Drive, Salt Lake City, UT 84113, USA

Developmental abnormalities of the cervical spine vary widely and are usually found as sporadic isolated cases. Others are found as part of a multi-organ-system syndromic anomaly. Many of these anomalies are asymptomatic and go undetected, but several types may result in biomechanical instability or compress neurologic structures, and thus place a patient at risk for neurologic injury or chronic pain from deformity. Identifying the lesions with significant clinical implications is important not only for treatment of the malformation itself but because they may be associated with other spinal and nonspinal faults of development. Here, the authors discuss the various congenital abnormalities and their clinical relevance.

Epidemiology of congenital disorders

Because many congenital abnormalities of the cervical spine are asymptomatic, the true incidence is likely largely underreported. It is estimated that up to 5% of fetuses have vertebral anomalies [1]. Indeed, the true incidence of even a relatively common congenital disorder of the cervical spine, Klippel-Feil syndrome (KFS), is unknown because of the asymptomatic nature of the disease and a lack of other consistent anomalies [2]. Some authors have reported that congenital anomalies of the cervical spine occur in approximately 1 in 40,000 to 42,000 births, with a slight female predominance [3,4].

The prevalence of congenital fusions of subaxial cervical vertebrae has been reported to be 0.71% on the basis of the study of skeletal specimens [5]. Congenital fusions can occur at any level of the cervical spine, although 75% occur in the region of the first three cervical vertebrae. Lower cervical fusions may occur in association with certain syndromes. Fetal alcohol syndrome has been associated with congenital neck fusions in up to 50% of patients affected by the disorder [4].

Although many developmental abnormalities of the cervical spine are asymptomatic and incidental, those that may require treatment, such as associated instability or spinal canal stenosis, must be recognized for appropriate care. These are the focus of this review.

Upper cervical spine abnormalities

The upper cervical spine is anatomically and biomechanically distinct from the remainder of the subaxial spine. Unlike the subaxial spine, in which axial weight is transferred primarily through the vertebral body, in C1 and C2, the weight of the skull is transferred by means of the occipital condyles to the lateral masses. There are no intervertebral discs at these levels. The primary motion at the occiput-C1 joint is flexion or extension (40%–50% of total flexion or extension), whereas the primary motion at C1 to C2 is rotation (40%–50% of total rotation). Several developmental abnormalities may occur at the craniovertebral junction.

Malformations of the occipital condyles

Anomalies of the occipital condyles are rare, and there have been few case reports in the

---

* Corresponding author.
  E-mail address: atomkpnk@yahoo.com (P. Klimo).

1042-3680/07/$ - see front matter © 2007 Elsevier Inc. All rights reserved.
doi:10.1016/j.nec.2007.04.005

literature. The proatlas, which is the fourth occipital sclerotome, eventually gives rise to the anterior rim of the foramen magnum and the occipital condyles. A third condyle is sometimes present in the midline (condylus occipitalis) [6]. Condylus occipitalis is usually a benign anomaly found at autopsy. Kotil and Kalayo [7] presented the only known case report of a 40-year-old woman with progressive myelopathy caused by this anomaly. Abnormally enlarged condyles have been reported. Halanski and colleagues [8] described a 22-month-old boy with torticollis who incurred a C1 fracture after a fall. Imaging revealed a large ipsilateral occipital condyle, termed a *coconut* condyle by the authors, who believed that this anomaly predisposed the patient to his fracture. Recently, Ohaegbulam and colleagues [9] presented a similar case of 10-year-old myelopathic girl with bilateral occipital condylar hyperplasia. The condyles were adequately resected through a midline dorsal approach.

Occipitalization of the atlas

Occipitalization of the atlas, which occurs in approximately 0.25% of the population, is characterized by fusion of the occiput to the atlas [10]. It can be complete, partial, unilateral, and bony or fibrous [11]. It is generally defined as a failure of segmentation between the last (fourth) occipital and first cervical sclerotomes. The condition has been associated with various syndromes, including achondroplasia, spondyloepiphyseal dysplasia, Larsen syndrome, and Morquio syndrome. Although it may be isolated, it usually occurs in conjunction with other anomalies, such as congenital fusion of the second and third cervical vertebrae, basilar invagination, Chiari I malformation, and KFS [12,13]. The original description of occipitalization of the atlas indicated that the atlas and occiput were fused anteriorly with hypoplastic or anomalous posterior atlantal elements in most cases [10,14]. Many of the afflicted patients were symptomatic, likely from instability attributable to a weakened or absent transverse atlantal ligament [15]. Symptoms described in these patients include weakness, numbness, or pain in the upper extremities with associated upper motor neuron signs, including hyperreflexia and spasticity. Clinically, these patients may present with a low hairline, restricted neck movements, and a short neck, all of which are also associated with KFS [12,16].

With assimilation of the atlas, the atlantoaxial segment can be abnormally taxed and can become unstable. This can then be followed by a reducible form of basilar invagination. During this time, pannus can develop around the odontoid process as the body tries to limit the amount of movement here. As the patient ages, the lesion becomes irreducible (usually when the child is older than 14 years of age) [17].

Treatment of occipitalization of the atlas is variable. In the case of an anterior arch of C1 fused to the occiput without associated translation of C1 relative to C2 (which may indicate an incompetent transverse ligament), the posterior elements of C1 can be resected. Associated atlanto-occipital or atlantoaxial instability should be treated with internal fixation and fusion. The first step is to determine whether atlantoaxial subluxation or basilar invagination is reducible by traction. If reduction is inadequate to reduce the spinal cord compression when visualized on MRI, ventral decompression, followed by fusion and stabilization, is required. If the abnormality is reducible, posterior stabilization alone is adequate [18]. Techniques for these particular scenarios are discussed elsewhere in this issue.

Atlantal anomalies

Various congenital anomalies affect the atlas. Patients with Down syndrome with occipitocervical instability have an absence of the concave C1 superior articular surface [19]. The arch can be fused to C2 or can be completely absent, or there may be a hemiring [20,21]. Various defects of the ring of C1 have been described, with posterior defects being much more common than anterior defects (Fig. 1) [22,23]. Anterior or posterior ring anomalies can often be misread as fractures on plain films, but evaluation using CT can delineate the difference [24]. These anomalies are usually without any clinical consequence, although they are sometimes associated with other anomalies or may themselves cause myelopathy [25,26]. If the defects result in hemirings, these can "spread" as the child develops (ie, the opening in the ring enlarges as the two hemirings migrate laterally), which can lead to progressive deformity, pain, basilar invagination, and myelopathy (Fig. 2). A well-described phenomenon of congenital partial aplasia of the posterior arch of the atlas has been described [27–30]. In this condition, a bony defect of the posterior arch of C1 is replaced

Type

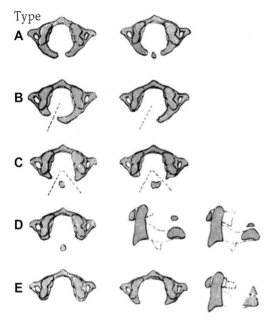

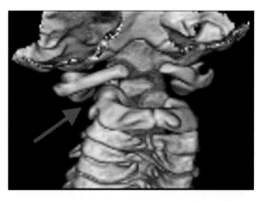

Fig. 2. Posterior view of a CT-derived three-dimensional model from a 2-year-old boy with multiple congenital anomalies, including a hemiring of C1. Note the "spreading" of the lateral masses of C1 compared with the superior articulating facet of C2 (*red arrow*).

Fig. 1. Classification of posterior arch defects of the atlas. Type A: failure of posterior midline fusion with a small gap remaining. Type B: unilateral clefts. Defects may range from a small gap to complete absence of the hemiarch. Type C: bilateral defects with preservation of the most dorsal part of the arch. Type D: complete absence of the posterior arch with a persistent isolated tubercle. Type E: complete absence of the entire posterior arch, including the posterior tubercle. (*From* Currarino G, Rollins N, Diehl JT. Congenital defects of the posterior arch of the atlas: a report of seven cases including an affected mother and son. AJNR Am J Neuroradiol 1994;15:253. Copyright © 1994 by American Society of Neuroradiology.)

with a dense fibrous band that is mobile and can repeatedly traumatize the posterior spinal cord.

Another well-described anomaly of the atlas that often causes progressive myelopathy is hypoplasia of the posterior arch [31–33]. In this condition, the posterior arch is abnormally small and the lamina is often bifid and turned inward [34], effectively decreasing the space available for the spinal cord. Interestingly, many patients do not present to medical attention with symptoms until later in life [35–38]. Treatment consists of simply removing the posterior arch.

The arcuate foramen, or posticus ponticus, represents anomalous ossification of the posterolateral surface of the atlas that creates complete bone encirclement of the vertebral artery. This is usually of no importance except in patients who need instrumentation of C1, particularly lateral

mass screws. Identification of this anomaly is important to prevent vertebral injury during placement of the screws [39].

Achondroplasia

Achondroplasia deserves special mention because of its significant association with craniocervical deformities. Although most cases are sporadic, a familial form is transmitted in an autosomal dominant fashion and is linked to the fibroblast growth factor receptor-3 gene [40]. Neurologic symptoms, including irregular respiratory patterns, may be seen in up to 85% of achondroplastic newborns [41,42]. The rate of sudden infant death in these children is significantly higher than that of the general population [43]. A narrowed foramen magnum and upper cervical stenosis may be seen with CT imaging in most patients [44,45]. The rate of growth of the foramen magnum is slowed during the first year of life, and this results in compression at the cervicomedullary junction (Fig. 3) [46]. Thus, the treatment for these patients includes suboccipital decompression and duraplasty to accommodate the lower brain stem and upper spinal cord. Subaxial cervical stenosis has also been associated with achondroplasia and is usually treated with laminectomy [47].

Basilar invagination

This condition is characterized by encroachment of the foramen magnum by the upper cervical spine, usually the odontoid process. The lower brain stem may be severely impacted by the dens because it is positioned aberrantly through

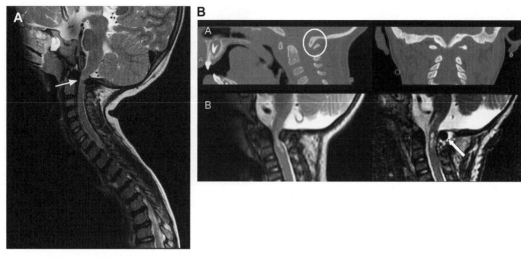

Fig. 3. (*A*) Compression at the craniocervical junction in achondroplasia. The white arrow indicates the area of compression of the cervicomedullary junction with signal changes in the spinal cord in this T2-weighted MRI scan. (*B*) Another example of cervicomedullary junction compression depicted with sagittal and coronal CT reconstructions (*A*) and pre- and postoperative MRI scans (*B*). In this 22-month-old boy who presented with apnea, aspiration pneumonia, and generalized hypotonicity, there was an unusual overgrowth of the opisthion ventral to the posterior ring of C1 (*red circle*). Note the degree of spinal cord compression with T2-hyperintense signal change before surgery. After bony resection only (*red arrow*), there is cerebrospinal fluid now ventral to the cord.

the foramen magnum and into the posterior fossa. Primary or true congenital basilar invagination is associated with other abnormalities, including atlanto-occipital fusion, hypoplasia of the atlas, hemirings of C1 with "spreading" of the lateral masses, odontoid abnormalities, KFS, and achondroplasia. Condylar hypoplasia elevates the position of the axis and atlas and often leads to basilar invagination. Acquired basilar invagination, or basilar impression, is caused by softening of the bone at the base of the skull as a result of degenerative disorders, such as Paget's disease of bone; osteogenesis imperfecta; Hurler syndrome; and severe rheumatoid arthritis or osteoarthritis, tumors, or infection.

The developmental cause of primary basilar invagination may be an insufficient amount of paraxial mesoderm, leading to underdevelopment of the occipital somites, subsequent shortening of the clivus, and an enlargement of the foramen magnum in the anteroposterior dimension [48]. During chondrification of the odontoid process, the cartilaginous dens may transiently reach into the foramen magnum [49]. Normally, the odontoid process descends to its normal position under the foramen magnum in the fetal period, but if this is incomplete, basilar invagination may result.

Generally, basilar invagination can be defined by the amount of protrusion of the odontoid

process through the foramen magnum. A general rule of thumb is that basilar invagination should be suspected if the C1-2 facet complex cannot be adequately visualized on a normal open-mouth anteroposterior view of the upper cervical spine. Several different methods to diagnose basilar invagination have been described. Common methods include use of the Chamberlain line, McRae line, or McGregor line (Fig. 4). All are based on lateral radiographs of the cervical spine. The Chamberlain line is drawn between the opisthion to the posterior aspect of the hard palate. The McGregor line is drawn from the posterior aspect of the hard palate to the base of the foramen magnum. The McRae line is drawn from the anterior to the posterior rim of the foramen magnum. Because The McRae line defines the opening of the foramen magnum, an odontoid process that projects above this line is likely to induce symptoms. McRae and Barnum [10] reported that a reduction of the opening of the foramen magnum to less than 19 mm was likely to produce neurologic deficits. Although plain radiographs have their utility as screening methods, the best imaging modality is MRI because it provides clinically useful information, such as the degree of impingement of neural structures.

Children with basilar invagination often present with a short neck and a limited painful range of

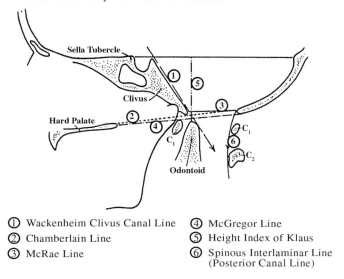

Lateral Craniometry with Points of Reference

① Wackenheim Clivus Canal Line   ④ McGregor Line
② Chamberlain Line   ⑤ Height Index of Klaus
③ McRae Line   ⑥ Spinous Interlaminar Line
                                       (Posterior Canal Line)

Fig. 4. The various methods (craniometry) used to assess basilar invagination, including the Wackenheim line, Chamberlain line, McRae line, height index of Klaus, and spinous interlaminar line.

motion. Basilar invagination has recently been separated into two distinct subtypes [50]. In one subtype, patients had only the radiographic finding of basilar invagination; in the other subtype, patients also had an associated Chiari I malformation. Symptoms are highly variable and often do not become apparent until the second or third decade of life. Symptoms may also be elicited by minor trauma. Patients may often present with muscle weakness, neck pain, posterior column dysfunction, and paresthesias [50]. Common presenting signs include localized torticollis, limited neck mobility, a low hairline, and a webbed and short neck [50].

Treatment of basilar invagination usually begins with the use of traction. This maneuver can reduce the compression of the neural structures by the odontoid (Fig. 5). Once the impression is reduced, a posterior occipitocervical stabilization procedure can be performed to maintain the reduction. If the invagination cannot be reduced, a transoral decompression, followed by a posterior occipitocervical fusion, may be required. Patients with an associated Chiari decompression may benefit from foramen magnum decompression with duraplasty, and a few require a stabilization procedure [50].

Iniencephaly

Iniencephaly consists of congenital cervical synostoses, fixed retroflexion or hyperextension of the head, severe cervical lordosis, and incomplete posterior neural closure (occipital defect or cervical spina bifida) [51–53]. Many patients with iniencephaly now survive into adulthood, but they are often incapacitated by cervical lordosis and hyperextension of the head. Treatment of this condition has included suboccipital release, gradual flexion of the head over several weeks in

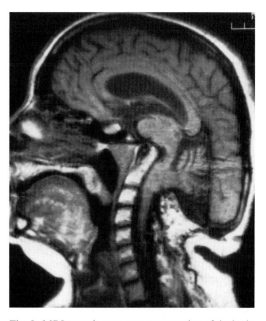

Fig. 5. MRI scan shows severe compression of the brain stem from basilar invagination.

a halo brace, and occipitocervical fusion to maintain the correction [54].

Posterior C2 arch anomalies

Although they are less common than defects of C1, posterior C2 arch defects often are more problematic. The reason for this is that they must be differentiated from traumatic spondylolisthesis, or hangman's fractures. In addition, fractures may be confused with a persistent neurocentral synchondrosis, so-called "primary spondylolysis" [55,56]. The neurocentral synchondrosis, which is the cartilaginous structure that joins the body of the axis to the two posterior centers of ossification, appears at birth and ossifies between 3 and 6 years of age but may persist and lead to confusion. If there is no sclerosis of the fragments that separate on flexion and the posterior arch of C2 is not malformed or underdeveloped, the defect likely represents a fracture [57].

Dysplastic or hypoplastic posterior arches of C2 may cause myelopathy. The clinical and radiographic picture is similar to that of a hypoplastic posterior arch of C1 in that the arch is often bifid and invaginating into the spinal canal, many patients present in adulthood, and treatment entails performing a laminectomy [58–60].

Anomalies of the odontoid

Congenital abnormalities of the second cervical vertebra often involve some malformation of the odontoid process. The degree to which the odontoid process may be affected ranges from hypoplasia to complete aplasia [16,61]. The resultant clinical picture may be one of atlantoaxial instability because of the fact that the normal anatomic and biomechanical complexes involving the transverse cruciate ligament and an intact odontoid process are not present. The true incidence of anomalies of the axis is unknown, but these anomalies are seen in association with Down syndrome, Morquio syndrome, and a variety of other skeletal dysplasias.

Os odontoideum is described as dissociation between the body of C2 and the dens, such that a disconnected ossicle takes the place of an intact odontoid process (Fig. 6). This should be differentiated from ossiculum terminale persistens, a condition whereby the tip of the dens, the ossiculum terminale, fails to fuse with the remainder of the dens. The ossiculum terminale usually is firmly bound to the main body of the dens by cartilage, and is consequently seldom the source of instability. Some believe that an os terminale becomes an os odontoideum when it enlarges in association with hypoplasia of the dens [57]. Historically, controversy existed regarding the cause of os odontoideum. Some authors favored a congenital cause, whereas others postulated that minor trauma in early childhood resulted in disruption of the vascular supply of the developing dens, causing it to dissociate from the axis [62–64]. Currently, most authors favor the latter explanation, as a chronic nonunited fracture of the odontoid process.

Patients with atlantoaxial instability from congenital malformations of the odontoid are at risk for significant neurologic injury. Many patients present with neck pain and headache from the instability, but instances of myelopathy and transient quadriparesis from minor trauma have been reported. If instability is suspected, dynamic imaging with flexion or extension films should be obtained. MRI should also be obtained to evaluate the spinal cord. Treatment for atlantoaxial instability resulting from os odontoideum or a maldeveloped odontoid process usually requires posterior stabilization. The highest success rates have been achieved with a C1-2 transarticular screw fixation method [65]. Some authors have also argued that even in the setting of asymptomatic instability, patients should undergo a fusion procedure, because even minor trauma may result in significant neurologic injury [66].

Subaxial spine abnormalities

Klippel-Feil syndrome

Perhaps the most commonly encountered congenital malformation of the cervical spine is KFS. In 1912, Klippel and Feil [67] reported the case of a patient with a short neck, a low hairline, and limited neck mobility (Fig. 7). At autopsy, the patient was found to have a spine consisting of only 12 discernible vertebrae. Although the triad of characteristics described is considered classic for the syndrome, it is now recognized that fewer than 50% of patients with congenital fusion of the cervical spine have all three signs [3]. The term Klippel-Feil syndrome refers to any congenital fusion of the cervical spine, with or without the classic triad, and is now commonly diagnosed in those patients with a congenital fusion of two or more cervical vertebrae (Fig. 8) [68]. The true incidence is impossible to know, but it is estimated that it occurs in approximately 1 in 40,000 to

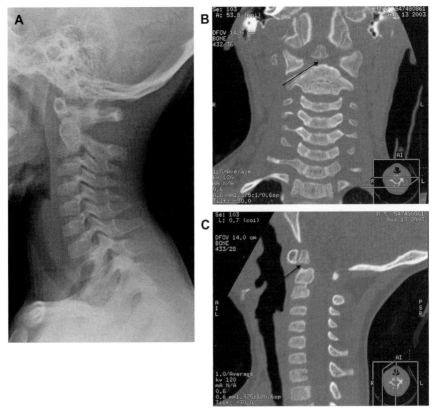

Fig. 6. Os odontoideum. Lateral radiograph (*A*), and CT coronal (*B*) and sagittal (*C*) reconstructions clearly show the disconnection of the dens from the body of C2 (*red arrow*).

42,000 births [3,69]. Several other abnormalities associated with KFS include congenital scoliosis, rib abnormalities, deafness, genitourinary abnormalities, Sprengel deformity, synkinesia, cervical ribs, and cardiovascular abnormalities [2,70–72].

The identification of a cause of KFS is complicated by the variable clinical presentation. In general, the syndrome is thought to result from the mutation or aberrant expression of genes involved in sclerotomal segmentation [73,74]. At least three distinct genetic forms of KFS have been described in the literature, each with associated birth defects [3]. An association with a mutation in the fibroblast growth factor receptor-3 gene in patients with autosomal dominant coronal synostosis, dysmorphic vertebrae and ribs, and Sprengel deformity has been described [75]; however, a similar phenotype has been observed without this particular mutation [76]. Recent pedigree analysis found that KFS and vocal cord impairment segregated with a paracentric inversion of chromosome 8q.

KFS has been characterized by several different classification schemes. In 1919, Feil divided the syndrome into three types on the basis of the site and extent of the congenital fusion. Type I described patients with fusion of cervical and upper thoracic vertebra. Type II described patients with only one or two cervical fusions. Type III included patients with fused cervical vertebra as well as lower thoracic or lumbar fusion. Some clinical correlations have been made with each type. Types I and III have shown a tendency toward association with scoliosis, and these types are typically inherited in an autosomal recessive manner [69,76–78]. Type II (the most common type) has been associated with other skeletal abnormalities, such as Sprengel deformity, and is generally inherited in an autosomal dominant fashion [76–78]. In general, however, this classification scheme has not proven clinically useful. A second scheme was used to describe three patterns of potentially unstable fusions [71,79]. Type I is characterized by fusion of C2 and C3 with

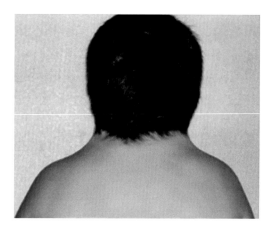

Fig. 7. Photograph of a patient with KFS. Note the short webbed neck and low-lying hairline.

occipitalization of the atlas. Type II describes a long cervical fusion with an abnormal craniocervical junction. Type III describes two segments of block fusion separated by a single nonfused interspace. Type III was thought to be the most susceptible to instability because of the theoretic strains on the nonfused interspace, but long-term clinical data have not confirmed this. Other authors have correlated various KFS deformities with dynamic imaging to create a classification scheme [80]. These authors showed that patients with hypermobility of the upper cervical spine

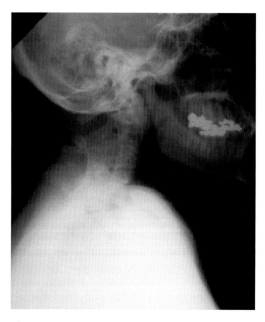

Fig. 8. Lateral radiograph of the cervical spine shows multiple cervical fusions in KFS.

were at the greatest risk of neurologic sequelae, whereas patients with hypermobility of the lower cervical spine were at higher risk for progressive degenerative disc disease. The most recent classification (reviewed by Tracy and colleagues [3]) separates KFS into four classes and incorporates the mode of inheritance [81]. Fusions at C1 with or without associated caudal fusions are Klippel-Feil type 1 (KF1) with an autosomal recessive inheritance pattern. KF1 is most often associated with other anomalies. KF2 describes patients with fusions no higher than C2-3. These patients have an autosomal dominant inheritance pattern and 100% penetrance of the C2-3 fusion. KF3 is defined as congenital fusions caudal to C2-3 and has autosomal recessive or dominant inheritance. KF4 is described as synonymous with Wildervanck syndrome, which is characterized by congenital cervical fusion, congenital hearing loss, and the Duane anomaly. It is thought to have an X-linked dominant inheritance pattern and is hemizygous lethal.

As mentioned previously, the classic triad of KFS is seen in fewer than 50% of patients. The most common clinical presentation of KFS is limited range of motion, particularly lateral bending. If fewer than three cervical vertebrae are fused, however, motion of the cervical spine may appear normal, because adjacent levels may compensate. Thus, patients with extensive neck fusions may present at an earlier age. Similarly, patients with higher fusions near the craniovertebral junction often present earlier (Fig. 9): patients with C1-2 fusions often present with pain in childhood, whereas those with lower cervical fusion present in the second or third decade of life or later, when symptomatic junctional degeneration develops [82]. Torticollis or neck webbing is seen in only 20% of patients with KFS [71,83–85]. Torticollis is not specific to any particular cervical spine anomaly. It may be a manifestation of a muscular condition or bony abnormalities [86]. Hemivertebra of the atlas is often seen in association with torticollis. Other conditions are associated with torticollis as well, including posterior fossa tumors, infections, and cervicothoracic scoliosis. In patients with severely limited neck mobility and a low posterior hairline, iniencephaly should be suspected.

Several other clinical presentations are associated with KFS. Facial asymmetry, such as that seen in the congenital craniosynostosis syndromes of Crouzon and Apert, may be associated with cervical spine anomalies [87]. Other associated

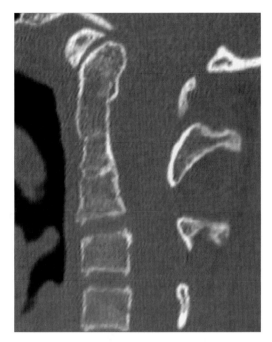

Fig. 9. Sagittal reconstruction CT scan shows congenital fusion of C2 and C3 in a young patient with KFS.

syndromes include Wildervanck, Rokitansky-Kuster-Hauser, or Goldenhar syndrome. Hearing loss can be present in up to 30% of patients with KFS, and hearing should be evaluated formally if the diagnosis is suspected [84,85]. Deafness may be the result of ankylosis of the ossicles, footplate fixation, an absent external auditory canal, or sensorineural hearing loss [88,89].

Numerous musculoskeletal anomalies are associated with KFS, with the most common being scoliosis (usually congenital), which occurs in up to 60% of patients. Sprengel deformity, a congenital elevation of the scapula, can be seen in 20% to 35% of patients with KFS. It is thought to arise from failure of descent of the scapula from the first embryologic cervical level to its normal position, just caudal to the first rib [90]. The time of descent coincides with cervical somite resegmentation, implying a connection between an anomalous scapular descent and aberrant fusion of cervical vertebral bodies. Other musculoskeletal anomalies include cervical ribs, rib anomalies, and hemivertebrae.

Cardiovascular abnormalities are reported to occur in up to 14% of patients with KFS. A ventricular septal defect, independently or in combination with other cardiac defects, is the most common associated abnormality [91,92]. Some authors recommend a baseline echocardiogram, especially for those patients undergoing surgery.

Various neurologic disturbances may be seen in patients with KFS. These include developmental abnormalities of the central nervous system, such as brain stem malformations; myelopathy as a result of long-standing spinal cord compression; radiculopathy as a result of nerve root irritation; and nonspecific symptoms of headache, weakness, and numbness. An unusual but not uncommon associated neurologic sign is synkinesis. This is a condition in which involuntary mirrored motions, primarily in the upper extremities, are observed. Although it may be seen in normally developed children, up to 20% of patients with KFS exhibit the condition [93,94]. Its cause is unknown, but autopsy results of two patients with KFS and synkinesia showed an incomplete pyramidal decussation. Synkinesia is generally effectively treated with occupational therapy, and the condition often subsides as the patient ages.

Genitourinary abnormalities are also associated with KFS. Up to 64% of patients have some defect in the genitourinary pathway, with the most common manifestation being unilateral renal agenesis [71,95,96]. The renal system begins its development at 28 to 30 days of embryologic life. An insult to the developing embryo between the fourth and eighth weeks of life may result in anomalies of the genitourinary system as well as those related to resegmentation of cervical somites. Other renal anomalies include malrotation of the kidney, absence of both kidneys, ureteral agenesis, hydronephrosis, and other malformations of the kidney [97–99]. Patients with KFS should receive an ultrasound scan of the renal system. Intravenous pyelography is suggested for patients with an abnormality detected on ultrasound or an inconclusive ultrasound study [95].

Abnormalities noted in the renal system may point to abnormalities of the reproductive system, particularly in women. An absent vagina, uterus, or ovaries have all been reported in association with KFS [97,100,101]. Male reproductive abnormalities, including dysplastic or undescended testes, have also been reported. In general, if abnormalities of the renal system are identified, a thorough ultrasonographic examination of the reproductive system should be performed as well.

Imaging of the cervical spine is important for an accurate diagnosis. Routine plain radiography consisting of anteroposterior, lateral, and

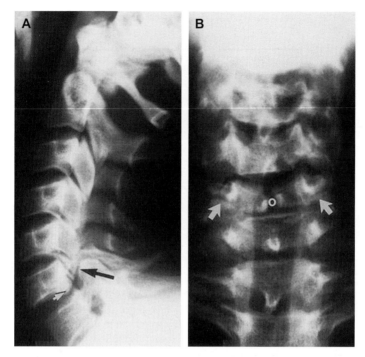

Fig. 10. Lateral (*A*) and anteroposterior (*B*) radiographs show spondylolysis of C6. On the lateral image, the black arrow shows the corticated cleft dividing the lateral masses, resulting in a small amount of anterolisthesis (*gray arrow*). The anteroposterior radiograph clearly shows the bilateral corticated clefts (*arrows*) and spina bifida occulta (o). (*From* Schwartz JM. Case 36: bilateral cervical spondylolysis of C6. Radiology 2001;220:192; with permission.)

open-mouth odontoid views is a useful initial study because it can be used to identify an obvious congenital fusion or cervical stenosis quickly. Flexion and extension views provide a dynamic snapshot of the cervical spine and can identify stability of the atlanto-occipital, atlantoaxial, and subaxial joints. In children younger than 8 years of age, radiography of the cartilaginous spine can be difficult to interpret. Patients with antero- or retrolisthesis of cervical vertebral bodies may have instability, although pseudosubluxation of C2 on C3 or C3 on C4 is physiologically normal in children [102–104]. Juvenile rheumatoid arthritis can mimic KFS, although additional clinical information easily distinguishes the two conditions [69].

MRI should be used in the setting of suspected compromise of the brain stem or spinal cord. Sagittal MRI allows for determination of the anteroposterior dimension of the spinal canal. Additionally, MRI allows for detection of other central nervous system lesions, such as syringomyelia, tethered cord, diastematomyelia, and Chiari malformation [3,105]. In addition to the imaging modalities that are useful for screening for associated systemic abnormalities (eg, renal ultrasound), further imaging of the thoracic and lumbar spine is warranted in patients with KFS because they may have abnormalities in these regions, such as scoliosis [69].

Treatment for KFS depends on the nature of the pathologic findings. Because many patients are asymptomatic throughout life, treatment must be individualized. Patients who are asymptomatic, have stable fusion patterns, and have an adequate spinal canal diameter may never develop symptoms [68,106]. Although many patients present with minor symptoms, it should be recognized that minor traumatic events have resulted in catastrophic spinal cord injuries leading to tetraplegia or even death [106–116]. For patients with atlanto-occipital instability, a technique for occipitocervical fusion should be used. Atlantoaxial instability is best approached with C1-2 transarticular screw fixation techniques. The operative details for these techniques are described elsewhere in the text. Patients with subaxial instability typically do not present with neurologic symptoms

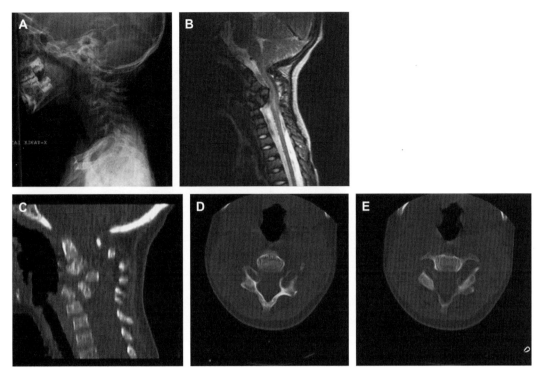

Fig. 11. Lateral radiograph (*A*) and sagittal CT scan (*C*) depict the "buckling" deformity of the neck with the spinal cord being compressed ventrally as shown in the sagittal MRI scan (*B*). The absence of an osseous bridge between the anterior and posterior elements and the enlarged and abnormally shaped foramen transversarium are seen in the axial CT scans (*D, E*).

but may have significant degenerative disc disease. These patients may be successfully treated with discectomy and fusion. Cervical stenosis is generally treated with posterior decompression and fusion if necessary [117,118].

Miscellaneous disorders

A variety of formation-segmentation anomalies can occur in the cervical spine as they do in other parts of the spine. These include midline vertebral body clefts, sagittal and coronal hemivertebrae, hypoplasia or complete absence of a vertebra, absence of a pedicle, and block vertebrae (most commonly between C2 and C3).

Cervical spondylolysis is a rare congenital spinal anomaly. It is defined as a cleft between the superior and inferior articular facets of the articular pillar or lateral mass, the cervical equivalent of the pars interarticularis of the lumbar spine (Fig. 10) [119,120]. Previously, cervical spondylolysis has only been described in adults [121,122]. Characteristic radiographic findings include well-corticated margins at the defect, a characteristic "bow-tie" deformity, and ipsilateral

dysplastic facets. Compensatory hypertrophic changes of the adjacent articular processes, spina bifida, and spondylolisthesis are frequently but not always seen [123]. Cervical spondylolysis most commonly occurs at a single level (the most common level is C6), but several cases of multilevel involvement have been reported [120,124–128].

Recently, an osseous disconnection between the anterior and posterior elements resulting in a severe kyphotic deformity and myelopathy has been described (Fig. 11) [129]. This has been described as congenital multilevel cervical disconnection syndrome. Patients with this disorder were treated with extensive anterior and posterior reduction, decompression, reconstruction, and stabilization or fusion procedures. It is hypothesized that this anomaly is a result of a failure of connecting chondrification centers to form (Fig. 12).

Summary

Developmental anomalies of the cervical spine vary widely. The development of the cervical spine

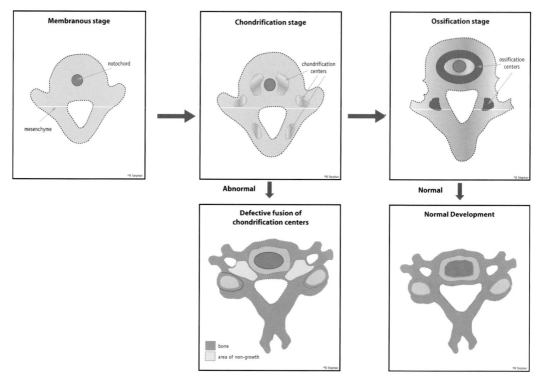

Fig. 12. The normal chondrification and ossification stages of spinal embryogenesis. The anomaly is attributable to improper fusion of chondrification or ossification centers.

depends on the interaction of several complicated genetic pathways. An alteration of these pathways may result in a malformation of the cervical spine, many of which are the result of a failure of segmentation of cervical somites. It is important to recognize that some of these malformations may be associated with other defects involving the cardiovascular, neurologic, renal, and reproductive systems.

The true incidence of these disparate anomalies is not known for certain, partly because of their frequent asymptomatic nature. Identifying the symptomatic anomalies requires adequate imaging. Patients may present with abnormalities as simple as two congenitally fused vertebrae requiring no treatment or as complex as craniocervical instability requiring occipitocervical fusion. Recognizing those congenital abnormalities that contribute to an unstable cervical spine or critical spinal stenosis may prevent a catastrophic spinal cord injury.

References

[1] Raimondi AJ, Choux M, Di Rocco C. The pediatric spine. New York: Springer-Verlag; 1989.

[2] Baba H, Maezawa Y, Furusawa N, et al. The cervical spine in the Klippel-Feil syndrome. A report of 57 cases. Int Orthop 1995;19(4):204–8.

[3] Tracy MR, Dormans JP, Kusumi K. Klippel-Feil syndrome: clinical features and current understanding of etiology. Clin Orthop Relat Res 2004; (424):183–90.

[4] Tredwell SJ, Smith DF, Macleod PJ, et al. Cervical spine anomalies in fetal alcohol syndrome. Spine 1982;7(4):331–4.

[5] Brown MW, Templeton AW, Hodges FJ 3rd. The incidence of acquired and congenital fusions in the cervical spine. Am J Roentgenol Radium Ther Nucl Med 1964;92:1255–9.

[6] Rao PV. Median (third) occipital condyle. Clin Anat 2002;15(2):148–51.

[7] Kotil K, Kalayci M. Ventral cervicomedullary junction compression secondary to condylus occipitalis (median occipital condyle), a rare entity. J Spinal Disord Tech 2005;18(4):382–4.

[8] Halanski MA, Iskandar B, Nemeth B, et al. The coconut condyle: occipital condylar dysplasia causing torticollis and leading to C1 fracture. J Spinal Disord Tech 2006;19(4):295–8.

[9] Ohaegbulam C, Woodard EJ, Proctor M. Occipitocondylar hyperplasia: an unusual craniovertebral junction anomaly causing myelopathy. Case report. J Neurosurg 2005;103(4 Suppl):379–81.

[10] McRae DL, Barnum AS. Occipitalization of the atlas. Am J Roentgenol Radium Ther Nucl Med 1953;70(1):23–46.

[11] Ryken TC, Menezes AH. Cervicomedullary compression by separate atlantal lateral mass. Pediatr Neurosurg 1993;19(3):165–8.

[12] Hensinger RN. Osseous anomalies of the craniovertebral junction. Spine 1986;11(4):323–33.

[13] Menezes AH, Ryken TC. Craniovertebral junction abnormalities in the pediatric spine. In: Weinstein SL, editor. The pediatric spine—principles and practice. Philadelphia: Lippincott Williams & Wilkins; 2004. p. 219–37.

[14] McRae D. Bony abnormalities in the region of the foramen magnum: correlation of the anatomic and neurologic findings. Acta Radiol 1953;40(2–3): 335–54.

[15] Wackenheim A. Occipitalization of the ventral part and vertebralization of the dorsal part of the atlas with insufficiency of the transverse ligament. Neuroradiology 1982;24(1):45–7.

[16] Guille JT, Sherk HH. Congenital osseous anomalies of the upper and lower cervical spine in children. J Bone Joint Surg Am 2002;84-A(2):277–88.

[17] Menezes AH, Ryken TC, Brockmeyer DL. Abnormalities of the craniocervical junction. In: McLone DG, editor. Pediatric neurosurgery—surgery of the developing nervous system. 4th edition. Philadelphia: W.B. Saunder Company; 2001. p. 400–22.

[18] Goel A, Kulkarni AG. Mobile and reducible atlantoaxial dislocation in presence of occipitalized atlas: report on treatment of eight cases by direct lateral mass plate and screw fixation. Spine 2004; 29(22):E520–3.

[19] Browd S, Healy LJ, Dobie G, et al. Morphometric and qualitative analysis of congenital occipitocervical instability in children: implications for patients with Down syndrome. J Neurosurg 2006; 105(1 Suppl):50–4.

[20] Mace SE, Holliday R. Congenital absence of the C1 vertebral arch. Am J Emerg Med 1986;4(4):326–9.

[21] Perez-Vallina JR, Riano-Galan I, Cobo-Ruisanchez A, et al. Congenital anomaly of craniovertebral junction: atlas-dens fusion with C1 anterior arch cleft. J Spinal Disord Tech 2002;15(1):84–7.

[22] Chambers AA, Gaskill MF. Midline anterior atlas clefts: CT findings. J Comput Assist Tomogr 1992; 16(6):868–70.

[23] Currarino G, Rollins N, Diehl JT. Congenital defects of the posterior arch of the atlas: a report of seven cases including an affected mother and son. AJNR Am J Neuroradiol 1994;15(2):249–54.

[24] Bonneville F, Jacamon M, Runge M, et al. Split atlas in a patient with odontoid fracture. Neuroradiology 2004;46(6):450–2.

[25] Garg A, Gaikwad SB, Gupta V, et al. Bipartite atlas with os odontoideum: case report. Spine 2004; 29(2):E35–8.

[26] Jodicke A, Hahn A, Berthold LD, et al. Dysplasia of C-1 and craniocervical instability in patients with Shprintzen-Goldberg syndrome. Case report and review of the literature. J Neurosurg 2006; 105(3 Suppl):238–41.

[27] Klimo P Jr, Blumenthal DT, Couldwell WT. Congenital partial aplasia of the posterior arch of the atlas causing myelopathy: case report and review of the literature. Spine 2003;28(12):E224–8.

[28] Sagiuchi T, Tachibana S, Sato K, et al. Lhermitte sign during yawning associated with congenital partial aplasia of the posterior arch of the atlas. AJNR Am J Neuroradiol 2006;27(2):258–60.

[29] Sharma A, Gaikwad SB, Deol PS, et al. Partial aplasia of the posterior arch of the atlas with an isolated posterior arch remnant: findings in three cases. AJNR Am J Neuroradiol 2000;21(6): 1167–71.

[30] Torreman M, Verhagen IT, Sluzewski M, et al. Recurrent transient quadriparesis after minor cervical trauma associated with bilateral partial agenesis of the posterior arch of the atlas. Case report. J Neurosurg 1996;84(4):663–5.

[31] Connor SE, Chandler C, Robinson S, et al. Congenital midline cleft of the posterior arch of atlas: a rare cause of symptomatic cervical canal stenosis. Eur Radiol 2001;11(9):1766–9.

[32] Nishikawa K, Ludwig SC, Colon RJ, et al. Cervical myelopathy and congenital stenosis from hypoplasia of the atlas: report of three cases and literature review. Spine 2001;26(5):E80–6.

[33] Sawada H, Akiguchi I, Fukuyama H, et al. Marked canal stenosis at the level of the atlas. Neuroradiology 1989;31(4):346–8.

[34] Devi BI, Shenoy SN, Panigrahi MK, et al. Anomaly of arch of atlas—a rare cause of symptomatic canal stenosis in children. Pediatr Neurosurg 1997;26(4):214–7 [discussion: 217–8].

[35] Komatsu Y, Shibata T, Yasuda S, et al. Atlas hypoplasia as a cause of high cervical myelopathy. Case report. J Neurosurg 1993;79(6):917–9.

[36] May D, Jenny B, Faundez A. Cervical cord compression due to a hypoplastic atlas. Case report. J Neurosurg 2001;94(1 Suppl):133–6.

[37] Phan N, Marras C, Midha R, et al. Cervical myelopathy caused by hypoplasia of the atlas: two case reports and review of the literature. Neurosurgery 1998;43(3):629–33.

[38] Tokiyoshi K, Nakagawa H, Kadota T. Spinal canal stenosis at the level of the atlas: case report. Surg Neurol 1994;41(3):238–40.

[39] Huang MJ, Glaser JA. Complete arcuate foramen precluding C1 lateral mass screw fixation in a patient with rheumatoid arthritis: case report. Iowa Orthop J 2003;23:96–9.

[40] Horton WA, Lunstrum GP. Fibroblast growth factor receptor 3 mutations in achondroplasia and related forms of dwarfism. Rev Endocr Metab Disord 2002;3(4):381–5.

[41] Reid CS, Pyeritz RE, Kopits SE, et al. Cervicome-dullary cord compression in young children with achondroplasia: value of comprehensive neuro-logic and respiratory evaluation. Basic Life Sci 1988;48:199–206.

[42] Reid CS, Pyeritz RE, Kopits SE, et al. Cervicome-dullary compression in young patients with achon-droplasia: value of comprehensive neurologic and respiratory evaluation. J Pediatr 1987;110(4): 522–30.

[43] Pauli RM, Scott CI, Wassman ER Jr, et al. Apnea and sudden unexpected death in infants with achondroplasia. J Pediatr 1984;104(3): 342–8.

[44] Hecht JT, Nelson FW, Butler IJ, et al. Computer-ized tomography of the foramen magnum: achon-droplastic values compared to normal standards. Am J Med Genet 1985;20(2):355–60.

[45] Wang H, Rosenbaum AE, Reid CS, et al. Pediatric patients with achondroplasia: CT evaluation of the craniocervical junction. Radiology 1987;164(2): 515–9.

[46] Hecht JT, Horton WA, Reid CS, et al. Growth of the foramen magnum in achondroplasia. Am J Med Genet 1989;32(4):528–35.

[47] Frigon VA, Castro FP, Whitecloud TS, et al. Iso-lated subaxial cervical spine stenosis in achondro-plasia. Curr Surg 2000;57(4):354–6.

[48] Marin-Padilla M. Cephalic axial skeletal-neural dysraphic disorders: embryology and pathology. Can J Neurol Sci 1991;18(2):153–69.

[49] O'Rahilly R, Muller F, Meyer DB. The human ver-tebral column at the end of the embryonic period proper. 2. The occipitocervical region. J Anat 1983;136(Pt 1):181–95.

[50] Goel A, Bhatjiwale M, Desai K. Basilar invagina-tion: a study based on 190 surgically treated pa-tients. J Neurosurg 1998;88(6):962–8.

[51] Georgopoulos G, Pizzutillo PD, Lee MS. Occipito-atlantal instability in children. A report of five cases and review of the literature. J Bone Joint Surg Am 1987;69(3):429–36.

[52] Morocz I, Szeifert GT, Molnar P, et al. Prenatal di-agnosis and pathoanatomy of iniencephaly. Clin Genet 1986;30(2):81–6.

[53] Nicholson JT, Sherk HH. Anomalies of the occipi-tocervical articulation. J Bone Joint Surg Am 1968; 50(2):295–304.

[54] Sherk HH, Shut L, Chung S. Iniencephalic defor-mity of the cervical spine with Klippel-Feil anoma-lies and congenital elevation of the scapula; report of three cases. J Bone Joint Surg Am 1974;56(6): 1254–9.

[55] van Rijn RR, Kool DR, de Witt Hamer PC, et al. An abused five-month-old girl: hangman's fracture or congenital arch defect? J Emerg Med 2005;29(1): 61–5.

[56] Smith JT, Skinner SR, Shonnard NH. Persistent synchondrosis of the second cervical vertebra simulating a hangman's fracture in a child. Report of a case. J Bone Joint Surg Am 1993;75(8): 1228–30.

[57] Swischuk LE. Imaging of the cervical spine in chil-dren. New York: Springer-Verlag; 2002.

[58] Asakawa H, Yanaka K, Narushima K, et al. Anomaly of the axis causing cervical myelopa-thy. Case report. J Neurosurg 1999;91(1 Suppl): 121–3.

[59] Koyama T, Tanaka K, Handa J. A rare anomaly of the axis: report of a case with shaded three-dimen-sional computed tomographic display. Surg Neurol 1986;25(5):491–4.

[60] Sakai S, Sakane M, Harada S, et al. A cervical my-elopathy due to invaginated laminae of the axis into the spinal canal. Spine 2004;29(4):E82–4.

[61] Dawson EG, Smith L. Atlanto-axial subluxation in children due to vertebral anomalies. J Bone Joint Surg Am 1979;61(4):582–7.

[62] Fielding JW, Hensinger RN, Hawkins RJ. Os odontoideum. J Bone Joint Surg Am 1980;62(3): 376–83.

[63] Hawkins RJ, Fielding JW, Thompson WJ. Os odontoideum: congenital or acquired. A case re-port. J Bone Joint Surg Am 1976;58(3):413–4.

[64] Ricciardi JE, Kaufer H, Louis DS. Acquired os odontoideum following acute ligament injury. Re-port of a case. J Bone Joint Surg Am 1976;58(3): 410–2.

[65] Gluf WM, Schmidt MH, Apfelbaum RI. Atlan-toaxial transarticular screw fixation: a review of surgical indications, fusion rate, complications, and lessons learned in 191 adult patients. J Neuro-surg Spine 2005;2(2):155–63.

[66] Clark CR. Cervical Spine Research Society. Edito-rial Committee. The cervical spine. 4th edition. Phil-adelphia: Lippincott Williams and Wilkins; 2005.

[67] Klippel M, Feil A. The classic: a case of absence of cervical vertebrae with the thoracic cage rising to the base of the cranium (cervical thoracic cage). Clin Orthop Relat Res 1975;(109):3–8.

[68] Theiss SM, Smith MD, Winter RB. The long-term follow-up of patients with Klippel-Feil syndrome and congenital scoliosis. Spine 1997;22(11): 1219–22.

[69] Thomsen MN, Schneider U, Weber M, et al. Scoli-osis and congenital anomalies associated with Klip-pel-Feil syndrome types I–III. Spine 1997;22(4): 396–401.

[70] Copley LA, Dormans JP. Cervical spine disorders in infants and children. J Am Acad Orthop Surg 1998;6(4):204–14.

[71] Hensinger RN, Lang JE, MacEwen GD. Klippel-Feil syndrome; a constellation of associated anomalies. J Bone Joint Surg Am 1974;56(6): 1246–53.

[72] Herman MJ, Pizzutillo PD. Cervical spine disor-ders in children. Orthop Clin North Am 1999; 30(3):457–66, ix.

[73] Clarke RA, Kearsley JH, Walsh DA. Patterned expression in familial Klippel-Feil syndrome. Teratology 1996;53(3):152–7.

[74] Clarke RA, Singh S, McKenzie H, et al. Familial Klippel-Feil syndrome and paracentric inversion inv(8)(q22.2q23.3). Am J Hum Genet 1995;57(6): 1364–70.

[75] Larson AR, Josephson KD, Pauli RM, et al. Klippel-Feil anomaly with Sprengel anomaly, omovertebral bone, thumb abnormalities, and flexion-crease changes: novel association or syndrome? Am J Med Genet 2001;101(2):158–62.

[76] Lowry RB, Jabs EW, Graham GE, et al. Syndrome of coronal craniosynostosis, Klippel-Feil anomaly, and Sprengel shoulder with and without Pro250Arg mutation in the FGFR3 gene. Am J Med Genet 2001;104(2):112–9.

[77] Gunderson CH, Greenspan RH, Glaser GH, et al. The Klippel-Feil syndrome: genetic and clinical reevaluation of cervical fusion. Medicine (Baltimore) 1967;46(6):491–512.

[78] Juberg RC, Gershanik JJ. Cervical vertebral fusion (Klippel-Feil) syndrome with consanguineous parents. J Med Genet 1976;13(3):246–9.

[79] Hensinger RN. Congenital anomalies of the cervical spine. Clin Orthop Relat Res 1991;(264): 16–38.

[80] Pizzutillo PD, Woods M, Nicholson L, et al. Risk factors in Klippel-Feil syndrome. Spine 1994; 19(18):2110–6.

[81] Clarke RA, Catalan G, Diwan AD, et al. Heterogeneity in Klippel-Feil syndrome: a new classification. Pediatr Radiol 1998;28(12):967–74.

[82] Dietz F. Congenital abnormalities of the cervical spine. In: Weinstein SL, editor. The pediatric spine—principles and practice. 2nd edition. Philadelphia: Lippincott Williams & Wilkins; 2004 p. 239–51.

[83] Gray SW, Romaine CB, Skandalakis JE. Congenital fusion of the cervical vertebrae. Surg Gynecol Obstet 1964;118:373–85.

[84] Stark EW, Borton TE. Hearing loss and the Klippel-Feil syndrome. Am J Dis Child 1972;123(3): 233–5.

[85] Stark EW, Borton TE. Klippel-Feil syndrome and associated hearing loss. Arch Otolaryngol 1973; 97(5):415–9.

[86] Ballock RT, Song KM. The prevalence of nonmuscular causes of torticollis in children. J Pediatr Orthop 1996;16(4):500–4.

[87] Sherk HH, Whitaker LA, Pasquariello PS. Facial malformations and spinal anomalies. A predictable relationship. Spine 1982;7(6):526–31.

[88] Jarvis JF, Sellars SL. Klippel-Feil deformity associated with congenital conductive deafness. J Laryngol Otol 1974;88(3):285–9.

[89] Palant DI, Carter BL. Klippel-Feil syndrome and deafness. A study with polytomography. Am J Dis Child 1972;123(3):218–21.

[90] Dolan KD. Cervical spine injuries below the axis. Radiol Clin North Am 1977;15(2):247–59.

[91] Morrison SG, Perry LW, Scott LP 3rd. Congenital brevicollis (Klippel-Feil syndrome) and cardiovascular anomalies. Am J Dis Child 1968;115(5):614–20.

[92] Nora JJ, Cohen M, Maxwell G. Klippel-Feil syndrome with congenital heart disease. Am J Dis Child 1962;102:858–64.

[93] Baird PA, Robinson GC, Buckler WS. Klippel-Feil syndrome. A study of mirror movement detected by electromyography. Am J Dis Child 1967; 113(5):546–51.

[94] Gunderson CH, Solitare GB. Mirror movements in patients with the Klippel-Feil syndrome. Neuropathologic observations. Arch Neurol 1968;18(6): 675–9.

[95] Drvaric DM, Ruderman RJ, Conrad RW, et al. Congenital scoliosis and urinary tract abnormalities: are intravenous pyelograms necessary? J Pediatr Orthop 1987;7(4):441–3.

[96] Moore WB, Matthews TJ, Rabinowitz R. Genitourinary anomalies associated with Klippel-Feil syndrome. J Bone Joint Surg Am 1975;57(3):355–7.

[97] Duncan PA. Embryologic pathogenesis of renal agenesis associated with cervical vertebral anomalies (Klippel-Feil phenotype). Birth Defects Orig Artic Ser 1977;13(3D):91–101.

[98] Duncan PA, Shapiro LR, Stangel JJ, et al. The MURCS association: mullerian duct aplasia, renal aplasia, and cervicothoracic somite dysplasia. J Pediatr 1979;95(3):399–402.

[99] Ramsey J, Bliznak J. Klippel-Feil syndrome with renal agenesis and other anomalies. Am J Roentgenol Radium Ther Nucl Med 1971;113(3):460–3.

[100] Baird PA, Lowry RB. Absent vagina and the Klippel-Feil anomaly. Am J Obstet Gynecol 1974; 118(2):290–1.

[101] Mecklenburg RS, Krueger PM. Extensive genitourinary anomalies associated with Klippel-Feil syndrome. Am J Dis Child 1974;128(1):92–3.

[102] Cattell HS, Filtzer DL. Pseudosubluxation and other normal variations in the cervical spine in children. A study of one hundred and sixty children. J Bone Joint Surg Am 1965;47(7):1295–309.

[103] Pollack CV Jr, Hendey GW, Martin DR, et al. Use of flexion-extension radiographs of the cervical spine in blunt trauma. Ann Emerg Med 2001; 38(1):8–11.

[104] Ralston ME. Physiologic anterior subluxation: case report of occurrence at C5 to C6 and C6 to C7 spinal levels. Ann Emerg Med 2004;44(5): 472–5.

[105] Ulmer JL, Elster AD, Ginsberg LE, et al. Klippel-Feil syndrome: CT and MR of acquired and congenital abnormalities of cervical spine and cord. J Comput Assist Tomogr 1993;17(2):215–24.

[106] Rouvreau P, Glorion C, Langlais J, et al. Assessment and neurologic involvement of patients with cervical spine congenital synostosis as in

Klippel-Feil syndrome: study of 19 cases. J Pediatr Orthop B 1998;7(3):179–85.

[107] Ducker TB. Cervical myeloradiculopathy: Klippel-Feil deformity. J Spinal Disord 1990;3(4):439–40 [discussion: 441–44].

[108] Elster AD. Quadriplegia after minor trauma in the Klippel-Feil syndrome. A case report and review of the literature. J Bone Joint Surg Am 1984;66(9): 1473–4.

[109] Epstein JA, Carras R, Epstein BS, et al. Myelopathy in cervical spondylosis with vertebral subluxation and hyperlordosis. J Neurosurg 1970;32(4): 421–6.

[110] Epstein NE, Epstein JA, Zilkha A. Traumatic myelopathy in a seventeen-year-old child with cervical spinal stenosis (without fracture or dislocation) and a C2-C3 Klippel-Feil fusion. A case report. Spine 1984;9(4):344–7.

[111] Hall JE, Simmons ED, Danylchuk K, et al. Instability of the cervical spine and neurological involvement in Klippel-Feil syndrome. A case report. J Bone Joint Surg Am 1990;72(3):460–2.

[112] Karasick D, Schweitzer ME, Vaccaro AR. The traumatized cervical spine in Klippel-Feil syndrome: imaging features. AJR Am J Roentgenol 1998;170(1):85–8.

[113] Sherk HH, Dawoud S. Congenital os odontoideum with Klippel-Feil anomaly and fatal atlanto-axial instability. Report of a case. Spine 1981; 6(1):42–5.

[114] Southwell RB, Reynolds AF, Badger VM, et al. Klippel-Feil syndrome with cervical compression resulting from cervical subluxation in association with an omo-vertebral bone. Spine 1980;5(5): 480–2.

[115] Strax TE, Baran E. Traumatic quadriplegia associated with Klippel-Feil syndrome: discussion and case reports. Arch Phys Med Rehabil 1975;56(8): 363–5.

[116] Torg JS, Pavlov H, Genuario SE, et al. Neurapraxia of the cervical spinal cord with transient quadriplegia. J Bone Joint Surg Am 1986;68(9):1354–70.

[117] Koop SE, Winter RB, Lonstein JE. The surgical treatment of instability of the upper part of the cervical spine in children and adolescents. J Bone Joint Surg Am 1984;66(3):403–11.

[118] Smith MD, Phillips WA, Hensinger RN. Fusion of the upper cervical spine in children and adolescents. An analysis of 17 patients. Spine 1991;16(7): 695–701.

[119] Raichel M, Lumelsky D, Tanzman M, et al. Congenital cervical spondylolisthesis [Hebrew]. Harefuah 2003;142(12):820–1, 879.

[120] Forsberg DA, Martinez S, Vogler JB 3rd, et al. Cervical spondylolysis: imaging findings in 12 patients. AJR Am J Roentgenol 1990;154(4):751–5.

[121] Dietz F. Congenital abnormalities of the cervical spine. In: Weinstein SL, editor. The pediatric spine. Principles and practice. 2nd edition. Philadelphia: Lippincott Williams & Wilkins; 2001. p. 239–51.

[122] Ganey TM, Ogden JA. Development and maturation of the axial skeleton. In: Weinstein SL, editor. The pediatric spine. Principles and practice. 2nd edition. Philadelphia: Lippincott Williams & Wilkins; 2001. p. 3–54.

[123] Poggi JJ, Martinez S, Hardaker WT Jr, et al. Cervical spondylolysis. J Spinal Disord 1992;5(3): 349–56.

[124] Kubota M, Saeki N, Yamaura A, et al. Congenital spondylolysis of the axis with associated myelopathy. Case report. J Neurosurg 2003;98(1 Suppl): 84–6.

[125] Garin C, Kohler R, Sales de Gauzy J, et al. Cervical spondylolysis in children. Apropos of 4 cases. Review of the literature [French]. Rev Chir Orthop Reparatrice Appar Mot 1995;81(7):626–30.

[126] Yochum TR, Carton JT, Barry MS. Cervical spondylolysis: three levels of simultaneous involvement. J Manipulative Physiol Ther 1995;18(6):411–5.

[127] Prioleau GR, Wilson CB. Cervical spondylolysis with spondylolisthesis. Case report. J Neurosurg 1975;43(6):750–3.

[128] Schwartz JM. Case 36: bilateral cervical spondylolysis of C6. Radiology 2001;220(1):191–4.

[129] Klimo P Jr, Anderson RCE, Brockmeyer DL. Multilevel cervical disconnection syndrome: initial description, embryogenesis, and management. J Neurosurg 2006;104(3 Suppl):181–7.

ELSEVIER
SAUNDERS

Neurosurg Clin N Am 18 (2007) 479–498

NEUROSURGERY
CLINICS
OF NORTH AMERICA

Congenital Abnormalities of the Thoracic and Lumbar Spine

Rod J. Oskouian, Jr, MD, Charles A. Sansur, MD,
Christopher I. Shaffrey, MD*

Department of Neurological Surgery, University of Virginia, Box 800212, Charlottesville, VA 22902, USA

Congenital spinal anomalies entail a wide spectrum of conditions that share in common some form of error during embryogenesis. Congenital disorders of the spine may not always be readily apparent at birth; they can present as a deformity with growth or with clinical signs of neurologic dysfunction early or later as an adolescent or adult. In this article the authors briefly summarize the embryology of the spine, which provides a background for understanding the pathophysiology of congenital spinal lesions. The discussion entails spine embryology and the developmental abnormalities commonly seen in the thoracolumbar spine.

Incidence

The incidence of congenital spinal anomalies is low and is usually seen as a sporadic entity. The incidence of congenital scoliosis in the general population is approximately 1/1000 to 1/2000 [1–3]. Certain conditions, such as spinal dysraphism, have a geographic epidemiology and have a 0.1% to 0.2% incidence in North America and a 10-fold increased incidence to 2.5% for subsequent offspring in the affected families [4]. Research on chromosomal analysis has linked a possible locus for certain types of deformities, such as hemivertebrae, to chromosome 17, whereas chromosome 18 has been associated with multiple vertebral segmentation defects [5–7].

Types of congenital abnormalities

Various types of congenital abnormalities of the thoracic, lumbar, and sacral spine are discussed in this article. The most noteworthy thoracolumbar congenital anomalies are congenital scoliosis and kyphosis. Lumbar spine anomalies discussed in this article include congenital lordosis, spinal stenosis, segmental spinal dysgenesis, dysplastic spondylolisthesis, spinal dysraphisms, diastematomyelia, neurenteric cysts, lipomas, dermal sinus tracts, dermoids, epidermoids, and tethered cord. The sacral spine disorders discussed in this article are sacral agenesis and teratomas.

Associated conditions

Congenital malformations of the spine are associated with other disorders affecting various organs that are developing during similar phases of embryogenesis. The most common organ system affected is the urologic system with as high as a 25% incidence being reported [8]. The next most common organ system to be affected is the cardiovascular system with a 10% incidence of ventricular septal defects, atrial septal defects, dextrocardia, or Fallot's tetralogy. Intraspinal abnormalities are also commonly found in patients who have congenital abnormalities of the vertebral column. These abnormalities are more common in patients who have congenital kyphosis and in patients who have scoliosis resulting from mixed and segmentation defects. Scoliosis patients who have cervical and thoracic hemivertebrae are also more likely to have intraspinal abnormalities [9]. In addition to imaging of the entire spine,

* Corresponding author.
  E-mail address: cis8z@virginia.edu (C.I. Shaffrey).

1042-3680/07/$ - see front matter © 2007 Elsevier Inc. All rights reserved.
doi:10.1016/j.nec.2007.04.004

renal, cardiac, and respiratory imaging should be performed when clinically indicated.

In a 2002 study from the United Kingdom, Basu and colleagues [10] analyzed a series of 126 consecutive patients who had congenital spinal deformity to assess the incidence of intraspinal anomaly and other organic defects. Intraspinal abnormalities were found in 47 patients (37%). In 55% of patients other organic defects were found. Cardiac defects were detected in 26% and urogenital anomalies in 21% of the patients.

Spine embryology

Embryogenesis

Embryogenesis is an intricately coordinated combination of cell proliferation, specification, and movement [11,12]. After induction of the germ layers, the blastula is transformed by gastrulation into a complex multilayer embryo. Gastrulation is marked by the formation of a blastopore, an opening in the blastula. The axial side is marked by the organizer, a signaling center that patterns the germ layers and regulates gastrulation movements. During internalization, endoderm and mesoderm cells move by way of the blastopore beneath the ectoderm.

Human spine development begins when the primitive streak develops. Before the primitive streak, the embryo is bilaminar consisting of the epiblast (primitive ectoderm) and hypoblast (endoderm). The primitive streak consists of a thickened linear band of epiblast that appears caudally in the dorsal aspect of the embryonic laminae. The streak elongates by adding cells caudally as the rostral end thickens to form the primitive knot. The primitive groove forms in the primitive streak that is continuous with the primitive pit in the primitive knot. The rostrocaudal axis of the embryo is defined when the primitive streak develops.

At day 16, epiblastic cells invade the primitive groove, separate from the epiblastic tissue, and migrate between the epiblast and hypoblast to form the embryonic mesoderm. This migration of cells transforms the bilaminar embryo into a trilaminar embryo, made up of ectoderm, mesoderm, and the endoderm that is made up of invading mesodermal cells and the laterally displaced remnants of the hypoblast. Gastrulation transforms the bilaminar embryo to a trilaminar embryo. Two groups of transcription factor genes, the homeobox and the zinc finger class, are believed to be vital for appropriate mesenchymal cell migration from the primitive streak. Any mutations in any of these genes can interfere with the process of formation of the mesoderm during gastrulation and of the neural crest from the neural tube and the development of the spine and spinal cord. A considerable number of congenital disorders of the spine involve malformations of tissues derived from these embryologic layers.

Neurulation and neurogenesis

The notochord is formed at day 16 in the midline at the rostral end of the embryo by mesoblastic cells that migrate cranially from Henson's node (primitive knot) between the ectoderm and endoderm. Henson's node is the organizing axis of the embryo and as it regresses caudally it leaves the notochord behind. The notochord and primitive streak play a crucial role in induction and development of future organ systems. During formation, the notochord induces the overlying ectoderm to form the neural plate. Primary neurulation involves the formation and infolding of the neural plate to form the neural tube that eventually becomes the spinal cord down to the level of the lumbosacral junction and occurs on days 18 to 27 after ovulation. On day 18, the neural plate invaginates to form the neural groove with neural folds bilaterally. By day 21, the neural folds have fused to form the neural tube. The neural tube then separates itself from the overlying ectoderm and the ectoderm fuses to become continuous over the dorsal aspect of the embryo.

The spinal cord distal to the second sacral vertebra develops by secondary neurulation. This secondary neurulation begins by having neural crest cells migrate into the dorsal midline of the mesoderm and become identifiable as ependyma and later evolving into neural cells. These cells then group together to form canals. They eventually fuse into one tubular structure that joins with the distal end of the spinal cord developing from the primary neurulation process. Closure of the neural tube begins in the cervical region at the sixth or seventh somite stage and closure spreads rostrally and caudally at this point.

Development of the spine, somite formation, and skeletogenesis

The formation of the spine around the notochord begins with the development of somites

[13]. The initial phase of this process is the mesenchymal phase followed by the cartilaginous development of the spine. By 9 weeks the final phase begins with osseous bone formation of the spine. The true development of the vertebral column begins with these somites. As the cells in the somites proliferate, distinct cell masses appear. The dermatome is the most lateral cell mass, destined to become the skin and subcutaneous tissue. The medial cell mass differentiates into two components. The myotome is the dorsal aspect of the medial cell mass and differentiates into a cell aggregate destined to become striated muscle. The sclerotome is the ventral aspect of the medial somite cell mass and becomes an aggregate of cells destined to become the skeletal system.

As the notochord and the neural tube develop, the intraembryonic mesoderm on both sides begins to thicken and form paraxial mesoderm. At approximately 20 days of gestation, the paraxial mesoderm divides into paired cuboidal structures called somites. The first pair of somites is near the rostral end of the neural tube and then they propagate in a rostral to caudal sequence. By day 30 there are 38 pairs of somites and eventually 42 to 44 pairs have formed: 4 occipital, 8 cervical, 12 thoracic, 5 lumbar, 5 sacral, and 8 to 10 coccygeal. Eventually, the first occipital and the last 5 to 7 coccygeal pairs disappear. The process of secondary neurulation results in the development of the spinal cord segments below the lumbosacral junction and occurs during days 28 to 48 after ovulation. The caudal eminence is responsible for the development of the terminal spinal cord, vertebral segments S2 through the last coccygeal segment, and portions of the hindgut and lower urogenital systems. Any malformation of the caudal eminence can lead to various disorders, including sacral agenesis, caudal regression, imperforate anus, cloacal exstrophy, and cloacal malformation.

Somites have regional and spatial specificity early in development. Somites destined to become vertebrae in the thoracic region can be transposed to the cervical region and vertebrae resembling thoracic vertebrae and extrathoracic ribs result. Some believe that the regional specificity of these somites is conferred by expression of homeobox or "Hox" genes. Additional developmental control of spinal development comes from paired box "Pax" genes [14]. In vertebrate embryos it has been shown that Pax gene expression has a critical role in sclerotome patterning and in the development of the perinotochordal tube and the development of the intervertebral discs during chondrification. Signals from the developing notochord are necessary for normal Pax-1 expression. Using antisense technology, researchers have shown that abnormal expression of Pax-1 during development results in complete loss or fusion of somites [15].

By 35 days, the cells of the sclerotome surround the notochord and neural tube forming mesenchymal vertebrae. The ventral collection of mesenchymal cells condenses to form the mesenchymal centrum, the primitive vertebral body. The ventral aspect of the mesenchymal condensation occurs slightly before the development of the dorsal aspect, thus longitudinally separating in time the origins of the primitive vertebral body and neural arch. Differentiation of the part of the sclerotome destined to become the vertebral body seems to be under the influence of the neural tube. While differentiation of the parts of the sclerotome destined to become the vertebral arch seems to be influenced by the neural crest; thus the vertebral body and vertebral arch are under different inductive control. Developmental abnormalities that occur during early gestation may independently affect the vertebral body or the developing vertebral arch. In addition, developmental abnormalities may be limited to the ventral and dorsal elements because of the difference in the time course of their development. The cells in each sclerotome form two distinct cell masses. There is a region of loosely packed cells in the rostral half of the sclerotome and a region of densely packed cells in the caudal half of each sclerotome. The densely packed cells evolve into intervertebral discs; the loosely packed cells eventually have chondrification centers develop within them and evolve into the bony elements of the spine.

As the vertebral canal expands, the notochord gradually regresses within these expansions. Notochord cells tend to cluster in the eventual intervertebral spaces. Notochord cells contribute significantly to the formation of the intervertebral disc, most notably the nucleus pulposus. Abnormal remnants of notochord can remain in the spinal axis most commonly in the coccygeal or basisphenoid regions and can give rise to chordomas. The vertebral matrix is conventionally understood to undergo three stages: membranous, chondrification, and ossification. Chondrification centers appear on day 42 in each mesenchymal vertebra; they appear on both sides of the small remnant of notochord and coalesce toward the center. A chondrification center forms laterally in each vertebral arch and propagates dorsally to form a cartilaginous arch. This chondrification expands dorsally to form the spinous process. Late chondrification centers form at the junction of the centrum and neural arch and extend laterally to form the transverse processes. Concurrently, the dense mesenchymal part of the somite that is to form the intervertebral disc condenses to form the annulus fibrosus.

Ossification of the vertebrae begins at about day 72, enhanced by embryonic movement. It is not complete, however, until early adulthood. Two primary ossification centers develop in the vertebral centrum and are located dorsal and ventral to the notochord, in contrast to the lateral chondrification centers. The dorsal and ventral ossification centers quickly fuse to form a single central ossification center. Ossification centers also form in each vertebral arch. The ossification center in each vertebral arch grows into three regions: the lamina, pedicle, and transverse process. At birth, each vertebra consists of three ossified bones connected by cartilage. The halves of the vertebral arch fuse between the ages of 3 and 5 years. The laminae fuse in the lumbar region and then progress rostrally. Five secondary ossification centers appear at puberty: one at the tip of the spinous process, one at the tip of each transverse process, and two rim epiphyses (superior and inferior) on the vertebral body. Ossification in the vertebral arch resembles diaphyseal ossification, whereas ossification of the centrum resembles epiphyseal ossification in long bones.

Each cartilage canal contains an artery, a vein, and associated surrounding capillary network. These end-artery systems have little or no anastomosis across the epiphyses. If a vascular network is compromised, rapid death of osteocytes occurs that can result in differential growth of the spine.

An adequate blood supply to the vertebrae is essential to the development and proliferation of the ossification centers. Cartilage canals are special structures that carry a vascular supply to the vertebral centrum. In contrast, the dorsal element vasculature enters from the peripheral periosteum.

The development of the thoracic and lumbar spine involves ossification of the neural arch and ventral segment corresponding to the 12 thoracic and 5 lumbar vertebrae. Vertebral ossifications are demonstrable by ultrasonography in the early second trimester. Most spinal defects are apparent by 20 to 22 weeks' menstrual age [16].

In 1977, Bagnall and colleagues [17,18] described the sequence of ossification centers in human fetal spine specimens. According to their studies, the sequence of neural arch ossification spreads from two basic regions: the lower thoracic and upper lumbar regions and the cervical region. They focused on T11, T12, and L1 ossification centers forming first, followed by the cervical spine, and that this differs from the traditional view that ossification occurs in a cranial to caudal fashion.

By the eighth postovulatory week, five cartilaginous sacral vertebrae are evident. Each of these vertebrae goes on to form a centrum and bilateral neural processes. The base of each neural process consists of a ventrolateral alar process and a dorsolateral element consisting of a costal and transverse element. At this point, the neural foramina face laterally. Much differential growth is required to turn these foramina to their eventual dorsal and ventral positions.

Ossification of the sacrum is unique in that two epiphyseal plates provide additional ossification to the rostral and caudal surfaces of each segment. The ossification centers in the first three sacral vertebrae are evident by the ninth embryologic week. The centers in the fourth and fifth segments appear after week 24. The vertebral arches of the sacral vertebrae have the conventional bilateral centers and six additional centers produce the sacral alae. The sacral vertebrae begin to fuse in the first postnatal year and the last two sacral vertebrae fuse by adolescence. By the age of 18 years the epiphyseal plates have formed on the auricular surfaces of the sacral alae and by the third decade the entire sacrum is fused.

Imaging

All patients afflicted with a congenital spinal disorder should receive a complete radiologic evaluation to determine the location and type of spinal deformity [19]. The age of the patient and the imaging required influence the choice of modality.

In the evaluation of a neonate, fetal ultrasonography is increasingly used as a primary screening tool for suspected congenital spinal anomalies and genitourinary abnormalities, beginning at about 18 to 22 weeks' gestational age. Ultrasonography images have improved significantly and have decreased the incidence of diagnostic amniocentesis needing to be performed and the risks associated with an invasive procedure. Despite the advancements made in ultrasonography equipment, it still remains operator-dependent, and accurate diagnosis depends on the skill and experience of the operator and the quality of the equipment. Ultrasonography has made it possible to evaluate the fetal spine in utero. Early detection of spinal anomalies allows for parental counseling and appropriate obstetrical and neurosurgical management. Real-time imaging allows the fetal spine to be examined in multiple dimensions and planes. Ultrasound enables viewing of the three ossification centers that form each fetal vertebra. This is crucial in detecting spina bifida defects. Ultrasonography of the fetal spine complements the use of alpha-fetoprotein levels in screening for neural tube defects.

As the child passes the neonatal period, plain films, CT, and MRI gain more usefulness and play specific roles. To reveal the flexibility and magnitude of the curves, standing upright plain films with flexion and extension views are superior to any other modality. The size of the spinal canal and bony spinal anatomy is best viewed using CT. The best way to image skeletal anomalies is by plain radiography and CT scans (Fig. 1).

MRI can provide exquisite information defining spinal cord anatomy and adjacent soft tissues. If spine imaging reveals the presence of a syrinx, then cranial imaging would be indicated to assess for the presence of a Chiari malformation. Various intraspinal abnormalities can be detected on MRI; these abnormalities are discussed in later sections of this article. Because the history and physical examination findings in patients who have congenital spinal deformity are not predictive of intraspinal anomalies, various studies support the use of MRI to image the entire spine. Patients who have an isolated hemivertebra and those who have a complex hemivertebral pattern have similar rates of intraspinal anomalies that are detected with MRI and similar rates of subsequent neurosurgical intervention. An MRI evaluation of the entire spine should therefore be considered for all patients who have congenital scoliosis, including those who have an isolated hemivertebra [20,21].

Thoracolumbar spine abnormalities

Congenital scoliosis

Congenital scoliosis is an abnormal curvature of the spine in the coronal plane that develops when anomalous vertebrae are present at birth.

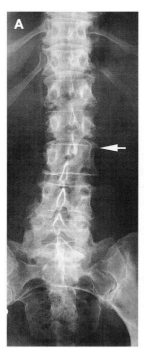
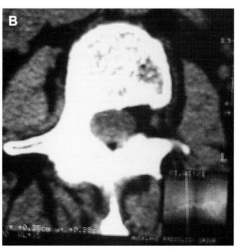

Fig. 1. (A) Plain standing radiograph demonstrating the absence of a pedicle (arrow) in a patient who presented with low back pain. (B) This finding was later confirmed with a CT scan.

Congenital scoliosis is distinct from infantile idiopathic scoliosis, although both present with deformity during childhood [22]. Infantile idiopathic scoliosis has no structural vertebral abnormality. Although vertebral abnormalities are present at birth in congenital scoliosis, the spinal deformity is rarely noticeable during infancy and usually presents during childhood or adolescence. Patients who have mild or compensated deformities are often diagnosed as adults when vertebral anomalies are discovered incidentally during routine radiographs. Congenital scoliosis can be associated with various cardiac, genitourinary, and skeletal abnormalities.

There is a wide spectrum of clinical presentations because of the range in number, location, and type of vertebral abnormalities that can exist in any individual. Certain vertebral anomalies result in rapidly progressive scoliosis during early childhood resulting in severe morbidity, whereas other anomalies cause little or no deformity at any time. In general, one quarter of all congenital scolioses do not progress, half of them progress slowly, and the remaining quarter progress rapidly. Major advancements have been made recently regarding congenital scoliosis with improved imaging of the spine by CT and MRI, classification by type of vertebral anomaly, improved understanding of the natural history, and clarification of the indications and timing of surgery.

Advances in imaging have aided the diagnosis of associated neural axis abnormalities, such as occult spinal dysraphism and tethering of the spinal cord. Up to 35% of all congenital scoliosis patients have some anomaly of the neural axis. Neural axis abnormalities include split cord malformations, Chiari malformations, lipomas, and spinal cord tethering [23]. Dorsal midline skin lesions (hairy patches or deep dimples), asymmetric foot deformities (cavus or flat feet), muscle weakness, or spasticity all suggest underlying nervous system abnormalities.

Normal spine growth is a result of the total growth that occurs at the endplates of the upper and lower surfaces of the vertebral bodies. Congenital vertebral anomalies can cause absence or functional deficiency of the growth plates on one or both sides of the spine. Asymmetric spine growth results from a difference in growth between the greater and lesser affected sides of the spine. In some cases, normal growth occurs on one side and no growth on the other, producing a large deformity. The rate of deterioration and the final severity of the congenital scoliosis are proportional to the degree of growth imbalance produced by the vertebral anomalies. The location of the deficient growth plates determines whether a pure scoliosis exists or if some component of sagittal plane deformity is present, resulting in kyphoscoliosis or lordoscoliosis.

Usually the vertebral abnormalities can be classified by the anomaly in the mesenchymal precursor that results in either a failure of formation or failure of segmentation. Failure of formation results from a defect in the developmental process that produces an absence of part or all of the vertebrae. The defects range from mild wedging to total absence of the vertebra. A hemivertebra occurs with the complete absence of half of a vertebra and is one of the most common causes of congenital scoliosis. The hemivertebra consists of a wedged vertebral body with a single pedicle and hemilamina.

Segmentation failure causes unilateral or bilateral bony fusion between vertebrae [5,6]. The defect can involve ventral elements, dorsal elements, or both (Fig. 2). The most common segmentation failure is the unilateral unsegmented bar, which results in a bony block that involves the disc spaces and facet joints. A combination of defects of formation and defects of segmentation can coexist in the same patient. An unsegmented bar with contralateral hemivertebrae can cause severe progressive scoliosis [24].

Three major types of hemivertebrae are classified by the positioning of the hemivertebra and whether the disc spaces above and below the hemivertebra are morphologically normal. A fully segmented hemivertebra has a normal disc space above and below the vertebral body that allows near-normal longitudinal growth. There is an absence of a portion of the vertebral body and growth plates on the side of the unformed vertebra that results in limited growth potential. Because of full growth potential on one side of the spine and none on the other side at the level of the hemivertebra, there is a potential for significant deformity development. The hemivertebra is located at the apex of the scoliosis in these cases (Fig. 3). The rate of progression and the need for treatment of the scoliosis caused by a fully segmented hemivertebra depends on its location in the spine, with the thoracolumbar and the lumbosacral junction being the most problematic. In general, these scoliotic curves progress at 1° to 2° per year.

The incarcerated hemivertebra is a variant of the fully segmented hemivertebra. This type of

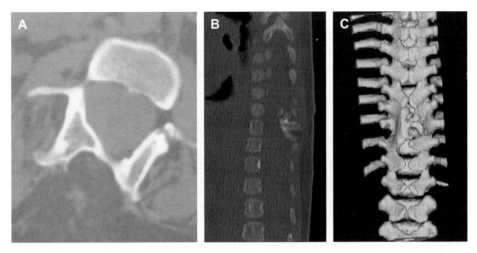

Fig. 2. (*A*) Axial multislice acquisition at 2-mm slice thickness was performed from T4 to L2 level with sagittal, coronal, and three-dimensional reconstructions performed. There is a fusion anomaly involving the posterior elements on the right at levels T9 to T11. (*B*) This anomaly is associated with expansion of the involved posterior elements and there is a bony spur (*C*) that protrudes in to the spinal canal causing narrowing at this level.

hemivertebra is set into defects in the vertebrae above and below it. The incarcerated hemivertebra is small and oval, with poorly formed disc spaces. The defects in the adjacent vertebrae tend to compensate for the hemivertebra and the poor potential growth of the malformed growth plates results in less scoliotic deformity compared with the standard fully segmented vertebrae.

A semisegmented hemivertebra is connected to either the vertebra above or below it and causes the absence of one disc space on the side of the hemivertebra with obliteration of two growth plates. Theoretically, this would result in similar growth on both sides of the spine because two active growth plates coexist on each side. The wedge shape of the hemivertebra and differences in growth between sides can result in some scoliosis, however.

A nonsegmented hemivertebra is connected to the vertebrae above and below, with no disc spaces and no growth potential. Although the wedge shape of the hemivertebra may cause some deformity, it is not progressive.

Another common cause of congenital scoliosis is a unilateral unsegmented bar. This condition results from a failure of segmentation of two or more vertebrae. The unsegmented bar contains no growth plates but the unaffected side of the spine continues to grow and the result is a significant spinal deformity. The imbalance in growth results in scoliosis with the unsegmented bar in the concavity. The rate of deterioration and final severity of scoliosis is determined by the number of vertebrae involved with the bar and the growth potential of the convexity. On average these curves deteriorate at a rate of 5° or greater per year and often result in a significant deformity.

A combination of hemivertebrae and unsegmented bars can coexist, often with a greater risk for progression than either condition alone. The total number and location of the congenital abnormalities determines the risk for progression. Knowledge of the natural history of these congenital deformities is essential because the natural history dictates the prognosis and treatment. The natural history of congenital scoliosis has been described in several excellent studies. In 1982, McMaster and colleagues [22,25], in a large study of 202 patients who had congenital scoliosis, reported that only 11% of cases were nonprogressive, 14% were slightly progressive, and the remaining 75% progressed significantly. The prognosis for congenital scoliosis with regard to its rate of deterioration and final severity depends on many factors. The type of anomaly that causes the most severe scoliosis is a unilateral unsegmented bar with contralateral hemivertebrae at the same level. This anomaly is followed by scoliosis resulting from a unilateral unsegmented bar alone, followed by two unilateral fully segmented hemivertebrae, a single fully segmented hemivertebra, and a wedge vertebra. The least severe scoliosis is caused by a block vertebra. Congenital scoliosis caused by unclassifiable anomalies can

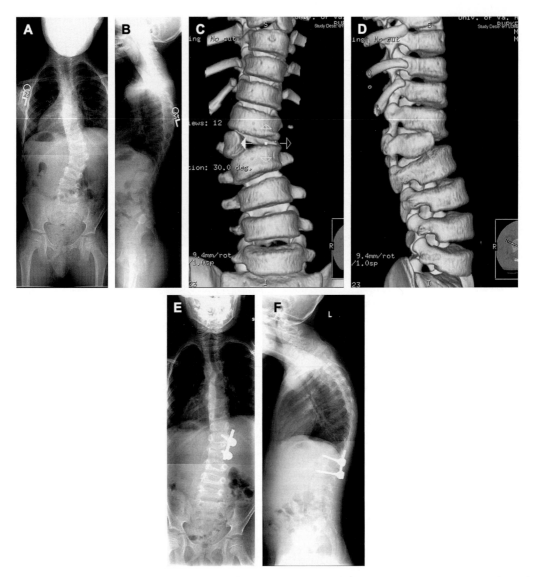

Fig. 3. A 6-year-old with known renal anomalies presented with progressive spinal deformity. (*A*) Posteroanterior and (*B*) lateral radiographs reveal an L2 hemivertebra with 53° of scoliosis and mild kyphosis. CT reconstruction anteroposterior (*C*) and lateral (*D*) demonstrates a fully segmented L2 hemivertebra with anterior failure of formation. Postoperative films 6 months following an anterior and posterior hemivertebra resection, instrumentation, and fusion. Unilateral instrumentation (*E*, *F*) with casting was used to prevent instrument crowding in this small patient.

be difficult to predict and requires careful monitoring. Scoliosis from a unilateral unsegmented bar with or without contralateral hemivertebrae should be treated immediately without waiting for a period of observation.

The level of the anomaly, the age of the patient, and the pattern of the curve play a role in the rate of deformity progression. The rate of deterioration is more significant in the thoracic and thoracolumbar regions, whereas cervicothoracic and lumbar regions are less severe. Congenital scoliosis seems to progress during the preadolescent growth spurt, after age 10 years. Scoliosis presenting as a clinical deformity in the first few years of life is associated with marked growth imbalance that results in severe deformity.

Multiple balanced anomalies throughout the spine do not progress, whereas the more unbalanced the anomalies, the more likely the scoliosis is to progress [22,25].

Surgery is the most effective treatment of severe or progressive congenital scoliosis. Many different forms of operative treatment exist for congenital scoliosis, and each treatment has different indications. The age of the patient, the site and type of vertebral anomaly, the size of the curvature, and the presence of other congenital anomalies dictate the type of procedure chosen. Progressive curves should be treated surgically, especially if they do not respond to orthotic treatment. The following are the main surgical options for the treatment of congenital scoliosis: hemivertebra excision, convex hemiepiphysiodesis, fusion in situ, spinal instrumentation, and thoracoplasty with vertical expansion prosthetic titanium rib (VEPTR).

Although a detailed description of each surgical technique is beyond the scope of this article, the indications for each of the above surgical options is discussed. Hemivertebra excision is indicated for patients younger than 5 years who have development of a structural secondary curve with a fixed decompensation in which adequate alignment cannot be achieved with other procedures [26]. Convex hemiepiphysiodesis, as the name implies, is a partial growth arrest procedure. For this procedure to be effective there must be little or no concave growth potential. The most common indication is a hemivertebra. The total correction obtained by performing a convex hemiepiphysiodesis varies because the younger the child at the time of the operation, the more potential that exists for correction over time. In general, this procedure should be reserved for children younger than 5 years who have mild to modest deformities [23]. Fusion in situ has been reported as the gold standard for progressive curves with minimal deformity, but reoperation may be needed in about 25% of cases. Fusion in situ requires the use of an appropriate cast or brace until the fusion is absolutely solid [27]. Instrumentation may be necessary to correct progressive curves with greater deformity and has become increasingly popular in recent times [28]. It has a greater risk for producing neurologic complications because of the effect of distraction on the spinal cord while the patient is anesthetized, however. Spinal cord monitoring using evoked potentials is becoming increasingly more common [23]. Patients who have progressive curves and congenital rib fusions require an expansion thoracostomy and VEPTR [29].

Congenital kyphosis

Congenital kyphosis is an uncommon sagittal plane deformity that, if left untreated, is often associated with neurologic deficit. As with congenital scoliosis, congenital kyphosis is caused by formation segmentation failure. Winter and colleagues [30] classified congenital kyphosis into three types: type I, failure of formation of the vertebral body; type II, failure of segmentation of the vertebral body resulting in a ventral unsegmented bar; and type III, mixed failure of formation and segmentation. The type I kyphosis is the most common and the most likely to develop severe deformity and neurologic compromise. The severity of type I kyphosis is directly proportional to the amount of vertebral body or bodies that fail to form. The type II kyphosis is less common, produces less severe deformity, and is much less frequently associated with neurologic compromise than type I. The amount of kyphosis produced is proportional to the discrepancy between the ventral vertebral growth and the growth of the dorsal elements. Type III kyphosis is rare and probably behaves like type I kyphosis.

If the defect is detected early, when the patient is younger than 5 years, with less than 55° of kyphosis, posterior fusion alone is recommended. When the deformity is larger than 55° or when the child is older than 5 years, a combined anterior and posterior arthrodesis is indicated [31]. The postoperative complications occurring in the treatment of congenital kyphosis can range from asymptomatic pseudarthrosis to paraplegia. In Kim and colleagues' [32] article on the treatment of congenital kyphosis, complications were more likely to occur in patients who had large deformities (greater than 60°) and those who had clinical or radiographic evidence of cord compression that underwent anterior surgery and posterior spinal arthrodesis.

Lumbar spine abnormalities

Congenital lordosis and spinal stenosis

Congenital lordosis is rarer than either congenital scoliosis or congenital kyphosis. This condition results from dorsal defects in segmentation, with normal ventral growth. Often it has some component of coronal plane deformity, leading to lordoscoliosis because of a dorsolateral location of the unsegmented bar. The most severe consequence of congenital lordosis is the development of impairment of pulmonary function when it occurs in the thoracic spine.

Congenital spinal stenosis occurs in a small number of patients who present with spinal stenosis. It results from a malformation present at birth that predisposes the patient to the development of stenosis, which often manifests itself later in life.

Verbiest [33–35] described three types of congenital spinal stenosis. The first is a stenosis as a part of spinal dysraphism. The signs and symptoms are usually the consequence not only of stenosis but also of myelodysplasia. Serious radicular neurologic deficit occurs frequently in this condition.

The second type of congenital spinal stenosis is a stenosis in an area of failure of vertebral segmentation. Stenosis in the area of the block vertebrae was determined by a reduction of the midsagittal diameters of the vertebral canal. The signs and symptoms did not differ from those observed with idiopathic developmental stenosis.

The third type of congenital spinal stenosis is an intermittent stenosis, De Anquin's syndrome, in which the spinous process of S1 is absent and the lamina of S1 has a large medial cleft. There may be a residual island of bone in the area of the cleft. This malformation is associated with a downward hooklike elongation of the spinous process of L5. The assumption of is that during an increased lordotic posture (ie, standing or walking), the tip of the hooklike spinous process of L5 presses directly on the ligamentum bridging the spina bifida occulta of S1 or on the rudimentary bony island in its central portion, thus reducing the midsagittal diameter of the upper sacral canal. This condition results in radicular pain during standing or walking, and is relieved by sitting.

Developmental spinal stenosis

Congenital spinal stenosis is differentiated from developmental spinal stenosis, which usually occurs as the result of an inborn chromosomal error or mutation that alters the fetal and postnatal spinal canal formation. Developmental spinal stenosis commonly occurs in conditions such as achondroplasia, hypochondroplasia, diastrophic dwarfism, Morquio's syndrome, and hereditary multiple exostoses. Idiopathic developmental spinal stenosis has been reported. This condition may involve only the lumbar spine, or can be associated with developmental stenosis of the cervical spine.

Segmental spinal dysgenesis

Segmental spinal dysgenesis is a localized congenital defect in which severe stenosis occurs with malalignment and focal agenesis or dysgenesis in the thoracolumbar or lumbar spine [7,36]. Neurologic deficits are often present at birth and may range from mild paresis to complete paraplegia. Patients may have congenital absence of nerve root or spinal cord segments. The spinal canal above and below the involved segment is usually normal and the sacrum is well formed, differentiating this condition from sacral agenesis with localized spinal stenosis as a universal finding.

Dysplastic spondylolisthesis

Congenital spondylolisthesis is the slippage of all or part of one vertebra in relation to another [37,38]. Several different causes have been identified. The role of upright posture contributing to this condition is well recognized. It has been stated that no known cases of spondylolysis or spondylolisthesis have been identified in nonambulatory patients. Spondylolisthesis is extremely rare during infancy. Spondylolysis has been associated with the onset of ambulation in early childhood. It has been suggested that spondylolisthesis results from a congenital defect or dysplasia that results in the development of a pars defect attributable to the stresses of upright posture and lumbar lordosis.

The most widely accepted classification of spondylolisthesis is by Wiltse and colleagues [39]. They divided spondylolisthesis into five types: type I, dysplastic spondylolisthesis; type II, isthmic spondylolisthesis; type III, degenerative spondylolisthesis; type IV, traumatic spondylolisthesis; and type V, pathologic spondylolisthesis. Wiltse later suggested a common congenital component in the cause of dysplastic and isthmic spondylolisthesis and further refined classification of spondylolisthesis.

Dysplastic spondylolisthesis accounts for 14% to 21% of the cases of spondylolisthesis with a 2:1 female to male ratio. This type is characterized by structural anomalies of the lumbosacral junction, including dysplasia of the lamina and facet joints. The lack of the normal facet buttress provided by normal facet joints predisposes toward a slippage of the rostral vertebra on its caudal counterpart. The dysplastic articular processes may be oriented in the axial or sagittal planes. In axial dysplasia, the articular processes have a horizontal orientation. This condition is often associated with spina bifida. In sagittal dysplasia, the facet joints are often asymmetric, but the neural arch is usually intact. High-grade slippage seldom occurs, therefore. Both types can present with hamstring spasm, back or leg pain, or neurologic deficit, including paresthesia, weakness, or rarely incontinence of the bowel or bladder. Neurologic deficits are usually associated with high-grade slips.

Axially oriented facet joints associated with spina bifida have an increased risk for high-grade spondylolisthesis. The pars interarticularis is often poorly developed and may elongate, develop a defect, or remain intact. If the pars interarticularis remains intact, neurologic symptoms usually occur only when the spondylolisthesis exceeds 35%. Progression of spondylolisthesis is more likely in younger or skeletally immature patients and patients who have wide spina bifida. Initial treatment should be nonoperative unless progression is documented in younger patients or slippage greater than 50% is observed at the time of the initial evaluation. The treatment options originally proposed are still valid and fusion in situ can be performed along with internal reduction and fixation with pedicle screws, especially with high-grade slips [40]. Spondylolisthesis in patients who have sagittally oriented facet joints and an intact L5 lamina is frequently treated with decompression with a fusion. Often, this results in a more rapid resolution of neuropathic pain and neurologic dysfunction.

Spinal dysraphism

Worldwide, the incidence of spinal dysraphism varies greatly and is highest in Northern Ireland where it approaches 8.7 per 1000 live births [4,41]. In the United States, the incidence of neural tube defects declined by 50% from 1.3 per 1000 births in 1970 to 0.6 per 1000 live births by 1989. Environmental factors that have been implicated include maternal hyperthermia; maternal deficiencies in folate, calcium, vitamin C, and zinc; and either lack of or overdose of vitamin A. The level of the spinal dysplasia depends on the embryologic age at which the malformation is obtained. It is generally believed that neural tube defects follow a multifactorial inheritance pattern that interacts with environmental factors. The risk for having a child who has spina bifida is approximately 0.1% but if there is a sibling with spina bifida the risk increases to 2.5% for subsequent children. There is also an increased risk for neural tube defects in the children of sisters and daughters of the mother who has a child who has a myelomeningocele.

Dysraphism refers to abnormal spinal cord and column development. Dysraphism is associated with malformations that arise from the failure of normal embryologic structures to fuse in the midline. Historically, dysraphism has been artificially divided into two groups: spina bifida aperta and spina bifida occulta. The first group involves midline lesions that are open, or might open, at birth. These lesions include myelomeningocele, meningocele, and myelodysplasia. The second group has malformations that are hidden by complete layers of dermis and epidermis. These lesions include lipomyelomeningocele, neurenteric cysts, lipoma, dermoid cysts, neurenteric cyst, dermal sinus tracts, tethered cord, and diastematomyelia.

The defect of spinal dysraphism occurs in the first 2 months of life. The neural tube develops from ectodermal cells, whereas the mesoderm by definition forms the bone, meninges, and muscle. The skin is separated from the neural tube by a layer of mesoderm. Incomplete separation of ectoderm from the neural tube results in cord tethering, diastematomyelia, or a dermal sinus. Premature separation of the cutaneous ectoderm from the neural tube results in incorporation of mesenchymal elements between the neural tube and skin, which may result in the development of lipomas. If the neural tube fails to fuse in the midline posterior spinal abnormalities, such as myelomeningoceles, occur.

In spinal dysraphism, the spinal column widens at the level of the defect. If the neural tube does not develop normally it causes a deficiency of dorsal element formation and the lateral and ventral displacement of the pedicles and lateral elements of the spine. In addition, other abnormalities of the vertebrae can be associated with spinal dysraphism, such as wedge vertebrae and hemivertebrae. Occasionally, patients who presented with what was believed to be idiopathic scoliosis have, in fact, some form of occult spinal dysraphism with multiple rib anomalies. Abnormal neural tube development prevents dermis and epidermis closure over the dorsal defect. Dura mater arises ventral to the deformed spinal cord but then stretches laterally over the expanded pedicles and facets to join the lateral margins of the epidermis. A thin layer of pia and arachnoid and the zona epithelioserosa, an extremely thin layer of epithelium, cover the dorsal defect.

Occult spinal dysraphism is not always immediately visible on the skin surface but there are classic clinical manifestations on the skin (Box 1). Spina bifida occulta occurs because of a dysembryogenesis of the dorsal neural arch structures (Fig. 4). Some believe that this occurs when an already closed neural tube ruptures. Increased pressure inside of the central canal of the neural tube can cause a rupture that spills proteinaceous fluid from the canal into the developing tissue. With the decrease in pressure, the defect in the neural tube reforms but the proteinaceous fluid inhibits normal development of the dorsal elements. Because the neural tube has closed, closure of the dermis and epidermis over the dorsal aspect of the spinal cord is not impeded. Malformations that begin before 28 days of gestation induce major defects in neurulation and cause a higher level of defects than malformations occurring after 28 days of gestation, when neurulation is complete; the higher the degree of dysplasia, the less survivable is the malformation. In one study of 510 infants surviving the first day of life approximately 10% of these lesions were cranial/cervical, 5% thoracic, 25% thoracolumbar, 65% lumbosacral. Anatomic studies have suggested a timetable for the formation of spinal dysraphism that ranges from 14 to 49 postovulatory days.

Hydromyelia can also occur and is a dilatation of the central canal lined by ependyma, usually in the lumbosacral region. Myelomeningocele or diastematomyelia is commonly associated with this condition. The central canal dilatation varies from oval to irregular or slit-shaped, projecting either bilaterally or dorsally. A hydromyelia should be differentiated from a syringomyelia, which is a fluid-filled cavity within the spinal cord not lined by ependyma. Syringomyelia is rare in children and usually related to trauma,

inflammation, tumor, or Chiari malformation. A myelocystocele is a hydromyelic dilatation of the central canal, the cystic cavity being within the cord and the spinal roots originating at the ventral and dorsal outer surface of the cyst wall.

Diastematomyelia

There are two types of split cord anomalies that have been described: diastematomyelia and diplomyelia [42–45]. Diastematomyelia actually causes the spinal cord to develop into two hemicords separated by a cartilaginous or bony septum and the two cords are contained in two separate dural sacs (Fig. 5). In a study of 60 patients, Hood and colleagues found that diastematomyelia occurs from the third thoracic to the fourth lumbar vertebrae. Approximately 50% of the lesions were associated with thoracic vertebrae and 50% were associated with lumbar vertebrae, in contrast to diplomyelia in which the two separate cords are contained in one dural sac without a spur present [43].

Pang and colleagues [46] presented a unified theory of diastematomyelia and diplomyelia embryogenesis that characterized these lesions as split cord malformations (SCMs). Type I SCMs consist of two hemicords, each contained in its own dural tube and separated by a dural sheathed rigid osseocartilaginous median septum. Type II SCMs consist of two hemicords housed in a single dural sheath and separated by a nonrigid, fibrous midline septum. In their study of 39 patients, Pang and associates [46] found 19 patients who had type I SCMs, 18 patients who had type II SCMs, and 2 patients who had composite SCMs in tandem.

Although it was long held that the presence or absence of medial nerve roots aided in distinguishing diastematomyelia from simple diplomyelia, Pang and colleagues [46] found that medial nerve roots occur in 75% of type I and type II SCMs. Notably, although most medial nerve roots were dorsal, ventral medial nerve roots were extremely rare. The SCM theory proposes that both types of SCMs originate from one embryologic error around the time of neural tube closure. The error occurs when the accessory neurenteric canal forms through the midline of the embryonic disc that maintains communication between endoderm and ectoderm [46]. While the abnormal fistula develops, mesenchyme condenses around it and the tract then splits the developing notochord and neural tube. The malformation phenotype depends on further spinal column/cord

---

Box 1. Cutaneous stigmata of underlying spinal dysraphism

Dermal dimple
Wayward gluteal fold
Hairy patch of skin
Midline visible or palpable mass
  overlying the spine (lipoma)
Dermal sinus
Capillary hemangioma
Rudimentary appendage

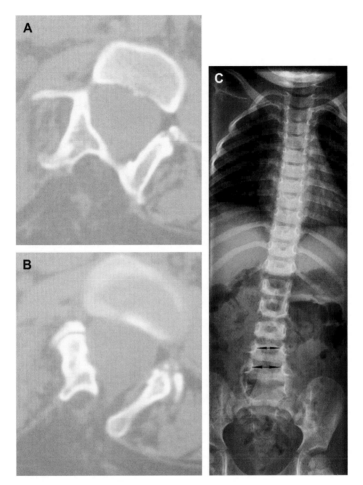

Fig. 4. (*A*) Axial CT scan demonstrating occult spinal dysraphism and a bifid spinous process without and (*B*) with a midline defect. (*C*) Plain radiographs indicating that the interpediculate distances are focally increased at L5 and S1, raising the possibility of occult spinal dysraphism. At L5 the distance is 3.0 cm and at S1, 3.9 cm. The expected upper limit at age 3 would be around 3.4 cm. The posterior elements are intact.

development. An SCM results if the embryo is able to heal around the tract. If the tract picks up primitive cells from the mesenchyme (destined to become the meninges), the two hemicords are each invested in dura mater. The dura mater can stimulate bone growth that results in a midline spur (type I SCM).

Neurenteric cysts

If there is retained endoderm in the tract between hemicords, a neurenteric cyst can result [12,46,47]. These rare lesions are retained cystic structures, ventrally located in the spinal canal, derived from embryonic foregut. These cysts occur most commonly in the thoracic and cervical spine. The epithelium of these cysts varies from ciliated columnar lining that suggests a respiratory origin to linings that can resemble gut mucosa. Because of embryonic gut rotation, neurenteric cysts tend to lie to the right of the vertebral column.

Most likely these lesions originate from communications between the yolk sac (foregut) and the dorsal surface of the embryo. Normally, such a neurenteric canal is located in the region of the coccyx. Accessory neurenteric canals, however, can occur rostral to the coccyx and if they persist, neurenteric cysts result. This persistent neurenteric tract can result in vertebral abnormalities, such as a widened vertebral body attributable to increased bone forming around the tract and

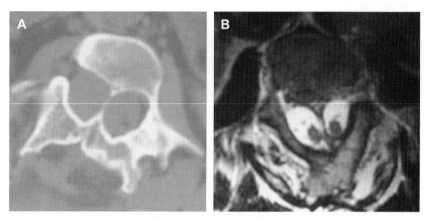

Fig. 5. (*A*) Axial CT scan demonstrating a classic bony spur seen in diastematomyelia with complete separation of the normal vertebral canal with (*B*) MRI axial images demonstrating the two separate dural sleeves for the spinal cord.

hemivertebrae. Neurenteric cysts can cause spinal cord compression usually presenting in childhood but also into adolescence and adulthood.

Lipomas

Lipomas of the spine are commonly observed in clinical practice, and may be considered a developmental abnormality [48]. The most common form is a lipoma associated with occult spinal dysraphism. They occur in the lumbosacral area 90% of the time. In contrast, intraspinal lipomas not associated with spina bifida account for 4.7% of intraspinal tumors in children and show a predilection for the thoracic spine. These lesions most likely result from inclusion of adipose cells from the overlying mesodermal tissue into the developing spinal canal or the folding neural tube. A tethered spinal cord occurs when these lesions transverse both the bony and neural elements of the spine.

Lipomas in the dura occur mainly in the caudal portion of the spine. Those in the region of the filum terminale are associated with congenital spinal anomalies. The lipoma is hyperintense on T1-weighted MRIs. Spinal lipomas are usually found in the extradural space in the thoracic region. The radiologic and MRI signal intensity characteristics are similar to those of intradural lipomas.

Lipomas associated with spinal dysraphism take three principal forms: dorsal, terminal, or transitional. In the dorsal form, the lipoma extends from the subcutaneous space through incomplete neural arches and attaches to the

dorsal spinal cord. It is rare for nerve roots to be contained within the substance of a dorsal lipoma. Terminal lipomas insert into the distal conus and may be entirely intraspinal, many times

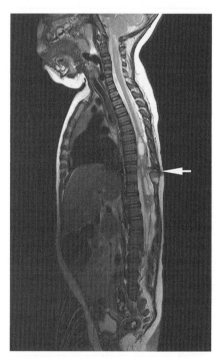

Fig. 6. The dermal sinus (*arrow*) is seen in sagittal images extending posteriorly from the posterior vertebral anomaly with no diastematomyelia identified. There is a syrinx measuring 1.3 cm in diameter immediately below the bony spur that is narrowing the spinal canal. There is a second syrinx above the anomaly that is 4 mm in diameter. The conus is at L1–L2 level.

containing nerve roots. Features of both dorsal and terminal lipomas appear in transitional lipomas. The embryology of caudal lipomas most likely arises during secondary neurulation. During secondary neurulation the caudal end of the neural tube blends with a large collection of undifferentiated cells, the caudal cell mass. The last phase of secondary neurulation involves regression of the previously formed tail structures, leaving the filum terminale, coccygeal ligament, and the terminal ventricle of the conus as its only remnants. Cell rests with the potential for differentiation may be left in these elements and account for the development of lipomas, hamartomas, teratomas, and the rare malignancy.

Epidermoids, dermoids, and dermal sinus tracts

Dermoids and epidermoids account for a small portion of all spinal tumors (1%–2%) at all ages [8,49]. They may be associated with a dermal sinus or occur in isolation. When not associated with dermal sinuses, they may occur with progressive compressive myelopathy or acute-onset chemical meningitis because of the rupture of the cyst and the spread of cholesterol crystals in the cerebrospinal fluid (CSF). The thoracic, lumbar, and sacral spine are affected, with a slight increase in incidence in the craniocaudal direction. CT and MRI characteristics are similar to those seen in epidermoids at other sites. Diffusion MRI is promising as an alternative to CT after an

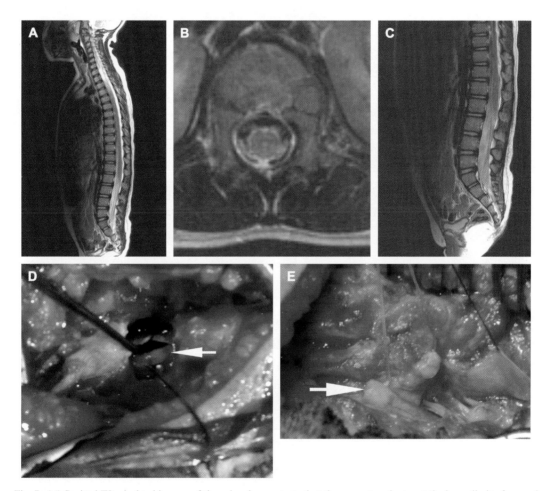

Fig. 7. (*A*) Sagittal T2-wieghted images of the spine demonstrate that the conus terminates at the lower limit of normal at the L2/L3 disc space. (*B*) Axial T2-weighted images of the lumbar spine show that the filum is slightly thickened with a fibrolipoma and 2.3-mm diameter in thickness. (*C*) Lumbar spine T2-weighted images show a borderline tethered cord especially given the slightly thickened fibrolipoma in the filum. (*D*) An intraoperative view of the thickened filum terminale (*arrow*) before sectioning (*E*) of the terminal portion of the filum (*arrow*).

intrathecal injection of contrast medium to detect and delineate the limits of the lesion.

Dermal sinus tracts are lined by squamous epithelium and may penetrate the spinal cord at any level in the midline from the lumbosacral spine to the occiput (Fig. 6). The incidence is said to be 1 in every 1500 births. Dermoid and epidermoid nodules can frequently accompany dermal

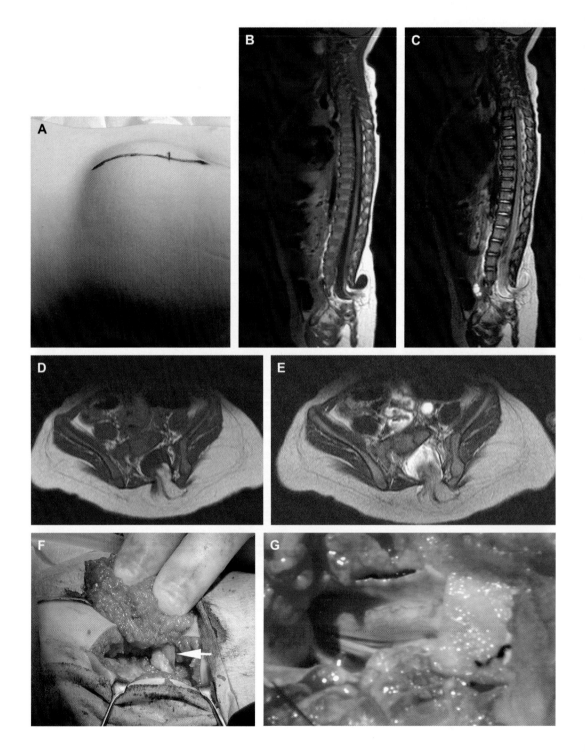

sinus tracts. Dermoid and epidermoid tumors may arise within the tract in approximately one half of all dermal sinuses. These tumors are also encountered within the subarachnoid space arising from isolated congenital rests of cells derived from the multipotential caudal cell mass.

The embryology of dermal sinus tracts and dermoids of the spine is probably a result of incomplete dysjunction of ectoderm from endoderm during the fourth week of embryologic development. The dermal tract becomes elongated during ascent of the spinal cord within the spinal canal, and may cross several layers of dermis and epidermal space before entering the subarachnoid space. Dermal sinus tracts may frequently be missed on initial examination of the infant and only become apparent when the child presents with recurrent meningitis (often *Staphylococcus aureus*) despite adequate antibiotic coverage. Definitive treatment of these lesions is complete surgical excision and there is no role for conservative therapy.

Tethered cord

Traditionally, tethered cord syndrome has been defined as a low-lying conus medullaris attributable to a short and thickened filum terminale (Fig. 7). Recently, the term has been expanded to include a spinal cord that is tethered by fibrous bands or adhesions or an intradural lipoma. The embryologic origin of the short and thickened fatty filum terminale is not known.

In filum terminal syndrome a thickened filum is attached to the dura, or an extradural band of connective tissue may anchor the cord. In some patients, the cord is bound down by lipomatous tumors or fibrous tissue, the sacral roots ascending. Lipomyelomeningoceles may attach dorsally to the conus and there can be a fatty filum that is anchoring the spinal cord (Fig. 8). The

pathophysiology of tethered cord syndrome has been postulated to involve hypoxic stress with vascular insufficiency on the stretched spinal cord. Clearly, these lesions can cause profound neurologic deficits with or without intervention and still carry high rate of neurologic deficit with surgery [50]. Spinal cord detethering is indicated in the presence of neurologic symptoms, which may include pain, bladder dysfunction, leg weakness with atrophy of the calf muscles, loss of deep tendon reflexes, and loss of sensation in a dermatomal distribution [51,52].

Disorders of the sacral spine

Sacral agenesis

Sacral agenesis has been defined as a group of disorders characterized by an absence of various portions of the caudal spine [53,54]. Sacral agenesis belongs within the spectrum of aplastic vertebral malformations that are loosely grouped under the entity of caudal regression syndrome. It can range from agenesis of the coccyx to absence of sacral, lumbar, and lower thoracic vertebrae.

The clinical severity parallels the number of spinal segments involved with the aplasia or dysplasia. With increasing severity there are often associated anomalies of the genitourinary, gastrointestinal, and urinary systems. Patients who have sacral agenesis usually lack motor function below the level of the last normal vertebra. Of interest in sacral agenesis, compared with other dysplastic syndromes of the lower spine (eg, myelomeningocele), is that sensation is relatively spared below the level of the lesion. In the development of the human embryo, the notochord induces the formation of the ventral spinal elements and cells derived from neural crest independently from the dorsal root ganglia. An insult specific to the

Fig. 8. (*A*) A 2-year-old child presented to the pediatrician with a lump on the back. An MRI was ordered and on the sagittal MRI sequences at the lumbosacral junction just below the fifth lumbar vertebra there is a large left-sided posterior bony defect. This measures approximately 14 mm in the sagittal plane and 8 mm across. The defect is filled with soft tissue of mixed signal on both T1 (*B*) and T2 (*C*). The terminal portion of the spinal cord can be seen passing through the spinal defect, which is intermediate signal on T2 and low signal on T1. A large tongue of fat can be seen filling the left side of the defect adjacent to the cord elements on axial images T1 (*D*) and T2 (*E*). There is no conus definitively identified and the spinal cord is seen to extend to the level of the defect below L5. The subcutaneous skin-covered mass extending from approximately L3 vertebral level to the midsacral level contains fat, spinal cord elements, and a well-circumscribed CSF collection measuring 14 × 11 × 12 mm that sits immediately adjacent to the bony defect in the midline and immediately superior to the tongue of fat and spinal cord. (*F*) An intraoperative photograph showing the lipomyelomeningocele and the relationship to the dura and conus. White arrow indicates the stalk of the lipomyelomeningocoele. (*G*) Intraoperative photograph demonstrating appearance after sectioning of stalk.

notochord/ventral spine could thus lead to the observed clinical picture in sacral agenesis.

The exact incidence of sacral agenesis is difficult to determine because mild caudal agenesis is often not clinically apparent and severe cases can result in stillbirth or neonatal death. Sacral agenesis is a relatively rare lesion. An incidence of 1 in 25,000 live births has been reported. Sacral agenesis is considered to have a sporadic, nonfamilial inheritance pattern, although cases of siblings who have the disorder have been reported. Maternal diabetes seems to increase the risk for sacral agenesis. Embryonal trauma producing longitudinal kinking of the long embryonic axis, dietary deficiencies, and teratogenic chemicals have caused caudal agenesis in experimental models. Caudal agenesis and other associated congenital anomalies, such as imperforate anus and cloacal exstrophy, result from alterations in the normal formation and development of the caudal eminence. The caudal eminence is a mass of undifferentiated cells at the caudal end of the embryo that gives rise to the distal spinal cord, the vertebral column, urogenital, and anorectal structures.

Sacral agenesis has been classified into four types by Renshaw [54], who based his classification on the amount of remaining sacrum and the orientation of the sacral articulation. Type I occurs in either partial or total unilateral agenesis of the sacrum. Type II is bilaterally symmetric partial agenesis of the sacrum, with a normal or hypoplastic first sacral vertebra and a stable articulation of the ilia with the first sacral vertebra. Type III is variable lumbar with total sacral agenesis. The ilia articulate with the lowest vertebra present in type III. Type IV lesions are like type III lesions, except that the caudal endplate of the lowest vertebra inserts on fused ilia or an iliac amphiarthrosis. Pang recently devised a new classification scheme that combined salient features from other classification schemes. By this method, lumbosacral agenesis is divided into five types, with some of these divided into subtypes. Type I is total sacral agenesis with some lumbar vertebrae also missing. Type II is total sacral agenesis with the lumbar vertebrae not involved. Type III is subtotal sacral agenesis with at least S1 present and the ilia articulate with the side of the rudimentary sacrum. Type IV is a hemisacrum, and type V is coccygeal agenesis [55].

The clinical features of sacral agenesis can be severe. Because of the lack of motor innervation of the lower limbs, intrauterine contractures develop. In severe forms of sacral agenesis, Renshaw III and IV, the malformation in the spine/pelvis articulation causes a severe kyphosis to develop. Affected children sit in the "Buddha" position with legs flexed and crossed and lean forward because of the kyphosis. Other spinal deformities develop in children who have sacral agenesis; congenital and developmental scoliosis and Klippel-Feil syndrome have been reported.

Multiple musculoskeletal deformities can present in patients who have sacral agenesis. Hip dysplasia, club foot, and knee flexion contractures are common. It seems that the causative factor responsible for sacral agenesis, such as an insult to the caudal eminence, occurs during the time of organogenesis. Children who have sacral agenesis can present with multiple abnormalities of the gastrointestinal, cardiac, and renal systems. There can be associated abnormalities of the terminal spinal cord associated with sacral agenesis. These include elongated conus medullaris with hydromyelia, tethering of the spinal cord by a thickened filum terminale, lipomas, split cord malformations, and terminal myelocystoceles. Neurogenic bladder almost always results in cases of sacral agenesis above S2.

Teratomas

Sacrococcygeal teratoma is the most common neoplasm in the newborn, with a reported incidence of 1 in 35,000 live births [56]. Seventy-five percent of affected infants are female. Most tumors are large, external, and cystic. Teratomas in the spine almost exclusively occur in the sacrococcygeal region. This is because of their origin from pluripotent tissue derived from the area around Hensen's node. This tissue migrates rostrally to lie in the coccyx. These usually benign tumors can undergo malignant transformation with delayed diagnosis or treatment. The tumor mass usually protrudes from between the anus and the coccyx, although some tumors are located predominantly in the presacral space of the pelvis. Although the diagnosis is often possible prenatally by ultrasound, small presacral tumors can be missed in the newborn. The tumors range in size but average approximately 8.5 cm. The cystic component is usually CSF, but is not connected with circulating spinal fluid within the thecal sac. The spinal fluid arises from choroid plexus contained within the tumor mass.

Sacrococcygeal teratomas have been classified into four types: type I tumors are totally external;

type II tumors are almost totally external; type III tumors are almost completely internal; and type IV tumors are completely internal [56–58]. Symptoms are largely related to the degree of displacement or obstruction of the bladder, urethra, or rectum.

Surgical therapy by midline or chevron incision is the mainstay for benign sacrococcygeal teratomas. After removal of the tumor with coccygectomy survival is 95%. Presacral tumors may require an abdominal approach combined with the usual sacral approach. Multiagent adjuvant chemotherapy is added to surgical therapy for malignant tumors with survival in up to 80% of cases reported.

Summary

Significant advances have been made in our understanding of the natural history and treatment of congenital spinal deformities. Early diagnosis remains the key to successful treatment.

References

[1] Giampietro PF, Blank RD, Raggio CL, et al. Congenital and idiopathic scoliosis: clinical and genetic aspects. Clin Med Res 2003;1:125–36.

[2] Shands AR Jr, Eisberg HB. The incidence of scoliosis in the state of Delaware; a study of 50,000 minifilms of the chest made during a survey for tuberculosis. J Bone Joint Surg Am 1955;37:1243–9.

[3] Wynne-Davies R. Congenital vertebral anomalies: aetiology and relationship to spina bifida cystica. J Med Genet 1975;12:280–8.

[4] Chatkupt S, Skurnick JH, Jaggi M, et al. Study of genetics, epidemiology, and vitamin usage in familial spina bifida in the United States in the 1990s. Neurology 1994;44:65–70.

[5] Christ B, Schmidt C, Huang R, et al. Segmentation of the vertebrate body. Anat Embryol (Berl) 1998; 197:1–8.

[6] Keynes RJ, Stern CD. Mechanisms of vertebrate segmentation. Development 1988;103:413–29.

[7] Scott RM, Wolpert SM, Bartoshesky LE, et al. Segmental spinal dysgenesis. Neurosurgery 1988;22: 739–44.

[8] Byrd SE, Darling CF, McLone DG, et al. MR imaging of the pediatric spine. Magn Reson Imaging Clin N Am 1996;4:797–833.

[9] Bradford DS, Heithoff KB, Cohen M. Intraspinal abnormalities and congenital spine deformities: a radiographic and MRI study. J Pediatr Orthop 1991; 11:36–41.

[10] Basu PS, Elsebaie H, Noordeen MH. Congenital spinal deformity: a comprehensive assessment at presentation. Spine 2002;27:2255–9.

[11] Dias MS, Walker ML. The embryogenesis of complex dysraphic malformations: a disorder of gastrulation? Pediatr Neurosurg 1992;18:229–53.

[12] Roessmann U. The embryology and neuropathology of congenital malformations. Clin Neurosurg 1983;30:157–64.

[13] Christ B, Wilting J. From somites to vertebral column. Ann Anat 1992;174:23–32.

[14] Smith CA, Tuan RS. Human PAX gene expression and development of the vertebral column. Clin Orthop Relat Res 1994;302:241–50.

[15] Smith CA, Tuan RS. Functional involvement of Pax-1 in somite development: somite dysmorphogenesis in chick embryos treated with Pax-1 pairedbox antisense oligodeoxynucleotide. Teratology 1995;52:333–45.

[16] Russ PD, Pretorius DH, Manco-Johnson ML, et al. The fetal spine. Neuroradiology 1986;28:398–407.

[17] Bagnall KM, Harris PF, Jones PR. A radiographic study of variations of the human fetal spine. Anat Rec 1984;208:265–70.

[18] Bagnall KM, Harris PF, Jones PR. A radiographic study of the human fetal spine. 2. The sequence of development of ossification centres in the vertebral column. J Anat 1977;124:791–802.

[19] Suh SW, Sarwark JF, Vora A, et al. Evaluating congenital spine deformities for intraspinal anomalies with magnetic resonance imaging. J Pediatr Orthop 2001;21:525–31.

[20] Belmont PJ Jr, Kuklo TR, Taylor KF, et al. Intraspinal anomalies associated with isolated congenital hemivertebra: the role of routine magnetic resonance imaging. J Bone Joint Surg Am 2004;86:1704–10.

[21] Prahinski JR, Polly DW Jr, McHale KA, et al. Occult intraspinal anomalies in congenital scoliosis. J Pediatr Orthop 2000;20:59–63.

[22] McMaster MJ, Ohtsuka K. The natural history of congenital scoliosis. A study of two hundred and fifty-one patients. J Bone Joint Surg Am 1982;64: 1128–47.

[23] Hedequist D, Emans J. Congenital scoliosis: a review and update. J Pediatr Orthop 2007;27:106–16.

[24] McMaster MJ. Congenital scoliosis caused by a unilateral failure of vertebral segmentation with contralateral hemivertebrae. Spine 1998;23:998–1005.

[25] McMaster MJ. Spinal growth and congenital deformity of the spine. Spine 2006;31:2284–7.

[26] Leatherman KD, Dickson RA. Two-stage corrective surgery for congenital deformities of the spine. J Bone Joint Surg Br 1979;61:324–8.

[27] Goldberg CJ, Moore DP, Fogarty EE, et al. Longterm results from in situ fusion for congenital vertebral deformity. Spine 2002;27:619–28.

[28] Hedequist DJ, Hall JE, Emans JB. The safety and efficacy of spinal instrumentation in children with congenital spine deformities. Spine 2004;29: 2081–6.

[29] Campbell RM Jr, Smith MD, Mayes TC, et al. The effect of opening wedge thoracostomy on thoracic

insufficiency syndrome associated with fused ribs and congenital scoliosis. J Bone Joint Surg Am 2004;86:1659–74.

[30] Winter RB, Moe JH, Wang JF. Congenital kyphosis. Its natural history and treatment as observed in a study of one hundred and thirty patients. J Bone Joint Surg Am 1973;55:223–56.

[31] Winter RB, Moe JH, Lonstein JE. The surgical treatment of congenital kyphosis. A review of 94 patients age 5 years or older, with 2 years or more follow-up in 77 patients. Spine 1985;10:224–31.

[32] Kim YJ, Otsuka NY, Flynn JM, et al. Surgical treatment of congenital kyphosis. Spine 2001;26: 2251–7.

[33] Verbiest H. Results of surgical treatment of idiopathic developmental stenosis of the lumbar vertebral canal. A review of twenty-seven years' experience. J Bone Joint Surg Br 1977;59:181–8.

[34] Verbiest H. Stenosis of the lumbar vertebral canal and sciatica. Neurosurg Rev 1980;3:75–89.

[35] Verbiest H. A radicular syndrome from developmental narrowing of the lumbar vertebral canal. 1954. Clin Orthop Relat Res 2001;384:3–9.

[36] Faciszewski T, Winter RB, Lonstein JE, et al. Segmental spinal dysgenesis. A disorder different from spinal agenesis. J Bone Joint Surg Am 1995;77:530–7.

[37] Wiltse LL. Spondylolisthesis in children. Clin Orthop 1961;21:156–63.

[38] Wiltse LL. Spondylolisthesis. West J Med 1975;122: 152–3.

[39] Wiltse LL, Newman PH, Macnab I. Classification of spondylolysis and spondylolisthesis. Clin Orthop Relat Res 1976;117:23–9.

[40] Wiltse LL, Hutchinson RH. Surgical treatment of spondylolisthesis. Clin Orthop Relat Res 1964;35: 116–35.

[41] Mitchell LE, Adzick NS, Melchionne J, et al. Spina bifida. Lancet 2004;364:1885–95.

[42] Gan YC, Sgouros S, Walsh AR, et al. Diastematomyelia in children: treatment outcome and natural history of associated syringomyelia. Childs Nerv Syst 2007;23(5):515–9.

[43] Hood RW, Riseborough EJ, Nehme AM, et al. Diastematomyelia and structural spinal deformities. J Bone Joint Surg Am 1980;62:520–8.

[44] Hori A, Fischer G, etrich-Schott B, et al. Dimyelia, diplomyelia, and diastematomyelia. Clin Neuropathol 1982;1:23–30.

[45] Winter RB, Haven JJ, Moe JH, et al. Diastematomyelia and congenital spine deformities. J Bone Joint Surg Am 1974;56:27–39.

[46] Pang D, Dias MS, hab-Barmada M. Split cord malformation: part I: a unified theory of embryogenesis for double spinal cord malformations. Neurosurgery 1992;31:451–80.

[47] Byrd SE, Darling CF, McLone DG. Developmental disorders of the pediatric spine. Radiol Clin North Am 1991;29:711–52.

[48] Rogers HM, Long DM, Chou SN, et al. Lipomas of the spinal cord and cauda equina. J Neurosurg 1971; 34:349–54.

[49] Guille JT, Sarwark JF, Sherk HH, et al. Congenital and developmental deformities of the spine in children with myelomeningocele. J Am Acad Orthop Surg 2006;14:294–302.

[50] Pang D, Wilberger JE Jr. Tethered cord syndrome in adults. J Neurosurg 1982;57:32–47.

[51] Warder DE, Oakes WJ. Tethered cord syndrome and the conus in a normal position. Neurosurgery 1993;33:374–8.

[52] Warder DE, Oakes WJ. Tethered cord syndrome: the low-lying and normally positioned conus. Neurosurgery 1994;34:597–600.

[53] Pang D, Hoffman HJ. Sacral agenesis with progressive neurological deficit. Neurosurgery 1980;7: 118–26.

[54] Renshaw TS. Sacral agenesis. J Bone Joint Surg Am 1978;60:373–83.

[55] Pang D. Sacral agenesis and caudal spinal cord malformations. Neurosurgery 1993;32(5):755–78; discussion 778–9.

[56] Valdiserri RO, Yunis EJ. Sacrococcygeal teratomas: a review of 68 cases. Cancer 1981;48:217–21.

[57] Ein SH, Adeyemi SD, Mancer K. Benign sacrococcygeal teratomas in infants and children: a 25 year review. Ann Surg 1980;191:382–4.

[58] Ein SH, Mancer K, Adeyemi SD. Malignant sacrococcygeal teratoma—endodermal sinus, yolk sac tumor—in infants and children: a 32-year review. J Pediatr Surg 1985;20:473–7.

ELSEVIER
SAUNDERS

Neurosurg Clin N Am 18 (2007) 499–514

NEUROSURGERY
CLINICS
OF NORTH AMERICA

Spinal Disorders Associated with Skeletal Dysplasias and Syndromes

Debbie Song, MD, Cormac O. Maher, MD*

Department of Neurosurgery, University of Michigan, 1500 East Medical Center Drive, Ann Arbor, MI 48109–0338, USA

Skeletal dysplasias are a heterogeneous group of disorders in which there is abnormal cartilage and bone formation, growth, and remodeling. More than 200 types of skeletal dysplasias have been described. Skeletal dysplasias may be classified as osteochondral dysplasias or dysotoses. Osteochondral dysplasias involve the whole skeleton. Achondroplasia is the most common type of osteochondral dysplasia. Dysostoses are those disorders that involve only a single group of bones. Skeletal dysplasias may also be categorized according to their pathogenesis. They may be idiopathic osteolytic syndromes, primary chromosomal abnormalities, or primary metabolic abnormalities. Skeletal dysplasias can affect the spine in variable ways, with corresponding diverse implications for diagnosis and treatment. Craniocervical junction abnormalities, atlantoaxial subluxation, and kyphoscoliotic deformities are among the common spinal problems that are found in certain skeletal dysplasias. This article focuses on key skeletal dysplasias and the neurosurgical implications of spinal involvement in children. Specific topics include foramen magnum and spinal stenosis in achondroplasia, vertebral dysplasia, vertebral segmentation and fusion abnormalities, atlantoaxial instability in Goldenhar's syndrome, spondyloepiphyseal dysplasia (SED), and Morquio's syndrome, dystrophic scoliosis and kyphosis in neurofibromatosis type 1 (NF1), and osteogenesis imperfecta (OI).

Achondroplasia

Achondroplasia is the most common form of rhizomelic dwarfism, characterized by a disproportionate shortening of the proximal limbs relative to the trunk. The condition occurs in 1 in every 26,000 to 28,000 births, with an estimated incidence of 0.03% to 0.05% of all live births [1–3]. Although it is the most common heritable skeletal dysplasia and is inherited in an autosomal dominant fashion, 80% of cases are attributable to spontaneous de novo point mutations in the fibroblast growth factor receptor 3 (*FGFR-3*) gene located on chromosome 4 [1,2,4]. In achondroplasia, there is a quantitative decrease in the rate of endochondral bone formation but rates of membranous bone formation, calcification, and remodeling are normal [4,5]. This results in a variety of skeletal manifestations that are recognizable at birth. These include shortened limbs and long bones, macrocephaly with frontal bossing and a low-set nasal bridge, genu varum abnormalities, and distinctive pelvic changes [5].

Neurologic manifestations of achondroplasia

Thirty-five percent to 47% of patients with achondroplasia have neurologic manifestations of their disease [1]. Neurologic conditions that are associated with achondroplasia include ventriculomegaly or hydrocephalus, compressive spinal syndromes, and developmental delay. In the pediatric population, foramen magnum stenosis with cervicomedullary compression is the most notable spinal condition that deserves attention. In older children and adults with achondroplasia, multisegment spinal stenosis involving the subaxial cervical or thoracolumbar spine may also be present.

---

* Corresponding author.
E-mail address: cmaher@umich.edu (C.O. Maher).

1042-3680/07/$ - see front matter © 2007 Elsevier Inc. All rights reserved.
doi:10.1016/j.nec.2007.05.004

Foramen magnum stenosis in pediatric patients with achondroplasia is a direct result of defective endochondral bone growth and an abnormal fusion pattern of the posterior basal synchondroses [3,6]. The foramen magnum is composed of the exoccipital, supraoccipital, and baso-occipital bones [7]. These bones of the skull base as well as bone of the neural arches normally enlarge by endochondral ossification [7,8]. Because of defective endochondral bone formation at the cranial base and craniocervical junction, an infant with achondroplasia may have a small foramen magnum, a short basicranium and clivus, a shallow posterior fossa with a horizontally oriented inferior occiput, an abnormal odontoid process, stenotic jugular foramina, and a narrow upper cervical canal [2,3,8].

In addition to defects in bone formation and growth, premature fusion and aberrant development of the two posterior synchondroses contribute to thickening of the rim of the foramen magnum, further contributing to its stenosis [2,8]. The hypertrophied margin of the foramen magnum can potentially project into the brain stem, causing severe angulation and pressure necrosis of the medulla or spinal cord [8]. Further compromise of the foramen magnum may be attributable to anterior extension of the squamous portion of the occipital bone into the foramen magnum, to abnormal fusion of the posterior neural arch of the atlas with the posterior margin of the foramen magnum, or to dense fibrotic epidural bands commonly found anterior to the posterior ring of the atlas [6]. In patients with achondroplasia, the odontoid process often projects posteriorly and superiorly into the small foramen magnum, resulting in medullary compression [7,8]. Autopsy studies and histologic analysis have demonstrated central cystic degeneration and necrosis, gliosis, and myelomalacia in the brain stem and upper cervical cord of patients with achondroplasia subject to chronic compression of the craniocervical junction because of foramen magnum stenosis [9].

Craniocervical stenosis secondary to foramen magnum narrowing is a radiographic diagnosis that is commonly found among pediatric patients with achondroplasia (Fig. 1). Wang and colleagues [10] found that 96% of pediatric patients with achondroplasia evaluated had sagittal and coronal foramen magnum dimensions at least 3 SDs less than those of age-matched controls. Kao and colleagues [11] used MRI to study the craniocervical junction in 10 children with achondroplasia, all of whom were found to have virtual obliteration of the subarachnoid space at the level of the foramen magnum. In all cases, the narrowed foramen magnum had a triangular shape [11]. Other abnormalities evident on craniocervical imaging of pediatric patients with achondroplasia may include larger tentorial angles with a more prominent and vertically directed straight sinus and upward displacement of the brain stem because of shortening of the basicranium at the skull base, resulting in a relatively vertical course of the optic nerves from the optic chiasm to the optic canal [6,7,11].

Cervicomedullary compression secondary to foramen magnum stenosis is a clinical diagnosis that can have protean manifestations in the achondroplastic child. Compression can affect the lower brain stem, high cervical cord, and associated spinal nerve roots, with neurologic sequelae that include myelopathy, hydrocephalus, respiratory disorders, and sudden death. Symptoms of cervicomedullary compression in infants include excessive hypotonia, poor head control, feeding or sleep difficulties, and apnea. Neurologic dysfunction in the youngest patients may be subtle and difficult to detect, because most patients with achondroplasia are significantly hypotonic during early infancy and may exhibit developmental delay in achieving motor milestones compared with unaffected children. Achondroplastic children usually sit unsupported at the age of 9 to 12 months and ambulate at the age of 18 months [4]. Most achondroplastic children gain normal strength and muscle tone and catch up with their unaffected peers on their motor skills by the age of 2 or 3 years [4].

Sudden death in infants with achondroplasia has been reported and is a catastrophic consequence of cervicomedullary compression. Based on a cohort of 781 individuals with achondroplasia, Hecht and colleagues [12] concluded there was a 7.5% risk of sudden death within the first year of life and a 2.5% risk of sudden death between 1 and 4 years of age. Pauli and colleagues [13] retrospectively studied 13 cases of infants with achondroplasia and sudden unexplained death or unexplained apnea. Of the 11 children who died suddenly, 5 had evidence of acute or chronic compression of the medulla and spinal cord at autopsy [13]. Postmortem assessments of other children with achondroplasia and sudden death have similarly found cystic degenerative changes of the lower brain stem and syrinx formation of the upper cervical cord [14].

Respiratory disturbances, including sleep apnea, are common among children with achondroplasia

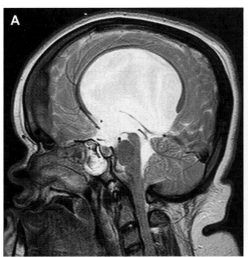
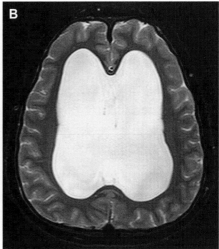

Fig. 1. (*A*) Sagittal T2-weighted MRI scan of a 13-year-old patient with achondroplasia. There is a short clivus and a small foramen magnum. A relatively narrow spinal canal is also seen. The sagittal (*A*) and axial (*B*) views demonstrate significant ventricular dilation without transependymal migration of cerebrospinal fluid. This patient had chronic macrocephaly without any neurologic symptoms of hydrocephalus.

and have a multifactorial etiology [11]. Damage to respiratory control centers in the medulla from foramen magnum stenosis likely contributes to central sleep apnea. Additionally, foramen magnum stenosis can lead to compression of lower motor neurons that innervate the diaphragm and other respiratory muscles, thereby causing weak or ineffective respirations [2]. Nonneurologic causes of respiratory dysfunction, including upper airway obstruction, a small thoracic cage, and midface hypoplasia, should also be addressed in the achondroplastic child. Apnea that is attributable to foramen magnum stenosis improves after decompression [6,11,15,16].

Crowding at the foramen magnum has also been implicated in the pathogenesis of communicating hydrocephalus in achondroplastic patients who exhibit dilated ventricles. Macrocephaly is a well-recognized feature of achondroplasia, but not all affected children have hydrocephalus [1,2]. The pathogenesis of hydrocephalus in children with achondroplasia is thought to involve obstruction of the cerebrospinal fluid (CSF) outflow pathways because of foramen magnum stenosis. Impaired CSF absorption because of jugular foramen stenosis and elevated venous sinus pressures may also contribute to the development of communicating hydrocephalus [7,11]. In cases of clinically asymptomatic mild to moderate ventricular dilatation, patients may be serially monitored without treatment, because ventriculomegaly usually arrests

over time [2,11,16]. Moreover, foramen magnum decompression usually does not relieve symptomatic hydrocephalus [2,3].

Although foramen magnum stenosis is a common radiologic finding in pediatric patients with achondroplasia, only a fraction of those patients exhibit symptoms of cervicomedullary compression [4,14]. In a prospective evaluation of 53 infants with achondroplasia, more than 70% of patients had foramen magnum stenosis and associated craniocervical abnormalities on MRI, ranging from narrowing or obliteration of the subarachnoid spaces to deformation of the spinal cord [14]. Despite this, only five of those patients demonstrated clinical symptoms of cervicomedullary compression necessitating surgical decompression [14]. Reid and colleagues [17] found evidence of foramen magnum stenosis in 60% of prospectively evaluated pediatric patients with achondroplasia, with 35% of the patients exhibiting clinical symptoms of cervicomedullary compression.

Testing the somatosensory evoked potentials (SSEPs) is occasionally useful in the evaluation of patients with achondroplasia. Although SSEP testing may show disruption of waveforms at the cervicomedullary junction, the lack of specificity of SSEP testing limits its utility in the pediatric achondroplastic population. One study showed that 44% of asymptomatic patients with achondroplasia had abnormal SSEP findings [18]. In another study, 11 children with achondroplasia

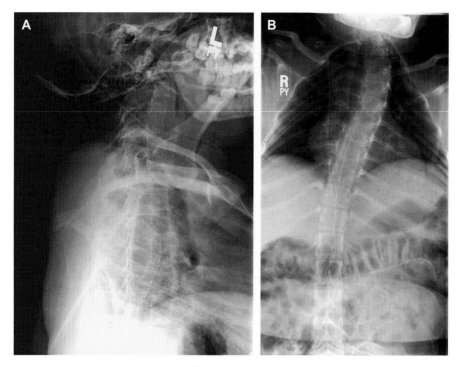

Fig. 2. Lateral (*A*) and anteroposterior (*B*) radiographs of a 14-year-old patient with osteogenesis imperfecta. There is diffuse osteopenia, scoliosis, compression of several cervical vertebral bodies, and a focal kyphosis at the midcervical level. All these findings are typical of this disease.

underwent SSEP testing as part of diagnostic evaluation [14]. Of the 7 children with clearly abnormal SSEP testing results, 5 were neurologically normal and remained without any clinical symptoms of cervicomedullary compression [14].

Surgical treatment of foramen magnum stenosis in achondroplasia

Prospectively determining which patients require surgical decompression can be difficult, given the variable natural history of foramen magnum stenosis in achondroplasia and the discrepancy that commonly exists between the degree of radiographic stenosis and the severity of clinical symptoms [7]. For this reason, treatment decisions should be based on signs or symptoms of neurologic dysfunction rather than on the radiologic evaluation alone. Clinical signs and symptoms of cervicomedullary compression, such as apnea, lower cranial nerve palsies, hyperreflexia, sustained clonus, and weakness, must be considered in conjunction with radiographic evidence of foramen magnum stenosis and compression of the neuraxis. MRI features that suggest

the need for foramen magnum decompression include intramedullary spinal cord changes on T2-weighted MRI scans, lack of CSF flow anteriorly and posteriorly at the foramen magnum, and the presence of a syrinx. In a prospective study of infants with achondroplasia, Pauli and colleagues [14] concluded that the signs and symptoms best predicting the need for surgical decompression were lower limb hyperreflexia or clonus, central hypopnea on polysomnography, and foramen magnum measurements lower than the mean for children with achondroplasia.

Early foramen magnum decompression is recommended in proven cases of symptomatic cervicomedullary compression. At the authors' institution, SSEP monitoring is used during patient positioning and throughout the entire operative procedure. A suboccipital craniectomy and removal of the posterior arch of the atlas are performed in a manner similar to a standard Chiari decompression. The authors prefer to access the underlying suboccipital bone through a chevron-shaped muscle-splitting incision just below the nuchal line. The posterior rim of the foramen magnum is often thickened. After bony removal, it is also common to find thickened fibrous epidural bands that need to be separated from the underlying dura. It is imperative that these thickened epidural bands be adequately removed, because they can be a source of significant cervicomedullary compression. Some surgeons have advocated the use of intraoperative ultrasound to assess the decompression and to look for adequate CSF pulsations around the brain stem before opening the dura. The authors prefer to open the dura and place a wide dural patch in every case. A pericranial patch graft or a commercially available dural substitute may be used, and the dura is closed in a watertight fashion.

Marked immediate improvement in neurologic function is often noted in symptomatic patients with achondroplasia after foramen magnum decompression, but permanent neurologic damage may result with delays in intervention [5,14]. Bagley and colleagues [2] have reported on a series of 43 symptomatic achondroplastic children who underwent foramen magnum decompression with complete or partial improvement in preoperative symptoms in all patients. In that series, the most common preoperative symptom was sleep apnea, which was present in 53% of the patients. There was a significant improvement in respiratory symptoms after surgical decompression in all patients [2]. In some of these cases, residual respiratory symptoms improved after treatment of nonneurologic causes of respiratory dysfunction [2]. Ryken and Menezes [3] identified 6 patients with achondroplasia and clinical and radiographic cervicomedullary compression who underwent surgical decompression. After surgery, all patients who presented with respiratory compromise or apneic spells improved, 75% of patients who presented with headaches had complete resolution of their pain, and all patients with preoperative myelopathy and ataxia improved [3]. Surgical decompression did not affect hypotonia that was present before surgery [3]. In another series, Aryanpur and colleagues [16] reported on 14 pediatric patients with achondroplasia who underwent surgical decompression. All these patients had improvement or resolution of their preoperative symptoms [16]. Nine of 10 patients in that report who presented with paresis had improvement in their strength after surgery. Six of 8 patients with hyperreflexia or hypertonia had resolution of these signs, and 6 of 8 patients who presented with cyanosis or apnea had total resolution of their respiratory problems after decompression [16]. Two patients who continued to have cyanosis or apneic episodes after foramen magnum decompression had additional surgery directed toward the cause of their obstructive apnea and went on to have resolution of their apnea [16].

Foramen magnum decompression can be performed with a relatively low expected rate of morbidity. The most common complication is CSF leak from the suboccipital incision or the site of a perioperatively placed externalized ventricular drain. Postoperative CSF leak was reported in 15.5% of cases by Bagley and colleagues [2] and in 4 of 15 patients by Aryanpur and colleagues [16]. Most case series report no surgical mortality [2,3,6,14,16]. For most children with achondroplasia, foramen magnum decompression in proven cases of cervicomedullary compression can provide excellent clinical benefit with minimal morbidity.

Spinal stenosis in achondroplasia

Spinal stenosis is a frequent finding in patients with achondroplasia. Premature fusion of the ossification centers of the vertebral bodies and posterior neural arches results in laminae and pedicles that are short and thick. In addition, the vertebral bodies have a reduced height, the neural foramina are smaller, and the interpedicular distance is narrowed [8,19]. The vertebral bodies assume a concave curvature posteriorly, with the inferior and superior end plates projecting into the spinal canal and further compromising the spinal subarachnoid space [19]. Patients may develop clinical signs and symptoms of subaxial cervical or thoracolumbar stenosis or nerve root compression. Although congenital stenosis usually becomes symptomatic when superimposed on degenerative changes in early adulthood, children and young adults with achondroplasia may develop clinically significant spinal stenosis or radiculopathy requiring treatment. Signs and symptoms that should prompt further investigation include paraparesis or quadriparesis, gait ataxia with frequent falls, spasticity, bowel or bladder dysfunction, intermittent claudication with paresthesias, or temporary deterioration of spinal cord function after seemingly minor trauma. Neurologic dysfunction from spinal stenosis, particularly when standing, is exacerbated by the excessive lumbar lordosis that is characteristic of teenagers and adults with achondroplasia. Neurologic compromise attributable to spinal stenosis or nerve root impingement usually responds well to standard posterior decompression, with consideration given to fusion if multiple-level laminectomies are required.

In preadolescent children with achondroplasia, thoracolumbar gibbus formation and kyphotic deformity can also produce neurologic dysfunction. Before ambulation, children with achondroplasia have a thoracolumbar kyphosis that is partially attributable to generalized hypotonia. Usually, the gibbus deformity and kyphosis of the thoracolumbar spine resolve with the onset of ambulation and an upright posture. An exaggerated lumbar lordosis develops thereafter into adulthood. In some children, however, the thoracolumbar kyphosis may persist or progress if there is severe anterior wedging of the vertebral bodies. This may result in compression of the conus medullaris or cauda equina. Typically, thoracolumbar kyphosis greater than 30° that persists after independent ambulation should be corrected. If the deformity is corrected before the age of 2 years, this may lead to hypoplastic vertebral bodies in the fused area; thus, some advocate correction around age of 4 or 5 years by means of decompression followed by an anterior and posterior fusion [20,21].

Goldenhar's syndrome

Goldenhar's syndrome, also known as oculoauriculovertebral dysplasia, is a clinically heterogeneous disorder characterized by hemifacial microsomia, epibulbar dermoid appendages, and spinal defects. Additional craniofacial, gastrointestinal, cardiac, renal, and ophthalmic anomalies may be associated with Goldenhar's syndrome. The syndrome occurs in 1 of every 3000 to 5000 live births [22]. Most cases are sporadic, and no underlying genetic mutation has been identified [22]. This syndrome is most likely attributable to a disruption in development of the first and second branchial arches as well as in the intervening first pharyngeal pouch and branchial cleft within the first 6 weeks of intrauterine life [22,23]. This is thought to be attributable to a disruption in the blood supply to this region by way of the primitive stapedial artery [22].

Spinal anomalies associated with Goldenhar's syndrome include vertebral hypoplasia, failure of segmentation, and failure of vertebral formation. Segmentation defects are more common in the cervical spine, whereas failure of vertebral formation more often occurs in the thoracolumbar spine [23,24]. Unbalanced hemivertebrae can produce scoliosis, often requiring surgical treatment [23,24]. Thoracolumbar kyphosis is also seen with segmentation anomalies [23,24]. Gibson and colleagues [23] identified vertebral anomalies in 21 (60%) of 35 children with Goldenhar's syndrome. Among the anomalies identified were block vertebrae (most often involving fusion of C3 and C4), unilateral hemivertebrae in the thoracolumbar spine, spina bifida occulta, butterfly vertebrae, and sacral agenesis [23]. Several patients had anomalies at multiple spinal levels. In all patients identified with scoliosis, an unbalanced hemivertebra was present and curvatures were in excess of 20° [23]. Although several subjects required surgical correction of their scoliosis, none of the children in that series demonstrated weakness or any other neurologic dysfunction [23]. Tsirikos and McMaster [24] identified Klippel-Feil anomalies in 40% of the patients in their series of children with Goldenhar's syndrome.

Several anomalies of the upper cervical spine have been identified in association with Goldenhar's syndrome. One group has reported a 12% incidence of platybasia and occipitalization of the atlas [23]. In addition, an increased frequency of odontoid hypoplasia with atlantoaxial instability has been reported in children with Goldenhar's syndrome. In the series of eight children with Goldenhar's syndrome reported on by Healey and colleagues [22], three had atlantoaxial instability greater than 5 mm with upward migration of the odontoid process. Two of the patients in that series had atlantoaxial instability greater than 7 mm and required surgical treatment [22]. Although atlantoaxial instability may remain clinically silent in children who have not yet reached skeletal maturity, Healey and colleagues [22] have advocated treatment in any child with instability greater than 6 mm to reduce the possibility of catastrophic spinal cord impingement. In cases in which instability is less than 6 mm, cervical flexion-extension films should be obtained every 6 months and the child should be advised against contact sports, which may threaten spinal cord injury [22]. Moreover, the relatively high frequency of cervical malformations may warrant an investigation into the possibility of cervical instability in any child with Goldenhar's syndrome who is to undergo induction with a general anesthetic [22].

Spondyloepiphyseal dysplasia

SED encompasses several disorders characterized by abnormal growth of the spinal vertebrae and epiphysis. Typically, individuals with SED have short-trunk dwarfism with shortened proximal and middle limbs but relatively normal-sized hands and feet. There are two major types of SED: SED congenita and SED tarda. SED congenita is the more severe form of the disorder, with recognizable features present at birth, and is commonly associated with serious spinal abnormalities in children. Delayed ossification of the vertebral bodies, coxa vara abnormalities of the hips, and retinal detachment are common manifestations of SED congenita [25]. Wynne-Davies and Hall [26] further classified SED congenita into a mild or severe clinical subtype, with the severe subtype associated with extremely short stature and severe coxa vara. SED congenita is inherited in an autosomal dominant fashion, but most cases result from new sporadic mutations in the *COL2A1* (type II collagen α_1 chain) gene on chromosome 12 [27]. Such mutations result in defective type II collagen, which is the major matrix protein in the nucleus pulposus, epiphyseal cartilage, and vitreous of the eye [27].

Atlantoaxial instability associated with odontoid hypoplasia or ligamentous laxity is the most common spinal manifestation of SED congenita in children. Although spinal cord compression is not present in all patients with atlantoaxial instability, the incidence of cervical myelopathy attributable to atlantoaxial subluxation may be as high as 35% in children with SED congenita [28]. Signs and symptoms of myelopathy may develop gradually and manifest as delayed motor development, slowly progressive weakness, spasticity, or sleep apnea and other respiratory abnormalities [29]. In other cases, however, sudden quadriplegia has resulted from minor trauma [29].

In a study of risk factors for myelopathy in patients with SED congenita, Nakamura and colleagues [29] found that atlantoaxial subluxation (defined as an atlantodental interval [ADI] of 5 mm or more in children) was present in most cases with myelopathy. Studies have also suggested that atlantoaxial subluxation progresses with age and with increasing ADIs [28]. Those patients whose sagittal canal diameter at the level of the atlas is 10 mm or less are at increased risk of spinal cord compression, as are patients with the severe subtype of SED congenita [28,29]. The sagittal axis diameter, measured between the posterior edge of the anterior arch of the atlas and the anterior edge of the posterior arch of the atlas, is small in most patients with SED congenita [28]. Os odontoideum, which is frequently present in these patients, is also associated with a narrowed

sagittal axis diameter. In a patient with a small sagittal axis diameter and atlantoaxial subluxation, reduction of the subluxation does not ensure an adequate sagittal canal diameter, even in extension [28]. In patients with a narrowed sagittal canal diameter that persists despite reduction in extension, removal of the posterior arch of the atlas in addition to a posterior occipitocervical fusion is recommended to reduce the subluxation and to decompress the spinal canal adequately [29]. Preoperative reduction and immobilization in a halo vest may be helpful [28]. Depending on the extent of the compression on preoperative imaging, additional procedures, such as a C2 laminoplasty and foramen magnum decompression, may be required [28]. Awake fiberoptic nasotracheal intubation should be performed to prevent spinal cord injury during induction.

Morquio's syndrome

Mucopolysaccharidosis (MPS) type IV, or Morquio's syndrome, is an autosomal recessive lysosomal storage disease characterized by an inability to metabolize keratan sulfate, a glucosaminoglycan found predominantly in cartilage and in the cornea. There are two subtypes of Morquio's syndrome: MPS IV type A is attributable to a deficiency in *N*-acetyl-galactosamine-6-sulfatase, and MPS IV type B is attributable to a deficiency in β-galactosidase [30]. Individuals with Morquio's syndrome have short-trunk dwarfism with skeletal features that may include pectus carinatum, thoracolumbar kyphosis, scoliosis, genus valgus, platyspondyly, flaring of the ribs, and joint hypermobility [30]. Corneal clouding is also common in patients with MPS IV. In contrast to patients with other MPSs, patients with Morquio's syndrome have normal intelligence. Although skeletal abnormalities are present and radiologically evident within the first year of life, patients with MPS IV appear healthy at birth and often have normal growth and development for the first 2 years of life [31]. Clinical and phenotypical abnormalities progress rapidly between 2 and 6 years of age. Morquio's syndrome occurs in 1 in 40,000 live births, and although patients may survive to adulthood, many patients die in early adulthood from cardiopulmonary disease or neurologic complications of their disorder [30,31].

As in SED congenita, the most common and serious condition associated with Morquio's syndrome is atlantoaxial subluxation with spinal cord compression. Odontoid dysplasia, which can include hypoplasia, aplasia, or os odontoideum, is a common finding in Morquio's syndrome, as is ligament laxity [32]. Both are contributing factors for atlantoaxial subluxation in these patients [31]. In the series of patients with Morquio's syndrome and radiographic atlantoaxial subluxation reported on by Stevens and colleagues [31], odontoid hypoplasia was present in every case. In normal development, most of the dens has ossified by birth. In the series reported by Stevens and colleagues [31], however, only the portion of the odontoid contained within the body of the axis had ossified by birth, and an os odontoideum was present in all skeletally mature individuals. Early detachment of the distal part of the dens, along with its delayed ossification, is attributable to articular hypermobility during development in patients with Morquio's syndrome [31]. Affected patients have a persistently narrowed internal diameter of the canal at the level of the atlas [32]. Atlantoaxial subluxation has been identified in up to 42% to 90% of cases of Morquio's syndrome [31,32].

Not all patients with atlantoaxial subluxation have spinal cord compression or require surgery. Symptomatic patients or patients with a 50% reduction in spinal cord diameter should be considered for surgical treatment, however [31]. The preferred time for an elective operation is between 3 and 8 years of age, when skeletal anomalies are well developed [31]. In patients who have undergone occipitocervical fusion, postoperative studies of the extradural compressive agents suggest regression of the extradural soft tissue and ossification of previously unossified cartilage [31]. Preoperative MRI is useful to assess extradural soft tissue elements and the degree of cord compression at the craniocervical junction. Intraoperative SSEP monitoring is essential.

Neurofibromatosis type 1

NF1 is the most common neurocutaneous syndrome, with an incidence of 1 in every 3300 individuals [33,34]. It is an autosomal dominant disorder caused by a mutation in the *NF1* tumor suppressor gene located on chromosome 17 [34]. NF1 is a multisystemic disease, with diagnostic criteria based on the presence of café-au-lait macules, Lisch nodules of the iris, axillary or inguinal freckling, familial inheritance patterns, and such distinct osseous lesions as cortical thinning of long bones or sphenoid wing dysplasia [34].

The most common spinal abnormality in children with NF1 is scoliosis. Scoliosis is present in approximately 10% to 20% of children with NF1 [34]. In patients with NF1, scoliosis has been postulated to occur because of mesodermal dysplasia, endocrine disturbances, or, in some cases, osteomalacia arising from infiltration of bone by tumors [34]. There are two main patterns of scoliosis in children with NF1: dystrophic scoliosis and nondystrophic scoliosis [34,35]. Nondystrophic scoliotic curves in children with NF1 resemble those in congenital idiopathic scoliosis. Typically, 8 to 10 vertebral segments are involved, and dysplastic changes in the bone are not prominent [35]. For idiopathic nondystrophic curves less than 20°, bracing can be offered. If the curve progresses to greater than 35° to 45°, posterior spinal fusion with segmental spinal instrumentation is usually indicated [35].

Dystrophic scoliosis, which involves short segments typically less than six vertebrae long, is characterized by dysplastic sharply angulated curves. The thoracic spine is most commonly affected [35]. Associated dysplastic abnormalities in the bones include severe wedging, rotation, and scalloping of the apical vertebral bodies; spindling of the transverse processes; apical rib penciling; and foraminal enlargement because of adjacent soft tissue paravertebral neurofibromas [35]. Dystrophic scoliosis in NF1 is progressive, and bracing is usually ineffective. In children with NF1 and dystrophic scoliotic curves less than 20°, Crawford [35] suggests checking for progression at 6-month intervals. For a dystrophic curve with greater than 20° of angulation, a posterior spinal fusion with segmental spinal instrumentation is usually recommended [35]. Because dystrophic scoliotic curves involve only short segments and the involved vertebrae have poor growth potential, early fusion does not cause significant stunting of trunk height; therefore, it need not be avoided in young children who are otherwise good candidates for fusion [36].

Dystrophic scoliosis may progress to kyphoscoliosis. Kyphoscoliosis in patients with NF1 involves dysplastic changes in the spine, with deformed vertebral bodies and an acute anteroposterior angulation, resulting in neurologic impairment in some cases [35,37,38]. Kyphoscoliosis secondary to encroachment of vertebral bodies by tumor growth has been associated with the development of paraplegia in patients with NF1 [28,29]. Patients with angular kyphosis respond poorly to a posterior fusion alone. Moreover, because the compression is usually anterior, a laminectomy alone for cord compression attributable to a kyphotic deformity is contraindicated because of the risk for instability with removal of posterior elements [35].

Spinal lesions that may occur in NF1 include spinal meningoceles, dural ectasia, and tumors [39–43]. Paraspinal neurofibromas are the most common spine tumors in patients with NF1 [40]. Such tumors arise from the dorsal roots in the cervical and lumbar regions, and most are intraforaminal and intracanalicular [40]. These lesions can grow, with resultant expansion of the foramina, enlargement of the spinal canal, and widening of the interpedicular distance, all of which can contribute to the development of instability and scoliosis [44]. These lesions are often asymptomatic. Khong and colleagues [40] reported on 53 children with NF1 and no neurologic symptoms. Approximately 13% of these patients were found to have spinal neurofibromas, including dumbbell, intradural, paraspinal, and plexiform neurofibromas. In that series, the incidence of scoliosis, localized cutaneous neurofibromas, and massive soft tissue neurofibromas was 71.4%, 71.4%, and 28.6%, respectively, in those children with spinal neurofibromas and 30.4%, 39.1%, and 8.7%, respectively, in those children without spinal neurofibromas [40]. Rarely, more malignant spinal tumors, such as malignant peripheral nerve sheath tumors (MPNSTs), and intramedullary tumors, such as astrocytomas and ependymomas, may occur [41,42]. Malignant transformation to MPNSTs is rare in children and is much more likely to occur during adulthood [40]. Surgical treatment with the goal of complete resection is indicated for symptomatic lesions, because partially resected tumors tend to recur [40].

Osteogenesis imperfecta

Osteogenesis imperfecta is a congenital disorder characterized by osteopenia, fragile bones susceptible to fracture, variable degrees of short stature, and progressive skeletal deformities (Fig. 2) [45]. This disease is attributable to mutations in one of two genes that code for the collagen type I α chains, COLA1A1 and COLA1A2 [46]. Type I collagen fibers are found in bone, organ capsules, fascia, cornea, sclera, tendon, meninges, and dermis [46]. Quantitative and qualitative defects in type I collagen have been reported in OI [46]. There are several classification schemes for subtypes of OI; the most common of these categorizes OI into four subtypes. Type I is a mild form with no long bone deformities, type II is lethal in the perinatal period with in utero fractures, type III is the most severe form in children who survive the perinatal period, and type IV is an undefined type with moderate bone deformities and variable short stature [46–48].

Kyphosis and scoliosis are the most common problems of the spine in children with OI. The incidence of scoliosis in OI has been reported to be as high as 80% in some series [49,50]. The degree of curvature is more severe in older children and in patients with more severe forms of OI. Benson and colleagues [49] found that the incidence of scoliosis is 26% in children younger than the age of 6 years and that the incidence of scoliosis rises significantly in children 6 years of age and older. There is a predictable, early progression of scoliotic curves in children with OI. The scoliotic curve in OI usually progresses despite bracing. In fact, brace therapy in severe forms of OI is usually not indicated because of poor therapeutic results and a high complication rate. Furthermore, the ribs of affected patients with OI type III and type IV are too fragile to transmit corrective forces to the spine with bracing, and bracing often causes further deformities of the rib cage, which can, in turn, compromise pulmonary function [49–51]. Children with OI and scoliosis have more than two times the risk of developing pathologic kyphosis [45]. Kyphosis, like scoliosis, is often associated with more severe forms of OI. Early spinal fusion in children with curves less than 40° has been advocated to halt or slow progression of spinal deformity and cardiopulmonary dysfunction [50].

Patients with OI are at risk for compression fractures and vertebral body collapse [49]. The vertebrae assume a biconcave shape, and microfractures adjacent to vertebral growth plates can interfere with growth and cause deformity [49]. Ishikawa and colleagues [52] found that in prepubescent children with six or more biconcave vertebrae present, severe scoliosis with a curve of more than 50° was likely to develop. Cyclic intravenous bisphosphonate pamidronate therapy has been found to have beneficial effects on vertebral morphometry in children and adolescents with severe forms of OI. With treatment, there is increased cortical long bone thickness and bone mineral density in the lumbar vertebral bodies, decreased fracture rates, and improved mobility [48]. Moreover, the effect is greatest in vertebral bodies that are more compressed [48]. Early treatment is advocated in children, and pretreatment may improve surgical outcomes for scoliosis.

A rare but potentially serious condition associated with OI is basilar impression attributable to repetitive microfractures of the base of the skull adjacent to the foramen magnum [47]. Janus and colleagues [47] reported on a series of 130 children with OI who were found to have basilar impression. None of these children displayed neurologic symptoms. The condition may progress slowly, and it is rare for children with OI to require surgical treatment. If neurologic compromise exists, however, a suboccipital decompression and upper cervical laminectomy are required. If there is significant anterior compression present, an anterior transoral approach for ventral clival-odontoid anterior atlas arch resection followed by posterior stabilization may be required.

Larsen's syndrome

Larsen's syndrome, first described in 1950, is a rare congenital disorder of connective tissue often characterized by the following anomalies: anterior dislocation of the knees; dislocations of the hips and elbows; equinovarus deformities of the feet; supernumerary ossification of the hands and feet; long fingers with shortened metacarpals; and dysmorphic facies with frontal bossing, hypertelorism, and a depressed nasal bridge [53–58]. Most cases occur sporadically, although autosomal recessive and dominant transmission has also been reported [57,58]. Spinal deformities are also commonly associated with Larsen's syndrome. The cervical spine is more often affected than the thoracic or lumbar spine, and typical vertebral anomalies include hypoplastic or flattened vertebral bodies or posterior elements, dysraphism, hemivertebrae, and wedged vertebrae [57,58].

Abnormal curvatures are also common, including cervical kyphosis, thoracic lordosis, lumbar kyphosis, scoliosis, and spondylolysis [57]. Dramatic midcervical kyphosis, most commonly at C4 to C5 and exaggerated with flexion, is often present and can lead to instability, progressive myelopathy, weakness, and even sudden death in Larsen's syndrome [54,55,58,59]. The incidence of cervical kyphosis is approximately 12% [57]. In a series of 38 patients with Larsen's syndrome, sudden death occurred in 14 patients with an average age at death of 1 year [54]. Micheli and colleagues [55] followed three children with Larsen's syndrome and cervicothoracic segmental abnormalities, one of whom developed progressive

instability and subluxation attributable to midcervical kyphosis and subsequently died from sudden cardiorespiratory arrest. Subsequent postmortem studies demonstrated C4-to-C5 subluxation in association with an area of cervicomedullary compression; histologic evaluation of the involved area revealed extensive gliosis and axonotmesis [55]. Forese and colleagues [59] also reported on one case of sudden death in a 6-month-old infant with Larsen's syndrome and severe midcervical kyphosis.

Anteroposterior dissociation associated with cervical kyphosis has also been reported in Larsen's syndrome [60,61]. This feature occurs because of the absence of pedicles and results in complete separation of the laminae and vertebral bodies at multiple levels, making operative fusion difficult and requiring extension of the fusion for several levels beyond the affected segments [61]. Katz and colleagues [60] described two such patients with cervical kyphosis, anteroposterior dissociation, and quadriparesis in Larsen's syndrome. One neonate was treated nonsurgically with early traction and cervicothoracolumbosacral orthosis and demonstrated clinical and radiographic improvement to at least 3 years of age [60]. Other surgeons favor early treatment of cervical kyphosis by posterior fusion in patients with Larsen's syndrome [62,63].

Although the natural history and optimal treatment of cervical spine anomalies have not been clearly established through long-term studies, patients with Larsen's syndrome require baseline radiographic films as well as serial surveillance imaging. Initially, cervical plain films in neutral, flexion, and extension positions should be obtained and can be supplemented with CT and MRI. Follow-up imaging may be done yearly in the absence of neurologic deterioration, and the decision to intervene surgically by means of decompression and surgical stabilization must be made on an individual case basis.

Down syndrome

Down syndrome, caused by trisomy of chromosome 21, is the most common inherited chromosomal disorder, with an estimated incidence of 1 in 700 live births. Atlantoaxial and occipitocervical instability is frequently encountered in patients with Down syndrome. Long-term studies on the natural history of craniovertebral instability in patients with Down syndrome are lacking, and controversy exists regarding optimal management in that subset of patients with Down syndrome and asymptomatic atlantoaxial subluxation. In 1983, the Special Olympics mandated screening all potential participants with Down syndrome for atlantoaxial subluxation and limiting the participation of those patients found to have radiographic evidence of instability [64]. Although these directives were supported by the Committee on Sports Medicine of the American Academy of Pediatrics, questions remain regarding the appropriate management of symptomatic and asymptomatic individuals found to have radiographic instability [65].

Stability at the C1-to-C2 joint results from the bony integrity of the odontoid process and the ligaments that support it—specifically, the transverse portion of the cruciate ligament and the alar ligaments [66,67]. Compromise in the bony or ligamentous components can lead to instability. Atlantoaxial instability in children with Down syndrome is thought to be related to excessive ligamentous laxity of the transverse ligaments [66–68]. Martel and Tishler [69] postulated that chronic endogenous trauma superimposed on congenitally weakened ligaments, as found in patients with Down syndrome, can lead to spondylitis with subsequent atlantoaxial dislocation. Others have proposed that ligamentous laxity may be related to an inflammatory process or to an intrinsic defect in collagen fibers that form ligaments [68]. Finally, osseous abnormalities, such as os odontoideum, odontoid hypoplasia, ossiculum terminale, or rotary atlantoaxial subluxation, are common in Down syndrome and can contribute to instability as well [66,68].

Cervical spine instability can be diagnosed using a variety of measurements and imaging studies. The ADI, measured between the posterior surface of the anterior arch of C1 and the anterior surface of the dens, is the most common parameter used to diagnose atlantoaxial instability. The ADI is a reflection of the space available for the cord (SAC), which can be better estimated by the neural canal width, as measured between the posterior surface of the dens and the anterior surface of the posterior arch of C1 [67,70]. In normal children, an ADI of 4 to 5 mm is considered the upper limit of normal [71,72]. Using those standards, radiographic atlantoaxial instability has been estimated to be present in 10% to 30% of patients with Down syndrome [66–68,70,73]. Only approximately 1% of patients with Down syndrome have symptomatic C1-to-C2 instability, however, and warrant operative treatment [71,74]. Ligamentous laxity has been

implicated in the development of atlantoaxial subluxation among patients with Down syndrome. The hypermobility that accompanies ligamentous laxity in Down syndrome, however, may not universally equate with instability. In most cases, radiographic abnormalities do not correlate with myelopathy or neurologic findings on examination. In a prospective study of 404 children with Down syndrome, Pueschel and Scola [68] found that 14.6% of patients had an ADI greater than or equal to 5 mm, and were thus described as having atlantoaxial instability. Only 6 patients from that cohort, or 1.5% of all the patients studied, were symptomatic and required an operation; 13.1% of the patients with Down syndrome had asymptomatic atlantoaxial instability [68]. Similarly, Roy and colleagues [73] studied 137 patients with Down syndrome and concluded that there was a 10.2% incidence of radiographic atlantoaxial instability, defined as an ADI greater than or equal to 3 mm on a lateral cervical spine radiograph in flexion. In the series of Elliott and colleagues [75], radiographic atlantoaxial instability, defined as an ADI greater than 4 mm on lateral radiographs, was present in 7 of 67 children with Down syndrome, none of whom were found to have clinical signs or symptoms of spinal cord compression. Finally, Ferguson and colleagues [76] found no difference in the incidence of neurologic compromise among patients with Down syndrome who had a normal ADI compared with those whose ADI ranged from 4 to 10 mm, leading some to conclude that traditional standards derived from radiographs of the general population may not be applicable to patients with Down syndrome [70].

In addition to atlantoaxial instability, instability at the occiput-to-C1 joint is also commonly present in children with Down syndrome. The occipitoatlantal joint is composed of the occipital condyles that are normally seated within the cup-shaped C1 articulation, supported by the capsular ligaments, tectorial membrane, and anterior and posterior atlantooccipital membranes [67]. Morphometric analyses of the occipital-to-C1 junction shape in children with Down syndrome and occipitocervical instability versus age-matched controls have demonstrated that the normal cup shape of the superior articular surface of C1 is flattened in the Down syndrome cohort [77]. This "rocker-bottom"-shaped joint cannot effectively prevent anterior or lateral subluxation, thus predisposing to instability [77]. In studies of patients with Down syndrome and symptomatic cranioverbal abnormalities, 40% to 50% of patients have been found to have occipitocervical instability; surgical treatment is recommended in any patient with greater than 8 to 10 mm of subluxation at the occiput-to-C1 level [66,67,77].

Patients with Down syndrome who have radiographic occipitocervical or atlantoaxial instability along with bony abnormalities at the craniovertebral junction, such as os odontoideum, odontoid hypoplasia, or abnormal ossification of the C1 arch, represent a subset of patients who are at increased risk for developing neurologic symptoms. Nader-Sepahi and colleagues [71] propose that ligamentous laxity results in hypermobility of the occiput-to-C1 and C1-to-C2 joints; this hypermobility, in turn, creates repetitive microtrauma and abnormal shearing forces that interfere with the normal ossification of C1 and C2. Repetitive minor trauma in the setting of an os odontoideum can lead to fractures of the odontoid, and segments of the apical portion of the dens may migrate upward under the pull of the alar and apical ligaments [66,71]. The transverse ligament, which normally maintains the position of the odontoid relative to the anterior arch of C1, becomes incompetent, and an irreducible subluxation may result [71]. In a study of pediatric patients with Down syndrome and symptomatic atlantoaxial instability, more than 80% of the children had an os odontoideum and 25% of the patients had ossification abnormalities of the C1 arch [71]. Braakhekke and colleagues [78] reviewed 20 patients with Down syndrome and myelopathy secondary to atlantoaxial instability and found that 9 patients had an odontoid abnormality consisting of odontoid hypoplasia or os odontoideum. In a prospective analysis by Menezes and Ryken [66] of 18 individuals with Down syndrome and symptomatic cervicomedullary compromise, 4 of 18 patients had an odontoid abnormality. In the study by Pueschel and Scolas [68] of 404 children with Down syndrome screened with lateral cervical spine radiographs, 21 patients were found to have osseous abnormalities of C1 or C2, which was likely an underestimation of the prevalence of osseous abnormalities, given the limited imaging modalities available. Vigilance must be maintained in managing children with Down syndrome and atlantoaxial instability with underlying craniovertebral junction osseous abnormalities, because they are at higher risk for spinal cord damage and neurologic deterioration.

The natural history of upper cervical spine instability in patients with Down syndrome has been widely debated. Conflicting reports exist on the progression of atlantoaxial instability. Burke and colleagues [79] studied 32 institutionalized patients with Down syndrome and found that the number of patients with radiographic atlantoaxial instability increased from 1 patient to 7 patients over a 13-year period. Six of the 7 patients found to demonstrate atlantoaxial instability had no neurologic symptoms; moreover, the single patient who demonstrated atlantoaxial instability initially had a normal radiographic examination 13 years later [79]. More recent studies have refuted the notion that atlantoaxial instability is a chronic and progressive condition in patients with Down syndrome. Pueschel and Scola [68] followed a population of 95 patients with Down syndrome for 3 to 6 years with lateral cervical spine radiographic examinations. They found that 7 of the 95 patients had progression of the ADI from less than 5 mm on the first radiograph to 5 mm or greater on the last radiograph; however, none of those 7 patients had any decline in their neurologic function [68]. Moreover, 19 of the 95 patients had an ADI of greater than or equal to 5 mm on initial examination but then were found to have an ADI of less than 5 mm on their most recent radiograph [68]. In a separate study of 141 patients with Down syndrome with serial follow-up imaging, Pueschel and colleagues [80] found that 92% of patients had minor changes of less than or equal to 1.5 mm in the ADI over time. Of the 8% of patients who had changes of the ADI between 2 and 4 mm over time, none had any neurologic symptoms [80]. In a longitudinal follow-up study of 90 children with Down syndrome, Morton and colleagues [81] found an overall reduction in the ADI and no new cases of radiographic atlantoaxial instability diagnosed at 5 years of follow-up. Thus, the correlation between the ADI and the risk of neurologic decline is tenuous. It has been noted that in children with Down syndrome and increased ADIs without any bony anomalies of the craniovertebral junction, the subluxation does not typically progress with time [67]. Such children should thus be managed conservatively with serial surveillance imaging.

Although it is difficult to predict who among those with radiographic instability are likely to go on to develop symptomatic atlantoaxial dislocation, there is no doubt that this does occasionally occur. Some studies have suggested that patients with an ADI of greater than or equal to 7 mm are at greater risk of developing symptomatic instability [80,82,83]. In the group of 9 patients with symptomatic C1-to-C2 dislocation reported on by Menezes and Rykens [66], the average predental space was 9 mm. Seven of the 12 patients in the cohort of children with Down syndrome and symptomatic atlantoaxial instability reported on by Nader-Sepahi and colleagues [71] had antecedent neck pain, torticollis, or progressive myelopathy, as manifested by gait deterioration, worsening spasticity or weakness, hyperreflexia, or clonus. Similarly, in a review of 31 cases of symptomatic atlantoaxial subluxation, 28 cases were preceded by a minimum of 1 month of neurologic signs and symptoms before serious neurologic compromise and frank dislocation [74]. Thus, a thorough neurologic examination is invaluable and may be more predictive than any radiographic criteria in determining which patients are at highest risk for developing symptomatic dislocation.

General management guidelines based on existing studies can be established for children with Down syndrome with respect to craniovertebral instability [67]. Screening cervical radiographs to assess for atlantoaxial instability should be done initially around the age of 3 years; before that, cartilage is still forming and radiographic interpretation of studies is difficult [80]. If such radiographs are normal, it is appropriate to repeat cervical spine radiographs every 5 years, including at the time of initial participation in the Special Olympics if applicable [68,80]. The activities of those children with normal imaging studies should not be limited. In patients with abnormal screening studies, including an ADI of 4.5 mm or greater or a neural canal width less than 14 mm as seen on cervical radiographs, an MRI scan should be obtained to assess for evidence of spinal cord injury. In such children, if there are findings on MRI, such as T2-weighted cord signal changes, or if neurologic signs and symptoms indicative of spinal cord injury are present, surgical correction is indicated. Operative stabilization is also indicated if an os odontoideum is present, which, by definition, constitutes clinical instability [67]. For asymptomatic patients with abnormal cervical spine radiographs but no clinical signs or symptoms and no MRI findings suggestive of spinal cord injury, close observation with at least yearly neurologic examinations and repeat cervical radiographs is indicated [67]. Such patients should avoid high-risk activities, such as contact sports, gymnastics, diving, high jump, and any other activities that favor neck flexion [68].

For patients with symptomatic atlantoaxial instability, cervical fusion is indicated. This can be accomplished using a variety of posterior fixation techniques. In some cases with persistent irreducible subluxation, a transoral resection of the odontoid may also be required. Reported complications of upper cervical spine stabilization in children with Down syndrome include infection, resorption of bone graft and pseudoarthrosis, incomplete reduction, adjacent segment instability, and new neurologic deficits [71,84–87]. In the past, fusion rates in children with Down syndrome had been reported to be as low as 40%, although this rate is improving with modern techniques [71]. The pseudoarthrosis rate may result from the frequent osseous abnormalities seen in Down syndrome, such as os odontoideum and an incomplete posterior C1 arch as well as the underlying ligamentous laxity [71]. Abnormalities in collagen leading to resorption of bone graft and deficient immunologic responses have also been postulated to play a role in pseudoarthrosis in Down syndrome [71,78]. More recently, posterior fusions using C1-to-C2 transarticular screws have achieved greater success compared with traditional Brooks or Gallie fusion operations. The use of transarticular screws obviates the need for an intact posterior C1 arch, and no instrumentation needs to be placed into the canal, risking injury. Reilly and Choit [88] used C1-to-C2 transarticular screws supplemented with autologous iliac crest autograft in 10 children, including 3 with Down syndrome. The children with Down syndrome were maintained after surgery in a halo, but all achieved good fusion with no loss of reduction and no adjacent segment disease when followed for 2 to 7 years [88]. A report by Gluf and Brockmeyer [89] on a series of 67 children with C1-to-C2 instability requiring fusion included 11 children with Down syndrome, who, in aggregate, had 19 transarticular screws placed, with the mean time to fusion achieved at 7.2 months in the cohort of children with Down syndrome. The authors reported a 100% fusion rate in patients with C1-to-C2 transarticular screws used as part of the fusion construct; moreover, halo immobilization was not required after surgery [71,89]. If the vertebral artery anatomy is not suitable for placement of a transarticular screw on one side, unilateral screw placement must be supplemented by an additional form of fixation, such as a Brooks fusion with posterior wiring [88]. In addition, newer techniques, such as C1 lateral mass screw–to–C2 pars screw constructs, are increasingly used for the treatment of C1-to-C2 instability. Fusion constructs should extend to the occiput when any of the following circumstances are present: atlanto-occipital subluxation or instability, cranial settling or basilar invagination, the need for concomitant transoral resection of an odontoid peg or anterior arch of C1, and an incomplete C1 ring or other congenital anomaly that compromises the structural integrity of the atlas in which only one transarticular screw is feasible [66,71]. With the appropriate fusion constructs, excellent surgical results can be attained in children with Down syndrome who require a high cervical fusion.

References

[1] Ruiz-Garcia M, Tovar-Baudin A, Del Castillo-Ruiz V, et al. Early detection of neurological manifestations in achondroplasia. Childs Nerv Syst 1997; 13(4):208–13.

[2] Bagley CA, Pindrik JA, Bookland MJ, et al. Cervicomedullary decompression for foramen magnum stenosis in achondroplasia. J Neurosurg 2006; 104(Suppl 3):166–72.

[3] Ryken TC, Menezes AH. Cervicomedullary compression in achondroplasia. J Neurosurg 1994;81(1):43–8.

[4] Rimoin DL. Cervicomedullary junction compression in infants with achondroplasia: when to perform neurosurgical decompression. Am J Hum Genet 1995;56(4):824–7.

[5] Frigon VA, Castro FP Jr, Whitecloud TS, et al. Isolated subaxial cervical spine stenosis in achondroplasia. Curr Surg 2000;57(4):354–6.

[6] Keiper GL Jr, Koch B, Crone KR. Achondroplasia and cervicomedullary compression: prospective evaluation and surgical treatment. Pediatr Neurosurg 1999;31(2):78–83.

[7] Yamada Y, Ito H, Otsubo Y, et al. Surgical management of cervicomedullary compression in achondroplasia. Childs Nerv Syst 1996;12(12):737–41.

[8] Hecht JT, Butler IJ. Neurologic morbidity associated with achondroplasia. J Child Neurol 1990; 5(2):84–97.

[9] Hecht JT, Butler IJ, Scott CI Jr. Long-term neurological sequelae in achondroplasia. Eur J Pediatr 1984;143(1):58–60.

[10] Wang H, Rosenbaum AE, Reid CS, et al. Pediatric patients with achondroplasia: CT evaluation of the craniocervical junction. Radiology 1987;164(2): 515–9.

[11] Kao SC, Waziri MH, Smith WL, et al. MR imaging of the craniovertebral junction, cranium, and brain in children with achondroplasia. AJR Am J Roentgenol 1989;153(3):565–9.

[12] Hecht JT, Francomano CA, Horton WA, et al. Mortality in achondroplasia. Am J Hum Genet 1987; 41(3):454–64.

[13] Pauli RM, Scott CI, Wassman ER, et al. Apnea and sudden unexpected death in infants with achondroplasia. J Pediatr 1984;104(3):342–8.

[14] Pauli RM, Horton VK, Glinski LP, et al. Prospective assessment of risks for cervicomedullary-junction compression in infants with achondroplasia. Am J Hum Genet 1995;56(3):732–44.

[15] Morgan DF, Young RF. Spinal neurological complications of achondroplasia: results of surgical treatment. J Neurosurg 1980;52(4):463–72.

[16] Aryanpur J, Hurko O, Francomano C, et al. Craniocervical decompression for cervicomedullary compression in pediatric patients with achondroplasia. J Neurosurg 1990;73(3):375–82.

[17] Reid CS, Pyeritz RE, Kopits SE, et al. Cervicomedullary compression in young patients with achondroplasia: value of comprehensive neurologic and respiratory evaluation. J Pediatr 1987;110(4):522–30.

[18] Stokes DC, Phillips JA, Leonard CO, et al. Respiratory complications of achondroplasia. J Pediatr 1983;102(4):532–41.

[19] Fortuna A, Ferrante L, Acqui M, et al. Narrowing of thoraco-lumbar spinal canal in achondroplasia. J Neurosurg Sci 1989;33(2):185–96.

[20] Sensenbrenner JA. Achondroplasia with hypoplastic vertebral bodies secondary to surgical fusion. Birth Defects Orig Artic Ser 1974;10(12):356–7.

[21] Tolo VT. Surgical treatment of kyphosis in achondroplasia. In: Nicoletti B, Kopits SE, Ascani E, et al, editors. Human achondroplasia: a multidisciplinary approach. New York: Plenum Press; 1988. p. 257–9.

[22] Healey D, Letts M, Jarvis JG. Cervical spine instability in children with Goldenhar's syndrome. Can J Surg 2002;45(5):341–4.

[23] Gibson JN, Sillence DO, Taylor TK. Abnormalities of the spine in Goldenhar's syndrome. J Pediatr Orthop 1996;16(3):344–9.

[24] Tsirikos AI, McMaster MJ. Goldenhar-associated conditions (hemifacial microsomia) and congenital deformities of the spine. Spine 2006;31(13): E400–7.

[25] Bethem D, Winter RB, Lutter L, et al. Spinal disorders of dwarfism. Review of the literature and report of eighty cases. J Bone Joint Surg Am 1981;63(9): 1412–25.

[26] Wynne-Davies R, Hall C. Two clinical variants of spondylo-epiphysial dysplasia congenita. J Bone Joint Surg Br 1982;64(4):435–41.

[27] Anderson IJ, Goldberg RB, Marion RW, et al. Spondyloepiphyseal dysplasia congenita: genetic linkage to type II collagen (COL2A1). Am J Hum Genet 1990;46(5):896–901.

[28] Miyoshi K, Nakamura K, Haga N, et al. Surgical treatment for atlantoaxial subluxation with myelopathy in spondyloepiphyseal dysplasia congenita. Spine 2004;29(21):E488–91.

[29] Nakamura K, Miyoshi K, Haga N, et al. Risk factors of myelopathy at the atlantoaxial level in

spondyloepiphyseal dysplasia congenita. Arch Orthop Trauma Surg 1998;117(8):468–70.

[30] Northover H, Cowie RA, Wraith JE. Mucopolysaccharidosis type IVA (Morquio syndrome): a clinical review. J Inherit Metab Dis 1996;19(3):357–65.

[31] Stevens JM, Kendall BE, Crockard HA, et al. The odontoid process in Morquio-Brailsford's disease. The effects of occipitocervical fusion. J Bone Joint Surg Br 1991;73(5):851–8.

[32] Takeda E, Hashimoto T, Tayama M, et al. Diagnosis of atlantoaxial subluxation in Morquio's syndrome and spondyloepiphyseal dysplasia congenita. Acta Paediatr Jpn 1991;33(5):633–8.

[33] Cnossen MH, de Goede-Bolder A, van den Broek KM, et al. A prospective 10 year follow up study of patients with neurofibromatosis type 1. Arch Dis Child 1998;78(5):408–12.

[34] Al-Otibi M, Rutka JT. Neurosurgical implications of neurofibromatosis Type I in children. Neurosurg Focus 2006;20(1):E2.

[35] Crawford AH. Neurofibromatosis in children. Acta Orthop Scand Suppl 1986;57(218):1–60.

[36] Winter RB, Moe JH, Bradford DS, et al. Spine deformity in neurofibromatosis. A review of one hundred and two patients. J Bone Joint Surg Am 1979; 61(5):677–94.

[37] Breig A. Biomechanics of the central nervous system; some basic normal and pathologic phenomena. Chicago: Year Book Publishers; 1960.

[38] Curtis BH, Fisher RL, Butterfield WL, et al. Neurofibromatosis with paraplegia: report of eight cases. J Bone Joint Surg Am 1969;51(5):843–61.

[39] Rockower S, McKay D, Nason S. Dislocation of the spine in neurofibromatosis. A report of two cases. J Bone Joint Surg Am 1982;64(8):1240–2.

[40] Khong PL, Goh WH, Wong VC, et al. MR imaging of spinal tumors in children with neurofibromatosis I. AJR Am J Roentgenol 2003;180(2): 413–7.

[41] Thakkar SD, Feigen U, Mautner VF. Spinal tumours in neurofibromatosis type 1: an MRI study of frequency, multiplicity and variety. Neuroradiology 1999;41(9):625–9.

[42] Lee M, Rezai AR, Freed D, et al. Intramedullary spinal cord tumors in neurofibromatosis. Neurosurgery 1996;38(1):32–7.

[43] Isu T, Miyasaka K, Abe H, et al. Atlantoaxial dislocation associated with neurofibromatosis. Report of three cases. J Neurosurg 1983;58(3):451–3.

[44] Pollack IF, Colak A, Fitz C, et al. Surgical management of spinal cord compression from plexiform neurofibromas in patients with neurofibromatosis 1. Neurosurgery 1998;43(2):248–55.

[45] Engelbert RH, Gerver WJ, Breslau-Siderius LJ, et al. Spinal complications in osteogenesis imperfecta: 47 patients 1-16 years of age. Acta Orthop Scand 1998;69(3):283–6.

[46] Rauch F, Glorieux FH. Osteogenesis imperfecta. Lancet 2004;363(9418):1377–85.

[47] Janus GJ, Engelbert RH, Beek E, et al. Osteogenesis imperfecta in childhood: MR imaging of basilar impression. Eur J Radiol 2003;47(1):19–24.

[48] Land C, Rauch F, Munns CF, et al. Vertebral morphometry in children and adolescents with osteogenesis imperfecta: effect of intravenous pamidronate treatment. Bone 2006;39(4):901–6.

[49] Benson DR, Donaldson DH, Millar EA. The spine in osteogenesis imperfecta. J Bone Joint Surg Am 1978;60(7):925–9.

[50] Widmann RF, Bitan FD, Laplaza FJ, et al. Spinal deformity, pulmonary compromise, and quality of life in osteogenesis imperfecta. Spine 1999;24(16): 1673–8.

[51] Hanscom DA, Winter RB, Lutter L, et al. Osteogenesis imperfecta. Radiographic classification, natural history, and treatment of spinal deformities. J Bone Joint Surg Am 1992;74(4):598–616.

[52] Ishikawa S, Niigata-Shi S, Kumar J, et al. Vertebral body shape as a predictor of spinal deformity in osteogenesis imperfecta. J Bone Joint Surg Am 1996;78(2):212–9.

[53] Larsen LJ, Schottstaedt ER, Bost FC. Multiple congenital dislocations associated with characteristic facial abnormality. J Pediatr 1950;37(4):574–81.

[54] Laville JM, Lakermance P, Limouzy F. Larsen's syndrome: review of the literature and analysis of thirty-eight cases. J Pediatr Orthop 1994;14(1):63–73.

[55] Micheli LJ, Hall JE, Watts HG. Spinal instability in Larsen's syndrome: report of three cases. J Bone Joint Surg Am 1976;58(4):562–5.

[56] Weisenbach J, Melegh B. Vertebral anomalies in Larsen's syndrome. Pediatr Radiol 1996;26(9): 682–3.

[57] Bowen JR, Ortega K, Ray S, et al. Spinal deformities in Larsen's syndrome. Clin Orthop Relat Res 1985; (197):159–63.

[58] Banks JT, Wells JC, Tubbs RS, et al. Cervical spine involvement in Larsen's syndrome: a case illustration. Pediatrics 2003;111(1):199–201.

[59] Forese LL, Berdon WE, Harcke HT, et al. Severe mid-cervical kyphosis with cord compression in Larsen's syndrome and diastrophic dysplasia: unrelated syndromes with similar radiologic findings and neurosurgical implications. Pediatr Radiol 1995;25(2):136–9.

[60] Katz DA, Hall JE, Emans JB. Cervical kyphosis associated with anteroposterior dissociation and quadriparesis in Larsen's syndrome. J Pediatr Orthop 2005;25(4):429–33.

[61] Luk KD, Yip DK. Congenital anteroposterior spinal dissociation in Larsen's syndrome: report on two operated cases with long-term follow-up. Spine 2002;27(12):E296–300.

[62] Johnston CE, Birch JG, Daniels JL. Cervical kyphosis in patients who have Larsen syndrome. J Bone Joint Surg Am 1996;78(4):538–45.

[63] Francis WR, Noble DP. Treatment of cervical kyphosis in children. Spine 1988;13(8):883–7.

[64] Special Olympics bulletin. Participation by individuals with Down syndrome who suffer from atlantoaxial dislocation condition. Washington (DC): Special Olympics; 1983.

[65] American Academy of Pediatrics Committee on Sports Medicine and Fitness. Atlantoaxial instability in Down syndrome. Pediatrics 1984;74(1): 152–4.

[66] Menezes AH, Ryken TC. Craniovertebral abnormalities in Down's syndrome. Pediatr Neurosurg 1992;18(1):24–33.

[67] Brockmeyer D. Down syndrome and craniovertebral instability: topic review and treatment recommendations. Pediatr Neurosurg 1999;31(2):71–7.

[68] Pueschel SM, Scola FH. Atlantoaxial instability in individuals with Down syndrome: epidemiologic, radiographic, and clinical studies. Pediatrics 1987; 80(4):555–60.

[69] Martel W, Tishler JM. Observations on the spine in mongolism. Am J Roentgenol Radium Ther Nucl Med 1966;97(3):630–8.

[70] Pizzutillo PD, Herman MJ. Cervical spine issues in Down syndrome. J Pediatr Orthop 2005;25(2):253–9.

[71] Nader-Sepahi A, Casey AT, Hayward R, et al. Symptomatic atlantoaxial instability in Down syndrome. J Neurosurg 2005;103(Suppl 3):231–7.

[72] Powers B, Miller MD, Kramer RS, et al. Traumatic anterior atlanto-occipital dislocation. Neurosurgery 1979;4(1):12–7.

[73] Roy M, Baxter M, Roy A. Atlantoaxial instability in Down syndrome—guidelines for screening and detection. J R Soc Med 1990;83(7):433–5.

[74] Davidson RG. Atlantoaxial instability in individuals with Down syndrome: a fresh look at the evidence. Pediatrics 1988;81(6):857–65.

[75] Elliott S, Morton RE, Whitelaw RA. Atlantoaxial instability and abnormalities of the odontoid in Down's syndrome. Arch Dis Child 1988;63(12): 1484–9.

[76] Ferguson RL, Putney ME, Allen BL Jr. Comparison of neurologic deficits with atlanto-dens intervals in patients with Down syndrome. J Spinal Disord 1997;10(3):246–52.

[77] Browd S, Healy LJ, Dobie G, et al. Morphometric and qualitative analysis of congenital occipitocervical instability in children: implications for patients with Down syndrome. J Neurosurg 2006;105(Suppl 1): 50–4.

[78] Braakhekke JP, Gabreels FJ, Renier WO, et al. Cranio-vertebral pathology in Down syndrome. Clin Neurol Neurosurg 1985;87(3):173–9.

[79] Burke SW, French HG, Roberts JM, et al. Chronic atlanto-axial instability in Down syndrome. J Bone Joint Surg Am 1985;67(9):1356–60.

[80] Pueschel SM, Scola FH, Pezzullo JC. A longitudinal study of atlanto-dens relationships in asymptomatic individuals with Down syndrome. Pediatrics 1992; 89(6 Pt 2):1194–8.

[81] Morton RE, Khan MA, Murray-Leslie C, et al. Atlantoaxial instability in Down syndrome: a five year follow up study. Arch Dis Child 1995;72(2): 115–8.

[82] Pueschel SM, Herndon JH, Gelch MM, et al. Symptomatic atlantoaxial subluxation in persons with Down syndrome. J Pediatr Orthop 1984;4(6):682–8.

[83] Pueschel SM, Findley TW, Furia J, et al. Atlantoaxial instability in persons with Down syndrome: roentgenographic, neurologic, and somatosensory evoked potential studies. J Pediatr 1987;110(4): 515–21.

[84] Doyle JS, Lauerman WC, Wood KB, et al. Complications and long-term outcome of upper cervical spine arthrodesis in patients with Down syndrome. Spine 1996;21(10):1223–31.

[85] Segal LS, Drummond DS, Zanotti RM, et al. Complications of posterior arthrodesis of the cervical spine in patients who have Down syndrome. J Bone Joint Surg Am 1991;73(10):1547–54.

[86] Smith MD, Phillips WA, Hensinger RN. Fusion of the upper cervical spine in children and adolescents: an analysis of 17 patients. Spine 1991;16(7):695–701.

[87] Nordt JC, Stauffer ES. Sequelae of atlantoaxial stabilization in two patients with Down's syndrome. Spine 1981;6(5):437–40.

[88] Reilly CW, Choit RL. Transarticular screws in the management of C1-C2 instability in children. J Pediatr Orthop 2006;26(5):582–8.

[89] Gluf WM, Brockmeyer DL. Atlantoaxial transarticular screw fixation: a review of surgical indications, fusion rate, complications, and lessons learned in 67 pediatric patients. J Neurosurg Spine 2005;2(2): 164–9.

ELSEVIER
SAUNDERS

Neurosurg Clin N Am 18 (2007) 515–529

NEUROSURGERY
CLINICS
OF NORTH AMERICA

Pediatric Scoliosis and Kyphosis

Mauricio A. Campos, MD[a,b], Stuart L. Weinstein, MD[a,*]

[a]Department of Orthopaedics and Rehabilitation, University of Iowa Hospitals and Clinics,
200 Hawkins Drive, JPP, Iowa City, IA 52242, USA
[b]Department of Orthopaedics, Pontificia Universidad Católica de Chile,
Marcoleta 352 interior, Santiago, Chile

Maladies affecting the maturing axial skeleton are multiple and may produce significant deformity of the spine. The etiologies are diverse encompassing congenital anomalies; neuromuscular conditions; developmental disorders; skeletal dysplasia; infectious, traumatic, and surgical sequelae; and, more rarely, neoplastic processes. The spine involvement can also be just one of the aspects of a more global condition that could diffusely affect the skeleton and other systems such as congenital anomalies of the cardiovascular or renal systems or central neural axis [1]. All these pathologic processes intermingle with the dynamics of growth, determining prognosis and adequate treatment in each case.

Normal development and growth of the spine

Somitogenesis takes place between days 20 to 30 after conception. The paraxial mesoderm adjacent to the notochord subdivides into somites (segmentation). As they mature, somites further subdivide into a sclerotome that will form the adult vertebrae and a myotome and a dermatome, the precursors of the axial musculature and part of the dermis, respectively [2]. The process of organogenesis occurs simultaneously to this phase of the development of the spine, which explains the frequent association between congenital defects of the axial skeleton and visceral anomalies [3,4]. The stage of primary ossification follows the process of chondrification of the mesenchymal

vertebral anlagen. Three primary centers of ossification are formed for every vertebra, except C1, C2, and the sacrum. These are located at the vertebral body (centrum) and one in each neural arch. The cartilaginous unions that separate these centers are two neurocentral synchondroses at the base of the pedicles and one posterior synchondrosis between the posterior arches. They ossify in a predictable manner at 3 to 6 and 2 to 4 years, respectively, and must not be confused with congenital defects (ie, spina bifida) [4]. On the other hand, the presence of these unions allows the progressive expansion of the spinal canal as the child grows, reaching its adult size by age 6 to 8 years [3].

Even in congenital cases, it is unusual for a deformity to be clinically evident at birth. These anomalies also may not be apparent on radiographs initially because of the incomplete ossification of the spine in the newborn [3]. Nevertheless, whatever the cause of the deformity, the risk of progression will be directly related to the spinal growth remaining [3,5–7] and the severity of the curve at presentation [8,9]. There are two periods of rapid spinal growth during childhood: between birth and 3 to 4 years and the adolescent growth spurt [10]. Chronological age, menarche in girls, serial height measurements, and Tanner staging are all useful and complementary clinical tools to estimate the remaining growth of the individual patient [6,10–14]. In general, the onset of the adolescent growth spurt occurs at 13 years in boys and 11 years in girls, before and after reaching Tanner stage two [10,12]. Menarche occurs in the declining phase of the growing peak and indicates a low risk of progression for curves under 30° [5,11,12] in idiopathic scoliosis. Skeletal maturity

* Corresponding author.
E-mail address: stuart-weinstein@uiowa.edu
(S.L. Weinstein).

1042-3680/07/$ - see front matter © 2007 Elsevier Inc. All rights reserved.
doi:10.1016/j.nec.2007.04.007

has also been correlated with radiological signs such as the Risser sign; triradiate cartilage closure; humeral head, elbow, and rib head epiphyseal closure; and carpal bone ossification [14–17]. Among them the most widely used is the Risser sign based on the appearance and fusion of the iliac apophysis (Fig. 1). In general, patients up to Risser 2 are considered immature. Furthermore, Lonstein and Carlson correlated this sign with the risk of curve progression in untreated patients with idiopathic scoliosis with curves up to 29°, showing an average risk of progression of 68% in patients who are Risser 0-1 with curves greater than 20° [5,15].

Clinical biomechanics

A well-balanced spine permits minimal energy expenditure during gait by keeping the trunk and the cranium centered over the pelvis. Spinal balance can be assessed clinically and radiographically by tracing a plumb line from the middle of the C7 vertebral body. This line should intersect the sacral midline ±1 cm in the coronal plane and posterior superior corner of S1 ± 2 cm in the sagittal plane [18–20]. Variations in positioning the patient for the radiograph can significantly alter these measurements [21]. There are also age-related changes with adolescents tending to stand in a greater negative balance than adults [22,23].

A delicate equilibrium exists between the alignment of the spine and the pelvis. The association between developmental hip dislocation and hyperlordosis has been long known [24,25]. A linear correlation has been described between the pelvic

incidence (the angle between the perpendicular to the midpoint of the sacral endplate and the axis of the hips) and the lumbar lordosis in healthy and scoliotic patients [26,27]. There is also a suggested relationship in the literature between other conditions affecting the lower extremities and changes of the lumbar spine such as limb length discrepancy [28–30], flexion or adduction-abduction hip contractures (windswept contractures) [31], and shortening of hamstrings [32]. This can be especially significant in neuromuscular patients, whose curves may be associated with pelvic obliquity resulting from spinal-femoral, pelvic-femoral, or spinal-pelvic muscle contractures [31,33,34].

When viewed in the frontal plane, the spine appears straight and symmetric. The sagittal plane reveals four normal curves: posteriorly convex in the thoracic and sacral regions (curves in kyphosis) and anteriorly convex in the cervical and lumbar regions (curves in lordosis). The last set of curves is called secondary as they are acquired once the child is beginning to assume bipedal stance [18]. The normal mature pattern of sagittal alignment is established by age 6 years. Because of the wide range of variation in normal sagittal curves between individuals, average values cannot be used as normatives. Thoracic kyphosis ranges between 20° and 40° from T5 to T12; lumbar lordosis from L1 to L5, 20° to 55° [35]. It's been noted on the other hand, that the average thoracic kyphosis increases with age from 20° in childhood to 40° in adulthood [36]. The apex of the thoracic kyphosis usually falls between T6 and T8 and the apex of the lumbar lordosis between L3 and L4 disc [18].

Patient evaluation

The detection of spinal deformities for some patients begins after birth during routine physical exam. Initial inspection of the newborn may identify early signs of spinal dysraphism such as midline sinuses, hairy patches, or other cutaneous lesions [13]. Truncal asymmetries can be detected within the first few years of life in cases of congenital deformities. Developmental changes marked by a delay in reaching milestones or abnormal gait may reflect early signs of neuromuscular diseases later associated with spinal deformity. Children with known congenital or acquired diseases associated with higher incidence of spinal deformities (ie, myelodysplasia) should be reviewed periodically with radiographs for early detection of spinal deformity. Other means of

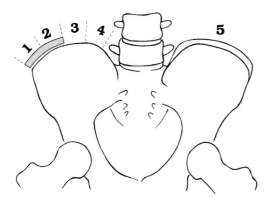

Fig. 1. The Risser Stage of iliac ossification. (*From* McCarthy RE. Evaluation of the patient with deformity. In: Weinstein SL, editor. The pediatric spine: principles and practice. Vol. 1. Philadelphia: Lippincot-Raven; 2001. p. 153; with permission.)

detection are school screening programs performed for the 10- to 12-year-old age group, based primarily on the observation of a significant paravertebral rotational deformity on the Adams forward bending test. However, the value of the screening programs has been questioned based on their cost-effectiveness, overreferral, low prevalence of curves that require active treatment, and little impact of nonoperative treatment on the natural history of the disease [37–39].

The spine surgeon must be aware that for many children the spinal deformity may be only a manifestation of a syndrome that has to be considered for planning an appropriate treatment. Abnormal perinatal history, affected family members, gait abnormalities, learning or hearing difficulties, visual problems, heart murmurs, extremity disorders, genitourinary problems, and certainly neurologic disorders can be parts of the puzzle to establish a diagnosis. General questions regarding general operations or illnesses can reveal disorders in other organ systems. Regarding the deformity itself, how it was detected, the age of presentation, previous treatments and compliance, and the apparent progression of the deformity are all important questions to estimate the future course of a disorder. Significant pain associated with the curve, as well as constitutional symptoms, should raise the suspicion of a destructive spinal lesion such as a tumor or infection [13,15]. The initial assessment of maturity can be performed with questions related to the onset of menarche in girls or the appearance of axillary or facial hair in boys, both facts that occur during the slowdown phase of velocity of growth. An important question is to understand how the curvature is affecting the child's life and development and what are the expectations that the patient and the patient's parents have regarding the results of treatment. What is the patient's normal functional capacity? Is the patient wheelchair bound? Does the patient use walking aids? Has the patient lost sitting abilities or hand use? Has there been any change in respiratory function or increased frequency of infections? All of these are important questions to consider in the evaluation of the functional impact of the deformity, especially in syndromic and neuromuscular patients.

The physical exam should begin with the observation of the patient's ability to walk while entering the room and his interaction with the caregivers and examiner. Body habitus must be noted. An extremely tall and thin patient could be part of the phenotype of Marfan syndrome [40–42]. Obesity in patients may hinder the detection of a curve or constitute also a trait of a genetic disorder (ie, Prader-Willi syndrome) [43]. Cutaneous inspection can reveal areas of skin breakdown related to the deformity or pelvic obliquity in neuromuscular patients. More than five café-au-lait spots may be observed in patients with neurofibromatosis [44]. Examination of the chest and rib cage and axillary and pubic areas can reveal chest wall deformities and also aid in Tanner staging. In patients with neuromuscular scoliosis and joint contractures, range of motion of each joint and, importantly, the hips should be performed.

The examination of the spine itself begins with the detection of asymmetries of the trunk including the shoulder level, a prominent scapula, or uneven waistline. In the standing position the head should be centered over the sacrum or the thorax over the pelvis in the sitting position for nonambulatory patients. Scoliosis secondary to limb-length discrepancy can be corrected with blocks placed underneath the shorter limb or examining the spine with the patient seated. The Adams forward bending test is accomplished by having the patient flex forward until the spine becomes parallel to the horizontal plane. Then the examiner searches for paravertebral deformity inspecting the patient from both the head and the bottom end. The patient should also be inspected from the side to assess the sagittal contour of the spine both standing and forward flexed. The flexibility of the curves can be also evaluated asking the patient to side-bend while he is in the forward bend position, observing if there's a change in the paravertebral deformity.

The most important part of the patient evaluation is the neurological exam. This may begin with watching the patient's gait and toe-and-heel walking. A complete neurological exam should be performed for the upper extremities when indicated, and full examination of the lower extremities including reflex testing, long tract signs, sensory testing, and motor testing must always be done. A thorough exam also includes abdominal cutaneous reflexes and gag reflex. Subtle findings may be present as cavus feet or asymmetric muscle trophism as a reflection of an underlying neurologic abnormality.

Radiographic evaluation

Initial radiographic evaluation is performed with posteroanterior and lateral full spine radiographs in a 36-inch film. This must be done in the patient's functional position: standing for ambulatory and sitting for wheelchair patients. For infants, supine films can be obtained. Any discrepancy in leg length should be corrected with a block placed under the patient's shorter leg when radiographs are taken [37]. The pattern of curvatures present must be noted; segmentation and congenital anomalies must be identified. The curve severity can be measured using the Cobb method [45]. For any given curve being measured, the most tilted vertebrae above and below the curve apex must be chosen. The angle between intersecting lines drawn perpendicular to the top of the top vertebrae and the bottom of the bottom vertebrae is the Cobb angle. Skeletal maturity should be estimated using the Risser sign [46] and observing other radiographical signs of bone maturity such as the closure of the triradiate cartilage [10]. Supine bending films or traction films should be obtained to determine curve flexibility in case surgery is considered [47–49]. Computed tomography can be used to better understand the anatomy of congenital defects of the spine [50,51]. In cases of syndromes associated with central nervous system (CNS) anomalies (ie, congenital scoliosis or myelomeningocele) or in patients with an abnormal neurological exam, an MRI should be done [1,7,15,37,50,52,53].

Scoliosis

Scoliosis is defined as a lateral curvature of the spine greater than 10° as measured by the Cobb method on a standing radiograph [9,54]. Scoliosis can be structural or nonstructural. A structural scoliosis is a fixed lateral curvature with rotation [55], whereas a nonstructural curve corrects in side-bending films and is reversible if the cause is addressed (ie, scoliosis secondary to radiculopathy). Structural scoliosis can be caused by various conditions. However, in most cases no cause is identified. These cases are termed idiopathic scoliosis.

Traditionally, idiopathic scoliosis has been categorized based on the age when the deformity was detected: infantile (younger than 3 years old), juvenile (between 3 and 9 years old), and adolescent (older than 10 years old) [55–57]. Because the cause of idiopathic scoliosis is unknown, the diagnosis should not be made until all other causes have been excluded [6,7,13,15,53,55].

Infantile and juvenile idiopathic scoliosis

Progressive curves occurring before age 5 years may produce significant thoracic deformities and life-threatening effects on the cardiopulmonary system [55,56]. This age range correlates with the postnatal phase of pulmonary development that could be hampered by the thoracic deformity, leading to restrictive pulmonary disease, pulmonary artery hypertension and cor pulmonale. Infantile scoliosis accounts for less than 1% of patients with idiopathic scoliosis in the United States [58]. It is more common in males producing curves with left convexities located in the thoracic or thoracolumbar regions. There are often associated anomalies such as plagiocephaly, bat ear deformity, congenital muscular torticollis, and hip dysplasia. In contrast with late-onset forms, a large number of patients have a spontaneous resolution of the curve ranging from 52% to 92% of the cases [59–61]. In most cases the curves are detected before the first year of life and usually they don't develop a compensatory curve. During initial evaluation, efforts should be made to rule out an underlying pathology and a neurogenic cause through a careful neurologic examination.

Radiographs are useful to detect congenital vertebral anomalies and to measure the curve severity. The incidence of occult central nervous system abnormalities in these patients is high even for those with a normal neurological exam. In a recent retrospective study of 46 patients with infantile idiopathic curves greater than 20° and normal neurological exam, 21.7% of CNS anomalies were found on MRI, 80% of them requiring neurosurgical intervention [62]. Based on these findings the authors recommended a total spine MRI for patients presenting with infantile curves measuring greater than 20°.

To differentiate between progressive and nonprogressive curves, measuring the rib-vertebral angle difference (RVAD) [59,63,64] has proven to be helpful for prognosis purposes (Fig. 2), although not replacing a 4- to 6-month clinical and radiographic follow-up [55]. The RVAD can be measured by tracing a perpendicular line to the endplates of the apical vertebra of the curve. Then a line parallel to the apical ribs is drawn. The difference between the two angles hence formed is the RVAD. An RVAD greater than 20° indicates a high likelihood of progression. Also, when one of the ribs overlaps the apical vertebra (phase 2 according to Mehta) the progression is certain and there is no need to obtain the RVAD. If curve progression is encountered, treatment should be instituted consisting of serial casting, bracing, or surgery if the conservative approaches fail [65].

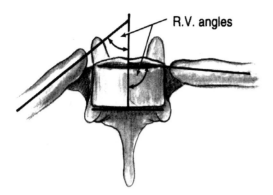

Fig. 2. Rib vertebral angle difference (RVAD) can be calculated by subtracting the convex value from the concave value at the apical vertebra. (*From* Warner WC. Juvenile idiopathic scoliosis. In: Weinstein SL, editor. The pediatric spine: principles and practice. Vol. 1. Philadelphia: Lippincot-Raven; 2001. p. 333; with permission.)

In contrast to infantile and adolescent idiopathic scoliosis, little is known about the curve patterns and natural history of juvenile scoliosis. This group accounts for 12% to 21% of the patients with idiopathic scoliosis in the United States [66]. As grouping of patients in this category is based mainly on arbitrary age cutoffs, they may consist actually of a mixed group of patients with late-onset infantile or early-onset adolescent idiopathic cases [55]. The reported overall female-to-male ratio ranges from 2:1 to 4:1 [55,67]. According to the study by Gupta and colleagues [68] the incidence of neural axis abnormalities in otherwise asymptomatic children in this group is 18% to 20%. They recommended an MRI to be performed at presentation. The predominant curve pattern may depend on the age analyzed, tending to be similar to infantile curves in younger patients, and to adolescent curves in older children. Robinson and McMaster [69] studied the curve patterns and prognosis of 109 patients with juvenile idiopathic scoliosis. Ninety-five percent of the cases showed progression despite brace treatment. They identified five curve patterns depending on the level of the apex of the main curve and the development of secondary curves. Thoracic curves with or without secondary lumbar curves were likely to progress. Lumbar and thoracolumbar curves were associated with a benign prognosis. This was confirmed by a recent retrospective study by Charles and colleagues [17] on 205 patients with juvenile idiopathic scoliosis, where they found three predictive factors of progression once the patients reached

the adolescent growth spurt: major thoracic curves curve patterns, Cobb angle at onset of puberty greater than 30°, and curve progression velocity greater than 10° per year. In contrast to infantile curves, in general, juvenile cases do not resolve spontaneously.

The surgical treatment for both the infantile and juvenile forms varies depending on the spinal growth remaining. Curve progression and increased rotation may occur with posterior spinal fusion alone if the anterior spinal growth continues and is tethered by the posterior fusion (crankshaft effect). Surgical alternatives for these patients can be divided into nonfusion and fusion techniques. The intent of the former is to achieve correction of the curve while at the same time allowing for spinal growth until definitive fusion is performed (ie, growing rods) [70–72]. Fusions in children younger than 10 years, Risser 0, and an open triradiate cartilage are at higher risk of crankshaft phenomenon, so an anterior fusion in these patients should be strongly considered [55,73].

Adolescent idiopathic scoliosis

The adolescent type (AIS) is by far the most common form of scoliosis seen in practice. Its prevalence and male:female ratio depends on the severity of the curves considered. Considering curves greater than 10° the prevalence is 2% to 3% and equal between boys and girls, whereas for curves greater than 40°, it is 0.1% and 10 times more prevalent in girls [6]. The natural history of this condition can be analyzed from two aspects: the risk of curve progression from diagnosis to skeletal maturity and the long-term effects of the condition in untreated adults [6,12]. In immature patients, factors associated with curve progression are greater curve magnitude at diagnosis and future growth potential, female sex, and thoracic curve pattern [5,6,9,15,46,74]. In an average 40.5-year follow-up of untreated patients, 68% of curves progressed after skeletal maturity [9,74,75]. Curves that reached 30° at maturity were unlikely to progress, in contrast with those that reached 50° to 75° at maturity that progressed steadily 1° per year. In late-onset disease, pulmonary function compromise in untreated patients is rare and is not seen until the curves measure at least 100° [76]. However, a 50° thoracic curve at skeletal maturity was a significant predictor of decreased pulmonary function in a cohort of 117 untreated patients followed for

50 years [77]. In general, it seems that untreated patients have slightly higher rates of back pain than controls in the long term, but this does not appear to cause them excessive disability.

Although extensively studied, the etiology of AIS remains obscure. Several theories exist including genetic factors, hormonal factors, growth abnormalities and biomechanical and neuromuscular theories, as well as different tissue disorders of bone, muscle, and fibrous tissue [6,7,15,53, 78–81]. The most accepted theory is the genetic, but the mode of inheritance is still unknown. Research into the etiology of AIS has been further difficult because many of the factors identified to play a role are secondary to the deformity rather than causative. Most of the authors suggest a multifactorial etiology.

Making the diagnosis of AIS implies ruling out other causes of scoliosis. Standing posteroanterior and lateral radiographs should be obtained to asses curve pattern, rule out congenital anomalies, determine Risser stage, and measure curve magnitude. Any element that deviates from the usual AIS presentation should raise the suspicion of an underlying cause. These elements include significant pain or stiffness associated with the curve, abnormal neurological exam, atypical curve patterns (ie, left thoracic curves), juvenile onset, severe curve despite immaturity, and rapid progression [7,15,37,82–84]. A patient with abnormal neurologic changes and a severe curve despite immaturity at presentation has an 86% chance of an MRI showing a neurogenic cause [83]. On the other hand, it has been shown that a typical AIS patient with a normal neurological exam has only a 3% probability of a positive MRI [85].

Since its introduction, King-Moe classification [47] has been widely used and accepted as the standard classification for AIS. This classification divided the curves into five types based on their number, flexibility, and deviation from the midline (Fig. 3). However, in 1997 Lenke and colleagues [86,87] presented a new classification system trying to address some shortcomings of the King-Moe classification such as not being comprehensive, not considering the 3-dimensional (3D) nature and sagittal plane of the deformity, failures in identifying curves amenable to selective fusion [88], lack of treatment guidance, and poor inter- and intraobserver reliability [89,90]. Lenke's classification consists of three parts (Fig. 4): the first assigns a curve type among six given; the curve type should be combined with a lumbar modifier to asses the deviation of the lumbar curve component from the midsacral line; and the third part addresses the sagittal profile of the curve. Despite its large number of curve possibilities (42 types), this classification has shown good intra- and interobserver reliability in studies with premeasured radiographs [86,87,91,92]. On the other hand, in studies with non-premeasured radiographs, its interobserver reliability has fallen to fair or poor

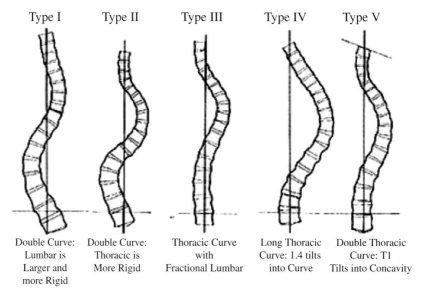

Fig. 3. King-Moe classification. (*From* King HA, Moe JH, Bradford DS, Winter RB. The selection of fusion levels in thoracic idiopathic scoliosis. J Bone Joint Surg Am 1983;65(9):1302–13; with permission.)

Curve Type			
Type	Proximal Thoracic	Main Thoracic	Thoracolumbar / Lumbar	Curve Type
1	Non-Structural	Structural (Major*)	Non-Structural	Main Thoracic (MT)
2	Structural	Structural (Major*)	Non-Structural	Double Thoracic (DT)
3	Non-Structural	Structural (Major*)	Structural	Double Major (DM)
4	Structural	Structural (Major*)	Structural	Triple Major (TM)
5	Non-Structural	Non-Structural	Structural (Major*)	Thoracolumbar / Lumbar (TL/L)
6	Non-Structural	Structural	Structural (Major*)	Thoracolumbar / Lumbar - Main Thoracic (TL/L - MT)

STRUCTURAL CRITERIA
(Minor Curves)

Proximal Thoracic: - Side Bending Cobb ≥ 25°
- T2 - T5 Kyphosis ≥ +20°

Main Thoracic: - Side Bending Cobb ≥ 25°
- T10 - L2 Kyphosis ≥ +20°

Thoracolumbar / Lumbar: - Side Bending Cobb ≥ 25°
- T10 - L2 Kyphosis ≥ +20°

*Major = Largest Cobb Measurement, always structural
Minor = all other curves with structural criteria applied

LOCATION OF APEX
(SRS definition)

CURVE	APEX
THORACIC	T2 - T11-12 DISC
THORACOLUMBAR	T12 - L1
LUMBAR	L1-2 DISC - L4

Modifiers

Lumbar Spine Modifier	CSVL to Lumbar Apex				Thoracic Sagittal Profile T5 - T12	
A	CSVL Between Pedicles				─ (Hypo)	< 10°
B	CSVL Touches Apical Body(ies)	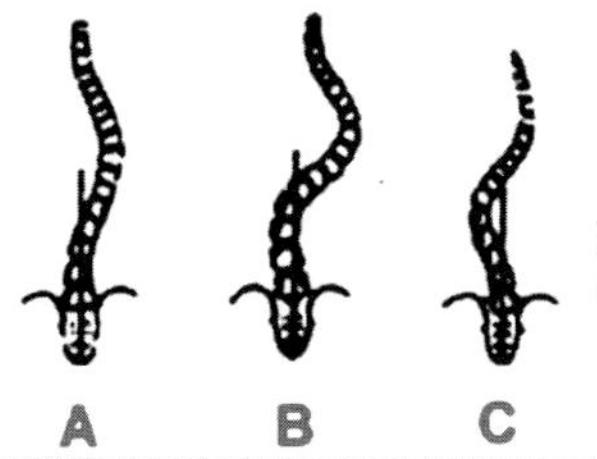 A	B	C	N (Normal)	10° - 40°
C	CSVL Completely Medial				+ (Hyper)	> 40°

Curve Type (1-6) + Lumbar Spine Modifier (A, B, or C) + Thoracic Sagittal Modifier (-, N, or +)
Classification (e.g. 1B+):_____

Fig. 4. Synopsis of Lenke's classification. (*From* Lenke LG, Betz RR, Harms J, et al. Adolescent idiopathic scoliosis: a new classification to determine extent of spinal arthrodesis. J Bone Joint Surg Am 2001;83-A(8):1169–81; with permission.)

[93,94]. One of the aims of this classification is to help in deciding which curves should be included in the fusion. In a retrospective study analyzing 183 idiopathic scoliosis patients surgically treated, Puno and colleagues [95] found that avoiding fusing unnecessary levels and better radiological results could be achieved following Lenke's classification guidelines. On the other hand, in a roundtable type of study, 28 selected surgeons agreed 84% to 90% of the time in classifying seven premeasured operative cases, but showed an average of nine levels of difference between fusion levels proposed and no agreement in the surgical approach [91]. Its utility as an instrument to detect curves amenable to selective fusion is limited as shown by a loose adherence to its guidelines to indicate a selective

fusion (67% to 94%) even among many of its own developers [96]. Additional elements should be taken into account to choose adequate candidates for selective fusion.

Treatment recommendations are observation for immature patients with curves under 25°, bracing for immature patients with curves between 25° and 40°, and surgery for immature patients with 40° curves or mature patients with curves over 50° [5,7,15,37,53]. The most frequently indicated surgery is an instrumented posterior spinal correction and fusion including the structural curves [97]. Some authors advocate an anterior spinal fusion for single thoracic and thoracolumbar/lumbar curves [98–100]. This can also be done via thoracoscopic approach in trained hands [101]. The instrumentation used for these purposes has evolved from nonsegmental systems such as Harrington rods, to current multisegmental systems including hooks and pedicle screws [102,103].

Congenital deformities

Congenital deformities are the result of abnormally formed vertebral elements that lead to an imbalanced spinal growth [104]. This group of malformations occurs during the embryonic period of intrauterine development in the first 6 weeks of life. By this time the mesenchymal anlage establishes a definitive anatomic pattern that will be followed by the cartilaginous and bony stages of the spinal development. Concomitantly, the mesenchymal molds for other organs are being formed, which explains a rate of associated anomalies up to 61% [50]. Among them, the most frequently affected organs are genitourinary (20% to 33%), cardiac (10% to 26%), neural axis (18% to 41%), auditory, and other musculoskeletal anomalies [1,7,50,105,106]. Six percent of the

patients in one study had life-threatening urologic problems and one third required active treatment in another [105,107]. It is thus extremely important that patients receive a complete evaluation for detection of these anomalies.

Congenital scoliosis classification is based on the embryologic development of the spine (Fig. 5). The anomalies are divided into failures of formation (wedged vertebrae or hemivertebrae), failures of segmentation (unsegmented bars or block vertebrae), and mixed anomalies. The resultant deformity depends then on the asymmetry of growth in opposite sides of the spine and its location around the spine (ie, a tethering unsegmented bar would produce kyphosis if it is located anteriorly or lordosis if posterior). Although the behavior of a specific patient's curve pattern is difficult to predict, some generalizations can be made. Most curves are progressive, and 10% to 25% are nonprogressive. Thoracic curves and thoracolumbar curves fare worse with an unsegmented bar with convex hemivertebrae having the poorest prognosis, followed by unsegmented bar alone

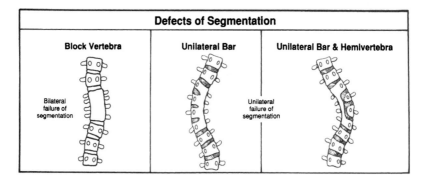

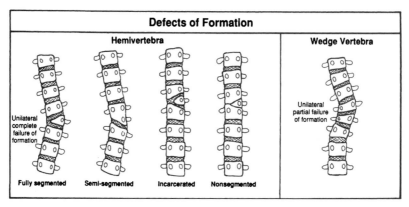

Fig. 5. Classification of congenital scoliosis. (*From* McMaster MJ. Congenital scoliosis. In: Weinstein SL, editor. The pediatric spine: principles and practice. Vol. 1. Philadelphia: Lippincot-Raven; 2001. p. 163; with permission.)

and double- or single-convex hemivertebrae [50, 108,109]. A single hemivertebra may or may not cause a progressive deformity, depending on its growth potential and location (ie, a lumbosacral hemivertebra will produce decompensation). The most likely times of progression match the phases of rapid spinal growth (the first 2 to 3 years of life and during the adolescent growth spurt) [110].

Congenital kyphosis is less common than scoliosis, but it can lead to serious consequences if left untreated, causing paraplegia [111]. It is classified into three types: type I being an anterior failure of formation (posterior hemivertebra), type II an anterior unsegmented bar, and type III being mixed defects. The worst prognosis is for upper thoracic type I defects.

Radiographic evaluation might be difficult in some cases because of incomplete ossification of the vertebral elements or complex patterns of deformity. Plain films should always include a lateral view to rule out the presence of a kyphotic component in the deformity. Interobserver variability up to 12° has been reported in measuring curve severity in these cases because of the difficulty in using the same landmarks for every measurement [50]. An MRI should be done in cases with abnormal neurological exam, findings suggesting spinal dysraphism, and progressive curves that are candidates for surgery [105]. Computed tomography and 3D reconstructions may be helpful to understand complex patterns of malformation.

In general, children with congenital deformities must be followed until the end of growth to prevent progression. Brace treatment has not been shown to be effective in managing the primary curve in congenital scoliosis. Surgery is indicated when there is documented progression or an anomaly is predicted to have a high risk of a poor outcome without treatment [104]. The surgical options are varied and include in situ fusions, convex growth arrest, hemivertebra excision, and correction and fusion with instrumentation with or without osteotomies [1,50]. Neurologic risk in this group of patients may be higher because of the stiffness of the curve elements, especially in kyphotic anomalies under distraction maneuvers.

On the other hand, nonoperative management has no place in the treatment of congenital kyphosis. Surgical alternatives are posterior fusion and casting for curves less than 40° in patients younger than 5 years old as a prophylactic surgery and anterior-posterior fusion with or without instrumentation for larger curves in older patients,

with decompression of the spinal cord in patients with neurological compromise [111].

Neuromuscular scoliosis

This group of deformities is driven by a disruption or alteration in the neural pathway through which the CNS controls and coordinates muscle activity [31,34]. Under this diagnosis are grouped several entities that share principles in the course of disease evaluation and management. All of them share a high rate of scoliosis prevalence ranging from 25% to 100% [31]. In general, the incidence of scoliosis development parallels the severity of the disorder. The Scoliosis Research Society (SRS) classifies neuromuscular scoliosis into neuropathic or myopathic, according to the elements within the myoneural path primarily affected. Both upper and lower motor neuron diseases are included in the first group (ie, cerebral palsy and spinal muscular atrophy, respectively). The second group is formed mainly by muscular dystrophy patients as cases with Duchenne muscular dystrophy.

Although some cases have similar curve patterns to AIS, others present with long C-shaped curves with marked pelvic obliquity. Moreover, in the sagittal plane they often present with either severe kyphosis or lordosis, in contrast to the relatively constant lordoscoliotic pattern in AIS. These curves tend to have an early onset, rapid progression during growth, and continued progression after maturity. In contrast to idiopathic patients, where the spinal curvature is the sole problem, these children often have additional comorbidities, such as mental retardation, seizure disorders, swallowing problems, nutritional deficits, joint contractures and dislocations, osteopenia, or insensate skin areas, emphasizing the necessity of a multidisciplinary approach especially in patients indicated for surgery.

Nonoperative treatment consists mainly of bracing, although it is generally accepted that it doesn't prevent curve progression in neuromuscular cases [112]. Nevertheless, many clinicians indicate bracing as a means to slow the curve progression and postponing the need of surgery in patients who are too young [34]. Usually during the adolescent growth spurt, curve control is lost and surgical stabilization is necessary. Better results of bracing have been reported in nonsevere flexible curves, immature children, and ambulatory patients, where a good correction of the curve has been achieved in the orthosis. Bracing can also be used together with other measures, such as sitting systems and wheelchair adaptations, to improve sitting balance, improve function, and reduce decubiti complications.

The surgical indication for patients with cerebral palsy and most upper and lower motor neuron conditions is a progressive curve greater than 40° to 50° that interferes with sitting balance [113]. In many centers treating patients with Duchenne muscular dystrophy, the surgical indication comes earlier, anticipating the deterioration in pulmonary function that occurs when the patients become wheelchair bound [114]. This usually occurs at approximately age 12 to 13 years, when patients have curves of 20° to 30°. The standard approach for neuromuscular scoliosis is an instrumented posterior spinal fusion from T2 to T3 stopping either in the lumbar spine or including the pelvis depending on the presence of pelvic obliquity and the ambulatory status of the patient. The instrumentation used has evolved from nonsegmental Harrington rods to multisegmental instrumentation currently; most frequently sublaminar wires or hook systems combined with Luque rods or a unit rod, which can distribute the corrective forces at all levels, appropriate for the osteoporotic bone frequently encountered in these cases. The technical goals of the surgery are to achieve a balanced trunk over the pelvis, a solid spinal fusion, and a level pelvis. The methods of pelvic fixation available are the Galveston technique with rods or iliosacral screws, S-contoured rods placed over the sacral ala, and transiliac fixation. In the case of rigid curves, immature patients, or absent posterior elements, an anterior release and fusion should be considered.

Postoperative complications occur more frequently in neuromuscular patients than in idiopathic scoliosis, ranging from 44% to 62% [115]. This difference stems from the multiple system compromise present in these patients and may include increased intraoperative blood loss [116], postoperative pneumonia (especially after combined procedures), surgical wound infection (greater risk for myelodysplastic patients) [117], prevalent urinary tract infections, skin pressure ulcers, and increased pseudoarthrosis rate and perioperative death.

Scheuermann kyphosis

Scheuermann kyphosis is defined as a structural deformity that presents in late childhood associated with thoracic wedged vertebral bodies [106].

Its reported incidence varies from 0.5% to 8% and its male-to-female ratio ranges from 1:2 to 7:1 [36,118–120]. Its etiology remains unknown, but various theories have been postulated. A genetic factor have been suggested, specifically a dominant autosomal inheritance [121]. In a study including 943 Danish twins with Scheuermann kyphosis, a 74% concordance between monozygotic twins was found, leading the authors to conclude a strong genetic influence in the disease [118]. Other causative factors cited are abnormal endochondral ossification, hormonal changes, mechanical factors, growth abnormalities, juvenile osteoporosis, and collagen alteration [122].

The natural history retains some controversial aspects. The disease onset occurs around 10 years. It is generally accepted that most often Scheuermann kyphosis has a benign course. Murray and colleagues [123] reported a study on 67 untreated patients with a mean kyphosis angle of 71°, evaluated at an average of 32 years after diagnosis, compared with an age-matched control group. The study demonstrated that patients with Scheuermann kyphosis had more intense back pain, jobs that tended to have lower physical requirements, weaker trunk extensor muscles, and different location of the pain compared with controls. However, no significant differences were found with controls regarding limitations on their activities secondary to the pain, days absent from work, social limitations, and, moreover, they showed little preoccupation with their physical appearance. Only the patients with thoracic kyphosis greater than 100° had restrictive lung disease. Others have reported that patients with untreated deformities above 75° can have severe pain and can be significantly limited with this condition [124]. Unfortunately, the likelihood of progression of any given curve is not known, although progression has been observed in some reports [36,106]. Neurological findings are rare.

There are two major forms of Scheuermann kyphosis: the more common thoracic type with an apex between T7 and T9, and a thoracolumbar/lumbar form with an apex at T10 to T12, generally presenting a less severe deformity. Usually patients seek medical attention mainly with deformity and cosmetic concerns in the adolescent population and because of pain, the latter occurring more often in adults. The physical exam is important to differentiate a structural hyperkyphosis from a postural roundback, being the second more flexible on extension and having a more rounded shape apex on forward bending rather than a sharply angulated bend of Scheuermann [120]. Hamstring tightness and normal neurological exam are usually found.

Abnormal thoracic kyphosis is more difficult to define than scoliosis, because of its wide normal range and normal age-related increase. The SRS considers a normal kyphosis of 20° to 40° in the growing adolescent. Although the specific radiological diagnostic criteria have varied in the literature, the most accepted are Sorensen's criteria that are increased kyphosis with greater than 5° of wedging in three or more consecutive thoracic vertebral bodies on the radiographs [125]. Other radiological features cited are endplate irregularities, Schmorl's nodes, and disk space narrowing. Hyperextension supine films over a bolster can be used to assess curve's flexibility. In cases of thoracolumbar Scheuermann, only endplate irregularities and disk space narrowing can be found.

Treatment modalities consist of observation, nonoperative treatment with bracing, and surgery. Bracing is regarded as an effective treatment in immature patients with curves between 45° and 60° [119], although the studies on this treatment are few, retrospective, lack control groups, and we currently cannot predict which patients are more likely to progress [36]. Sachs and colleagues [126] reported on the treatment of 120 patients with a Milwaukee brace showing an initial 50% of correction, followed by a 20° loss of correction at the 5-year follow-up. Sixty-nine percent of the compliant patients had a successful treatment, defining success as a 3° decrease in thoracic kyphosis, which is below the intraobserver variance according to one study [127].

Surgical treatment is reserved generally for curves greater than 75° in mature patients, those who progressed despite brace treatment, and in the rare cases with pain unresponsive to nonoperative measures or patients with neurological derangement [36,106,119,120,122,125,127]. Most reports center success rates on deformity correction, whereas pain relief is more or less consistently achieved after surgery in the different series. Initially the standard surgical approach was a posterior spinal fusion using Harrington compression instrumentation, which obtained a very good correction initially, but was followed by loss of correction over time [128,129]. Therefore, an anterior release and fusion, followed by a posterior instrumented spinal fusion was proposed to avoid loss of correction, especially in stiff curves that do not bend out to less than 50° and

adult patients [130,131]. With the advent of new techniques of shortening spinal ostetomies done through the posterior approach and the increased use of segmental pedicle screws in thoracic deformities, the question of the need for an anterior approach is being reformulated [125,132]. However, long-term follow-up studies with these techniques are not available.

References

[1] Lonstein JE. Congenital spine deformities: scoliosis, kyphosis, and lordosis. Orthop Clin North Am 1999;30(3):387–405, viii.

[2] Tracy MR, Dormans JP, Kusumi K. Klippel-Feil syndrome: clinical features and current understanding of etiology. Clin Orthop Relat Res 2004; (424):183–90.

[3] Ganey TM, Ogden JA. Development and maturation of the axial skeleton. In: Weinstein SL, editor. The pediatric spine: principles and practice. 2nd edition. New York: Lippincott Williams & Wilkins; 2001. p. 3–54.

[4] Ogden JA. Skeletal injury in the child. 3rd edition. New York: Springer; 2000.

[5] Lonstein JE, Carlson JM. The prediction of curve progression in untreated idiopathic scoliosis during growth. J Bone Joint Surg Am 1984;66(7):1061–71.

[6] Miller NH. Cause and natural history of adolescent idiopathic scoliosis. Orthop Clin North Am 1999; 30(3):343–52, vii.

[7] Wiggins GC, Shaffrey CI, Abel MF, et al. Pediatric spinal deformities. Neurosurg Focus 2003;14(1):1–14.

[8] Bunnell WP. The natural history of idiopathic scoliosis before skeletal maturity. Spine 1986;11(8): 773–6.

[9] Weinstein SL. Idiopathic scoliosis. Natural history. Spine 1986;11(8):780–3.

[10] Dimeglio A. Growth in pediatric orthopaedics. J Pediatr Orthop 2001;21(4):549–55.

[11] Little DG, Song KM, Katz D, et al. Relationship of peak height velocity to other maturity indicators in idiopathic scoliosis in girls. J Bone Joint Surg Am 2000;82(5):685–93.

[12] Lonstein JE. Scoliosis: surgical versus nonsurgical treatment. Clin Orthop Relat Res 2006;443:248–59.

[13] McCarthy RE. Evaluation of the patient with deformity. In: Weinstein SL, editor. The pediatric spine: principles and practice. 2nd edition. New York: Lippincott Williams & Wilkins; 2001. p. 133–57.

[14] Song KM, Little DG. Peak height velocity as a maturity indicator for males with idiopathic scoliosis. J Pediatr Orthop 2000;20(3):286–8.

[15] Roach JW. Adolescent idiopathic scoliosis. Orthop Clin North Am 1999;30(3):353–65, vii–viii.

[16] Hoppenfeld S, Lonner B, Murthy V, et al. The rib epiphysis and other growth centers as indicators

of the end of spinal growth. Spine 2004;29(1): 47–50.

[17] Charles YP, Daures JP, de Rosa V, et al. Progression risk of idiopathic juvenile scoliosis during pubertal growth. Spine 2006;31(17):1933–42.

[18] Bernhardt M. Normal spinal anatomy: normal sagittal plane alignment. In: Bridwell KH, Dewald RL, editors. The textbook of spinal surgery, vol. 1. 2nd edition. Philadelphia: Lippincott-Raven; 1997. p. 185–91.

[19] McGlashen K, Ashton-Miller JA, Green M, et al. Trunk positioning accuracy in the frontal and sagittal planes. J Orthop Res 1991;9(4):576–83.

[20] Betz RR. Kyphosis of the thoracic and thoracolumbar spine in the pediatric patient: normal sagittal parameters and scope of the problem. Instr Course Lect 2004;53:479–84.

[21] Horton WC, Brown CW, Bridwell KH, et al. Is there an optimal patient stance for obtaining a lateral 36 radiograph? A critical comparison of three techniques. Spine 2005;30(4):427–33.

[22] Schlenk RP, Kowalski RJ, Benzel EC. Biomechanics of spinal deformity. Neurosurg Focus 2003; 14(1):1–15.

[23] Vedantam R, Lenke LG, Keeney JA, et al. Comparison of standing sagittal spinal alignment in asymptomatic adolescents and adults. Spine 1998; 23(2):211–5.

[24] Wedge JH, Wasylenko MJ. The natural history of congenital dislocation of the hip: a critical review. Clin Orthop Relat Res 1978;(137):154–62.

[25] Weinstein SL. Natural history of congenital hip dislocation (CDH) and hip dysplasia. Clin Orthop Relat Res 1987;(225):62–76.

[26] Legaye J, Duval-Beaupere G, Hecquet J, et al. Pelvic incidence: a fundamental pelvic parameter for three-dimensional regulation of spinal sagittal curves. Eur Spine J 1998;7(2):99–103.

[27] Mac-Thiong JM, Labelle H, Berthonnaud E, et al. Sagittal spinopelvic balance in normal children and adolescents. Eur Spine J 2007;16(2):227–34.

[28] Jones KB, Sponseller PD, Hobbs W, et al. Leg-length discrepancy and scoliosis in Marfan syndrome. J Pediatr Orthop 2002;22(6):807–12.

[29] Papaioannou T, Stokes I, Kenwright J. Scoliosis associated with limb-length inequality. J Bone Joint Surg Am 1982;64(1):59–62.

[30] Stanitski DF. Limb-length inequality: assessment and treatment options. J Am Acad Orthop Surg 1999;7(3):143–53.

[31] Lonstein JE. Neuromuscular spinal deformities. In: Weinstein SL, editor. The pediatric spine: principles and practice. 2nd edition. New York: Lippincott Williams & Wilkins; 2001. p. 789–96.

[32] Glard Y, Launay F, Viehweger E, et al. Hip flexion contracture and lumbar spine lordosis in myelomeningocele. J Pediatr Orthop 2005;25(4):476–8.

[33] Shook JE, Lubicky JP. Paralytic scoliosis. In: Bridwell KH, Dewald RL, editors. The textbook

of spinal surgery, vol. 1. 2nd edition. Philadelphia: Lippincott-Raven; 1997. p. 839–80.

[34] McCarthy RE. Management of neuromuscular scoliosis. Orthop Clin North Am 1999;30(3): 435–49, viii.

[35] Pizzutillo PD. Nonsurgical treatment of kyphosis. Instr Course Lect 2004;53:485–91.

[36] Wenger DR, Frick SL. Scheuermann kyphosis. Spine 1999;24(24):2630–9.

[37] Greiner KA. Adolescent idiopathic scoliosis: radiologic decision-making. Am Fam Physician 2002; 65(9):1817–22.

[38] Bunnell WP. Selective screening for scoliosis. Clin Orthop Relat Res 2005;(434):40–5.

[39] Dickson RA, Weinstein SL. Bracing (and screening)—yes or no? J Bone Joint Surg Br 1999;81(2): 193–8.

[40] Di Silvestre M, Greggi T, Giacomini S, et al. Surgical treatment for scoliosis in Marfan syndrome. Spine 2005;30(20):E597–604.

[41] Lipton GE, Guille JT, Kumar SJ. Surgical treatment of scoliosis in Marfan syndrome: guidelines for a successful outcome. J Pediatr Orthop 2002; 22(3):302–7.

[42] Sponseller PD, Bhimani M, Solacoff D, et al. Results of brace treatment of scoliosis in Marfan syndrome. Spine 2000;25(18):2350–4.

[43] Kroonen LT, Herman M, Pizzutillo PD, et al. Prader-Willi Syndrome: clinical concerns for the orthopaedic surgeon. J Pediatr Orthop 2006; 26(5):673–9.

[44] Gutmann DH, Aylsworth A, Carey JC, et al. The diagnostic evaluation and multidisciplinary management of neurofibromatosis 1 and neurofibromatosis 2. JAMA 1997;278(1):51–7.

[45] Moe JH, Bradford DS. Moe's textbook of scoliosis and other spinal deformities. 2nd edition. Philadelphia: Saunders; 1987.

[46] Risser JC, Norquist DM, Cockrell BR Jr, et al. The effect of posterior spine fusion on the growing spine. Clin Orthop Relat Res 1966;46:127–39.

[47] King HA, Moe JH, Bradford DS, et al. The selection of fusion levels in thoracic idiopathic scoliosis. J Bone Joint Surg Am 1983;65(9):1302–13.

[48] Large DF, Doig WG, Dickens DR, et al. Surgical treatment of double major scoliosis. Improvement of the lumbar curve after fusion of the thoracic curve. J Bone Joint Surg Br 1991;73(1):121–4.

[49] McCall RE, Bronson W. Criteria for selective fusion in idiopathic scoliosis using Cotrel-Dubousset instrumentation. J Pediatr Orthop 1992;12(4): 475–9.

[50] Hedequist D, Emans J. Congenital scoliosis. J Am Acad Orthop Surg 2004;12(4):266–75.

[51] Newton PO, Hahn GW, Fricka KB, et al. Utility of three-dimensional and multiplanar reformatted computed tomography for evaluation of pediatric congenital spine abnormalities. Spine 2002;27(8): 844–50.

[52] Sarwark JF. Kyphosis deformity in myelomeningo-cele. Orthop Clin North Am 1999;30(3):451–5, viii–ix.

[53] Reamy BV, Slakey JB. Adolescent idiopathic scoliosis: review and current concepts. Am Fam Physician 2001;64(1):111–6.

[54] Kane WJ. Scoliosis prevalence: a call for a statement of terms. Clin Orthop Relat Res 1977;(126): 43–6.

[55] Dobbs MB, Weinstein SL. Infantile and juvenile scoliosis. Orthop Clin North Am 1999;30(3): 331–41, vii.

[56] James JI. Idiopathic scoliosis; the prognosis, diagnosis, and operative indications related to curve patterns and the age at onset. J Bone Joint Surg Br 1954;36(1):36–49.

[57] Gillingham BL, Fan RA, Akbarnia BA. Early onset idiopathic scoliosis. J Am Acad Orthop Surg 2006;14(2):101–12.

[58] James JI, Lloyd-Roberts GC, Pilcher MF. Infantile structural scoliosis. J Bone Joint Surg Br 1959;41: 719–35.

[59] Ferreira JH, de Janeiro R, James JI. Progressive and resolving infantile idiopathic scoliosis. The differential diagnosis. J Bone Joint Surg Br 1972; 54(4):648–55.

[60] Lloyd-Roberts GC, Pilcher MF. Structural idiopathic scoliosis in infancy: a study of the natural history of 100 patients. J Bone Joint Surg Br 1965;47: 520–3.

[61] Ceballos T, Ferrer-Torrelles M, Castillo F, et al. Prognosis in infantile idiopathic scoliosis. J Bone Joint Surg Am 1980;62(6):863–75.

[62] Dobbs MB, Lenke LG, Szymanski DA, et al. Prevalence of neural axis abnormalities in patients with infantile idiopathic scoliosis. J Bone Joint Surg Am 2002;84(12):2230–4.

[63] Mehta MH. The rib-vertebra angle in the early diagnosis between resolving and progressive infantile scoliosis. J Bone Joint Surg Br 1972;54(2): 230–43.

[64] Thompson SK, Bentley G. Prognosis in infantile idiopathic scoliosis. J Bone Joint Surg Br 1980;62(2): 151–4.

[65] Dickson RA. Early-onset idiopathic scoliosis. In: Weinstein SL, editor. The pediatric spine: principles and practice. 2nd edition. New York: Lippincott Williams & Wilkins; 2001. p. 321–8.

[66] Ponseti IV, Friedman B. Prognosis in idiopathic scoliosis. J Bone Joint Surg Am 1950;32(2):381–95.

[67] Warner WCJ. Juvenile idiopathic scoliosis. In: Weinstein SL, editor. The pediatric spine: principles and practice. 2nd edition. New York: Lippincott Williams & Wilkins; 2001. p. 329–45.

[68] Gupta P, Lenke LG, Bridwell KH. Incidence of neural axis abnormalities in infantile and juvenile patients with spinal deformity. Is a magnetic resonance image screening necessary? Spine 1998; 23(2):206–10.

[69] Robinson CM, McMaster MJ. Juvenile idiopathic scoliosis. Curve patterns and prognosis in one hundred and nine patients. J Bone Joint Surg Am 1996; 78(8):1140–8.

[70] Akbarnia BA, Marks DS, Boachie-Adjei O, et al. Dual growing rod technique for the treatment of progressive early-onset scoliosis: a multicenter study. Spine 2005;30(17 Suppl):S46–57.

[71] Klemme WR, Denis F, Winter RB, et al. Spinal instrumentation without fusion for progressive scoliosis in young children. J Pediatr Orthop 1997; 17(6):734–42.

[72] Moe JH, Kharrat K, Winter RB, et al. Harrington instrumentation without fusion plus external orthotic support for the treatment of difficult curvature problems in young children. Clin Orthop Relat Res 1984;(185):35–45.

[73] Sanders JO, Herring JA, Browne RH. Posterior arthrodesis and instrumentation in the immature (Risser-grade-0) spine in idiopathic scoliosis. J Bone Joint Surg Am 1995;77(1):39–45.

[74] Weinstein SL. Bristol-Myers Squibb/Zimmer award for distinguished achievement in orthopaedic research. Long-term follow-up of pediatric orthopaedic conditions. Natural history and outcomes of treatment. J Bone Joint Surg Am 2000; 82(7):980–90.

[75] Weinstein SL, Ponseti IV. Curve progression in idiopathic scoliosis. J Bone Joint Surg Am 1983; 65(4):447–55.

[76] Weinstein SL, Zavala DC, Ponseti IV. Idiopathic scoliosis: long-term follow-up and prognosis in untreated patients. J Bone Joint Surg Am 1981;63(5): 702–12.

[77] Weinstein SL, Dolan LA, Spratt KF, et al. Health and function of patients with untreated idiopathic scoliosis: a 50-year natural history study. JAMA 2003;289(5):559–67.

[78] Machida M. Cause of idiopathic scoliosis. Spine 1999;24(24):2576–83.

[79] Miller NH. Adolescent idiopathic scoliosis: etiology. In: Weinstein SL, editor. The pediatric spine: principles and practice. 2nd edition. New York: Lippincott Williams & Wilkins; 2001. p. 347–54.

[80] Lowe TG, Edgar M, Margulies JY, et al. Etiology of idiopathic scoliosis: current trends in research. J Bone Joint Surg Am 2000;82(8):1157–68.

[81] Parent S, Newton PO, Wenger DR. Adolescent idiopathic scoliosis: etiology, anatomy, natural history, and bracing. Instr Course Lect 2005;54: 529–36.

[82] Bridwell KH. Adolescent idiopathic scoliosis: surgery. In: Weinstein SL, editor. The pediatric spine: principles and practice. 2nd edition. New York: Lippincott Williams & Wilkins; 2001. p. 385–411.

[83] Morcuende JA, Dolan LA, Vazquez JD, et al. A prognostic model for the presence of neurogenic lesions in atypical idiopathic scoliosis. Spine 2004; 29(1):51–8.

[84] Benli IT, Uzumcugil O, Aydin E, et al. Magnetic resonance imaging abnormalities of neural axis in Lenke type 1 idiopathic scoliosis. Spine 2006; 31(16):1828–33.

[85] Winter RB, Lonstein JE, Heithoff KB, et al. Magnetic resonance imaging evaluation of the adolescent patient with idiopathic scoliosis before spinal instrumentation and fusion. A prospective, double-blinded study of 140 patients. Spine 1997; 22(8):855–8.

[86] Lenke LG, Betz RR, Harms J, et al. Adolescent idiopathic scoliosis: a new classification to determine extent of spinal arthrodesis. J Bone Joint Surg Am 2001;83(8):1169–81.

[87] Lenke LG, Edwards CC 2nd, Bridwell KH. The Lenke classification of adolescent idiopathic scoliosis: how it organizes curve patterns as a template to perform selective fusions of the spine. Spine 2003; 28(20):S199–207.

[88] Lenke LG, Bridwell KH, Baldus C, et al. Preventing decompensation in King type II curves treated with Cotrel-Dubousset instrumentation. Strict guidelines for selective thoracic fusion. Spine 1992;17(8 Suppl):S274–81.

[89] Cummings RJ, Loveless EA, Campbell J, et al. Interobserver reliability and intraobserver reproducibility of the system of King, et al. for the classification of adolescent idiopathic scoliosis. J Bone Joint Surg Am 1998;80(8):1107–11.

[90] Lenke LG, Betz RR, Bridwell KH, et al. Intraobserver and interobserver reliability of the classification of thoracic adolescent idiopathic scoliosis. J Bone Joint Surg Am 1998;80(8):1097–106.

[91] Lenke LG, Betz RR, Haher TR, et al. Multisurgeon assessment of surgical decision-making in adolescent idiopathic scoliosis: curve classification, operative approach, and fusion levels. Spine 2001; 26(21):2347–53.

[92] Ogon M, Giesinger K, Behensky H, et al. Interobserver and intraobserver reliability of Lenke's new scoliosis classification system. Spine 2002;27(8): 858–62.

[93] Niemeyer T, Wolf A, Kluba S, et al. Interobserver and intraobserver agreement of Lenke and King classifications for idiopathic scoliosis and the influence of level of professional training. Spine 2006; 31(18):2103–7 [discussion: 2108].

[94] Richards BS, Sucato DJ, Konigsberg DE, et al. Comparison of reliability between the Lenke and King classification systems for adolescent idiopathic scoliosis using radiographs that were not premeasured. Spine 2003;28(11):1148–56 [discussion: 1156–7].

[95] Puno RM, An KC, Puno RL, et al. Treatment recommendations for idiopathic scoliosis: an assessment of the Lenke classification. Spine 2003; 28(18):2102–14 [discussion 2114–5].

[96] Newton PO, Faro FD, Lenke LG, et al. Factors involved in the decision to perform a selective versus nonselective fusion of Lenke 1B and 1C (King-Moe II) curves in adolescent idiopathic scoliosis. Spine 2003;28(20):S217–23.

[97] Coe JD, Arlet V, Donaldson W, et al. Complications in spinal fusion for adolescent idiopathic scoliosis in the new millennium. A report of the Scoliosis Research Society Morbidity and Mortality Committee. Spine 2006;31(3):345–9.

[98] Betz RR, Harms J, Clements DH 3rd, et al. Comparison of anterior and posterior instrumentation for correction of adolescent thoracic idiopathic scoliosis. Spine 1999;24(3):225–39.

[99] Lowe TG, Betz R, Lenke L, et al. Anterior single-rod instrumentation of the thoracic and lumbar spine: saving levels. Spine 2003;28(20):S208–16.

[100] Betz RR, Shufflebarger H. Anterior versus posterior instrumentation for the correction of thoracic idiopathic scoliosis. Spine 2001;26(9):1095–100.

[101] Newton PO. The use of video-assisted thoracoscopic surgery in the treatment of adolescent idiopathic scoliosis. Instr Course Lect 2005;54: 551–8.

[102] Lenke LG. Debate: resolved, a 55 degrees right thoracic adolescent idiopathic scoliotic curve should be treated by posterior spinal fusion and segmental instrumentation using thoracic pedicle screws: pro: thoracic pedicle screws should be used to treat a 55 degrees right thoracic adolescent idiopathic scoliosis. J Pediatr Orthop 2004;24(3): 329–34 [discussion: 338–8].

[103] Suk SI, Lee CK, Kim WJ, et al. Segmental pedicle screw fixation in the treatment of thoracic idiopathic scoliosis. Spine 1995;20(12):1399–405.

[104] McMaster MJ. Congenital scoliosis. In: Weinstein SL, editor. The pediatric spine: principles and practice. 2nd edition. New York: Lippincott Williams & Wilkins; 2001. p. 161–77.

[105] Basu PS, Elsebaie H, Noordeen MH. Congenital spinal deformity: a comprehensive assessment at presentation. Spine 2002;27(20):2255–9.

[106] Fardon DF. North American spine society. Orthopaedic knowledge update. Spine 2. 2nd edition. Rosemont (IL): American Academy of Orthopaedic Surgeons; 2002.

[107] MacEwen GD, Winter RB, Hardy JH. Evaluation of kidney anomalies in congenital scoliosis. J Bone Joint Surg Am 1972;54(7):1451–4.

[108] McMaster MJ, Ohtsuka K. The natural history of congenital scoliosis. A study of two hundred and fifty-one patients. J Bone Joint Surg Am 1982; 64(8):1128–47.

[109] Winter RB, Lonstein JE, Boachie-Adjei O. Congenital spinal deformity. Instr Course Lect 1996; 45:117–27.

[110] McMaster MJ. Spinal growth and congenital deformity of the spine. Spine 2006;31(20):2284–7.

[111] McMaster MJ, Singh H. The surgical management of congenital kyphosis and kyphoscoliosis. Spine 2001;26(19):2146–54 [discussion: 2155].

[112] Miller A, Temple T, Miller F. Impact of orthoses on the rate of scoliosis progression in children with cerebral palsy. J Pediatr Orthop 1996;16(3): 332–5.

[113] McCarthy JJ, D'Andrea LP, Betz RR, et al. Scoliosis in the child with cerebral palsy. J Am Acad Orthop Surg 2006;14(6):367–75.

[114] Sussman M. Duchenne muscular dystrophy. J Am Acad Orthop Surg 2002;10(2):138–51.

[115] Murphy NA, Firth S, Jorgensen T, et al. Spinal surgery in children with idiopathic and neuromuscular scoliosis. What's the difference? J Pediatr Orthop 2006;26(2):216–20.

[116] Edler A, Murray DJ, Forbes RB. Blood loss during posterior spinal fusion surgery in patients with neuromuscular disease: is there an increased risk? Paediatr Anaesth 2003;13(9):818–22.

[117] Banta JV, Drummond DS, Ferguson RL. The treatment of neuromuscular scoliosis. Instr Course Lect 1999;48:551–62.

[118] Damborg F, Engell V, Andersen M, et al. Prevalence, concordance, and heritability of Scheuermann kyphosis based on a study of twins. J Bone Joint Surg Am 2006;88(10):2133–6.

[119] Ascani E, La Rosa G, Ascani C. Scheuermann kyphosis. In: Weinstein SL, editor. The pediatric spine: principles and practice. 2nd edition. New York: Lippincott Williams & Wilkins; 2001. p. 413–31.

[120] Lowe TG. Scheuermann's disease. Orthop Clin North Am 1999;30(3):475–87, ix.

[121] Halal F, Gledhill RB, Fraser C. Dominant inheritance of Scheuermann's juvenile kyphosis. Am J Dis Child 1978;132(11):1105–7.

[122] Tribus CB. Scheuermann's kyphosis in adolescents and adults: diagnosis and management. J Am Acad Orthop Surg 1998;6(1):36–43.

[123] Murray PM, Weinstein SL, Spratt KF. The natural history and long-term follow-up of Scheuermann kyphosis. J Bone Joint Surg Am 1993;75(2):236–48.

[124] Lowe TG, Kasten MD. An analysis of sagittal curves and balance after Cotrel-Dubousset instrumentation for kyphosis secondary to Scheuermann's disease. A review of 32 patients. Spine 1994;19(15):1680–5.

[125] Arlet V, Schlenzka D. Scheuermann's kyphosis: surgical management. Eur Spine J 2005;14(9):817–27.

[126] Sachs B, Bradford D, Winter R, et al. Scheuermann kyphosis. Follow-up of Milwaukee-brace treatment. J Bone Joint Surg Am 1987;69(1):50–7.

[127] Stotts AK, Smith JT, Santora SD, et al. Measurement of spinal kyphosis: implications for the management of Scheuermann's kyphosis. Spine 2002; 27(19):2143–6.

[128] Bradford DS, Moe JH, Montalvo FJ, et al. Scheuermann's kyphosis. Results of surgical treatment by posterior spine arthrodesis in twenty-two patients. J Bone Joint Surg Am 1975;57(4):439–48.

[129] Soo CL, Noble PC, Esses SI. Scheuermann kyphosis: long-term follow-up. Spine J 2002;2(1):49–56.

[130] Lim M, Green DW, Billinghurst JE, et al. Scheuermann kyphosis: safe and effective surgical treatment using multisegmental instrumentation. Spine 2004;29(16):1789–94.

[131] Bradford DS, Ahmed KB, Moe JH, et al. The surgical management of patients with Scheuermann's disease: a review of twenty-four cases managed by combined anterior and posterior spine fusion. J Bone Joint Surg Am 1980;62(5):705–12.

[132] Lee SS, Lenke LG, Kuklo TR, et al. Comparison of Scheuermann kyphosis correction by posterior-only thoracic pedicle screw fixation versus combined anterior/posterior fusion. Spine 2006;31(20): 2316–21.

ELSEVIER
SAUNDERS

Neurosurg Clin N Am 18 (2007) 531–547

NEUROSURGERY
CLINICS
OF NORTH AMERICA

Tethered Cord Syndrome

Pankaj K. Agarwalla, BS, Ian F. Dunn, MD,
R. Michael Scott, MD, Edward R. Smith, MD*

Department of Neurosurgery, Children's Hospital of Boston, 300 Longwood Avenue, Boston, MA 02115, USA

Definition—what is a "tethered cord?"

A tethered spinal cord is best defined as an abnormal attachment of the spinal cord to the tissues that surround it. The term has acquired a number of different meanings over time. This label has been applied to descriptions of radiographic findings and to varied constellations of clinical signs and symptoms. For example, in 1976 Hoffman and colleagues [1] used the phrase "tethered spinal cord" to define a radiographic diagnosis—a spinal cord "with a low conus medullaris and a thickened filum terminale measuring 2 mm or more in diameter," excluding other conditions such as "lipomyelomeningoceles, meningoceles, myelomeningoceles, diastematomyelia, and intraspinal space-occupying dysraphic conditions such as dermoid tumors, intraspinal meningoceles, neurenteric cysts, and teratomatous cysts" [1]—many of which today are considered typically representative of tethering of the spinal cord.

The radiographic diagnosis of tethered spinal cord is distinct from the clinical diagnosis of tethered cord syndrome, that is, the signs and symptoms believed to result from excessive tension on the spinal cord. The spinal cord most frequently is tethered in the lumbosacral region [2,3]. Ascribed clinical manifestations include pain (especially with flexion), bowel and bladder dysfunction, weakness, sensory changes, gait abnormalities, and musculoskeletal deformities of the feet and spine, such as scoliosis or clubfoot [1,2,4–11]. Cutaneous stigmata signifying an underlying congenital defect of the spinal cord also are common [12].

Over time, the term "tethered cord" has been used interchangeably to include both the radiographic and clinical findings described here. Although the incidental radiographic finding of an asymptomatic tethered spinal cord is becoming increasingly common, more often some combination of clinical signs and symptoms results in a patient's coming to the attention of the neurosurgeon. Therefore this article focuses primarily on the clinical entity of tethered cord syndrome, with discussion of its history, pathophysiology, diagnosis, and treatment.

Brief history

Review of the early literature related to tethered cord syndrome reveals a gradual awareness that myriad causes can contribute to a similar presentation. Reports often had two common themes, a clinical scenario of progressive lower-extremity symptoms and recovery following surgical intervention. In one of the first recorded cases documenting the diagnosis and treatment of tethered cord syndrome, an 1857 report describes a young child who presented with worsening right-sided lower extremity weakness and twitching [13]. The child underwent surgical exploration of his spine, and a lesion consistent with a spinal lipoma was found. At surgery, the spinal cord was freed from its attachments to the dura, and the symptoms resolved [13].

In 1891, Jones [14] described what probably is the first true "untethering" operation in a 22-year-old patient who had developed talipes equinovarus deformities, weakness and atrophy of the lower limbs, difficulty with micturition, and pain in his feet. At operation, Jones [14] performed

* Corresponding author.
  E-mail address: edward.smith@childrens.harvard.edu (E.R. Smith).

1042-3680/07/$ - see front matter © 2007 Elsevier Inc. All rights reserved.
doi:10.1016/j.nec.2007.04.001

a successful division of a "dense adventitious fibrous band" within the spinal canal. Six months
postoperatively, the patient was able to walk
freely without pain, had improved micturition,
and regained leg muscle size and strength.

Another important development in the history
of tethered cord syndrome was the recognition
that symptoms may be exacerbated by activity. In
1916, Spiller [15], a neurologist, described two adolescent patients who presented with symptoms of
tethered cord syndrome that developed subsequent to strenuous activity. Two boys, 14 and 18
years of age, presented with leg weakness and
enuresis after exercise, including flexion related to
training for rowing. This new understanding—
that there may be a dynamic component to the
development and progression of tethered cord
syndrome—resulted in an impetus for earlier
identification of affected patients so they could
avoid activities that could lead to spinal cord
stretching, presumably the cause of the neurologic
deficits [15].

In addition to a growing recognition of the
distinct clinical entity of tethered cord syndrome,
the literature also reflected a progressive evolution
in the debate regarding timing of treatment of
affected patients. As early as 1918, a correlation
between prompt treatment and improved outcome
was acknowledged [16]. The benefit of early treatment, coupled with increasing awareness of findings on physical examination associated with
tethered cord syndrome, led to a proposal to treat
asymptomatic patients prophylactically, "in the
hope of obviating the development of symptoms
during adolescence" [16]. Although the expeditious treatment of symptomatic patients has
been accepted generally, the debate surrounding
asymptomatic patients who have anatomically
tethered spinal cords continues.

Tethered cord syndrome, attributed to a wide
spectrum of causes and poorly understood mechanistically, remained vaguely defined for several
decades [17]. In the 1950s, however, reports began
to recognize the connection between disparate
pathophysiologic entities, particularly diastematomyelia, spinal lipomas, and thickened fila termina-
lia, and a common clinical presentation [13,14,16,
18–20]. In 1953, Garceau [21] conceived the terms
"filum terminale syndrome," and "cord-traction
syndrome," proposing a causal relationship between a thickened filum found on exploration of
patients who presented clinically with spinal
deformities and progressive neurologic deterioration. The distinction between the clinical "tethered

cord syndrome" and the radiographic "tethered
spinal cord" continued with Hoffman's [1] definition of a "tethered spinal cord" made in the
1970s.

Despite the creation of the distinct term
"tethered cord syndrome" to encompass the signs
and symptoms thought to be the clinical manifestations of a tethered spinal cord, the wide range of
causes reported in association with this tethered
cord syndrome, coupled with the continued lack
of consensus regarding what constitutes the tethered cord syndrome, has resulted in the admission
by one group that tethered cord syndrome constitutes, at best, "a loose diagnosis" [17,22]. In future efforts in this area, it will be important to
make clear distinctions between clinical and radiographic findings.

Embryologic considerations

Although a lengthy discussion of embryology
is not within the scope of this article (for a more
thorough review, see Dias and McLone [23]), understanding the varied clinical manifestations of
tethered spinal cord is enhanced by an apprecia-
tion of the relevant embryology. A considerable
number of developmental errors can result in conditions that functionally tether the spinal cord.
These congenital conditions, distinct from acquired causes of tethering (such as infection, tumor, or scar), can present in myriad ways and at
different stages of a child's maturation. A working
knowledge of the embryologic processes underlying these conditions can aid the neurosurgeon in
understanding and avoiding the potential hazards
intrinsic to the treatment of these children.

Notochordal development

In the first few weeks of development, neurulation begins with the formation of the notochord
arising from the primitive pit [23]. The primitive
pit subsequently recedes caudally while the notochord elongates cranially [23]. The notochord
then undergoes intercalation, fusing with the underlying endoderm to form the notochordal plate.
This plate is continuous with the yolk sac and also
is continuous with the amniotic sac [23].

Primary neurulation

The notochord induces formation of the neural
tube dorsally from the overlying ectoderm by
means of the neural groove from days 18 to 24
after ovulation [24]. This process gives rise to the
cervical, thoracic, and lumbar neural tube [25].

Somites develop from the paraxial mesenchyme and represent the majority of the future vertebral column at these levels as well [25]. Most relevant to the tethered cord in primary neurulation is the closure of the neural groove. The level of final closure of the caudal neuropore corresponds to the second sacral vertebral level (S2) [24], suggesting that spinal malformations arising from S2 or above probably result from disordered primary neurulation [23].

Secondary neurulation

During the time of primary neurulation, the primitive streak regresses to form the axial mesenchyme of the caudal eminence (also known as end-bud [24]), which extends from the site of the neurenteric canal to the cloacal membrane [25]. The caudal eminence provides the cells for the formation of the neural tube caudal to somite 31, corresponding to the future S2 level. Once primary closure is complete, secondary neurulation from the caudal eminence begins but not in the form of a folding neural plate as in primary neurulation. Rather, a "neural cord" forms with a central canal continuous with the more rostrally formed primary neural tube; this distinct process of secondary neurulation helps explain the clinically relevant pathophysiologic entity of caudal agenesis [24,26,27].

Ascent of conus and relationship with meninges

Beginning at postovulatory day 43 to 48, the conus medullaris "ascends" relative to the vertebral bodies through two mechanisms: (1) differential growth of bony vertebrae compared with the neural tissue of the spinal cord and (2) retrogressive differentiation during which the caudal cord loses much of its thickness and character [23]. The conus does not ascend throughout childhood and remains at approximately its birth position of L1-2; a cord at L2-3 or above is considered within normal range [28]. Wolf and colleagues [29], using ultrasound, found that the conus is still "ascending" from L2-4 to L1-2 during postmenstrual week 30 to 40 and generally achieves its normal position of L1-2 after postmenstrual week 40. The clinical relevance of these data is that any patient who has a conus found at L3 or below should be considered for evaluation of tethered cord syndrome.

In addition to the formation of the neural tube, the spinal cord must be invested with membranes and a vasculature. These generally are considered to be derived from the mesodermal layer, although there has been debate on their origins [30–32]. In both open and closed spinal dysraphisms, it is clear that the usual meningeal stratification often is abnormal, with the potential for improperly located tissue (eg, subdural extension of adipose tissue in lipomyelomeningocele). In abnormal development, therefore, the surgeon must be aware of unusual meningeal arrangements, both between the dura and the leptomeninges and between the dura and the conus.

This overview of the embryology helps explain the development of the abnormal anatomy that results in a tethered spinal cord. Although this information can be invaluable to understanding and interpreting physical findings and imaging studies, it is important to appreciate a distinction between the anatomic findings of a tethered spinal cord and the functional problems that produce the symptoms of tethered cord syndrome. Some of the symptoms that are part of the clinical presentation of these patients may be caused by intrinsic, congenital defects in the nerves and spinal cord, and, as such, cannot be remedied by surgical intervention. In contrast, some symptoms are secondary to reversible causes that are amenable to surgical treatment. It therefore is important for the treating physician to establish and document a baseline examination before undertaking any potential intervention to help distinguish between pre-existing and recurrent problems.

Causes

Any process that tethers the spinal cord can result in a patient who has tethered cord syndrome. Children can be born with normal anatomy and develop a tethered cord through an acquired process, such as infection, scarring, or tumor. Although these acquired (secondary) causes are important, this section focuses on congenital (primary) causes of tethered cord. The previous review of the embryology of the developing spinal cord provides a context for presenting the more commonly encountered congenital causes of tethered spinal cord discussed in this article.

Abnormal secondary neurulation and disorders of caudal eminence

Because the filum terminale and the caudal spinal cord are formed from the caudal eminence through secondary neurulation, disorders in this process can lead to conditions in which the caudal cord might be tethered. The simplest form of such conditions is a filum terminale, which can be thickened, potentially with lipomatous tissue (the so-called "fatty filum"). Hoffman and colleagues [1] have suggested that a diameter of 2 mm or greater should be considered an abnormally thickened filum. Impaired canalization of the growing secondary neural tube (the neural cord) with cells capable of growth and differentiation, particularly preadipose tissue, is believed to be the cause of both the thickened and fatty filum terminale [33]. The fatty filum commonly is associated with cases of imperforate anus, suggesting a common timing of pathogenesis during development [33].

Terminal myelocystoceles, also thought to arise from disordered secondary neurulation, are found at the terminal end of the developing neural tube. These myelocystoceles usually contain two sacs, one a dilation of the embryologic terminal ventricle and another a dilated and ectatic dural and arachnoid sleeve [23]. They often are associated with a lipoma (lipomyelocystocele), and, because the mesenchyme of the caudal eminence also forms many of the structures of the hindgut, terminal myelocystoceles also are found commonly with abnormalities of other caudal systems, particularly in the complex of omphalocele, extrophy, imperforate anus, and spinal malformations (OEIS syndrome) [23]. The disorder is believed to be mesenchymal, and the surface ectoderm and skin usually are intact. The finding of dorsal bony dysraphism is common also.

Abnormal secondary neurulation can lead to a variety of other complex spinal dysraphisms in the caudal region. Termed "caudal agenesis" or "dysgenesis," these congenital malformations involve abnormal or incomplete formation of caudal elements of the embryo. They arise from problems with canalization of the caudal neural cord (the secondary neural tube) or in the process of retrogressive differentiation during the ascent of the conus [34]. Because the filum terminale forms as a glioependymal strand during retrogressive differentiation, caudal agenesis (especially the simplest form, sacral agenesis, which affects coccygeal spinal levels) often leads to an elongated and tethered conus.

Caudal agenesis often is accompanied by other caudal hindgut and genitourinary malformations. This process can be viewed as a spectrum, ranging from a simple imperforate anus to complete caudal agenesis with sirenomelia (mermaid syndrome), which shows malformation of limb buds, genitourinary apparatus, caudal neural tube, and anorectal system [23]. In between are a host of syndromes associated with caudal agenesis, congenital abnormalities, and tethering of the spinal cord. In particular, a tethered spinal cord is a common finding in patients who have OEIS, vertebral, anal, transesophageal, radial, and renal abnormalities (VATER syndrome), or the Currarino triad [34].

OEIS syndrome is defined by the presence of an omphalocele, extrophy of the cloaca, an imperforate anus, and spinal malformations, often including a tethered spinal cord. VATER syndrome refers to a presentation with the combination of vertebral anomalies, an imperforate anus, a tracheoesophageal fistula, and renal-radial anomalies. The Currarino triad, caused by a genetic defect in a homeobox gene at 7q36, includes three findings: an anorectal malformation, a presacral mass (usually an anterior myelomeningocele), and sacral bone abnormalities [35]. Patients who have Currarino triad also have distinct clinical features, including a narrow pelvis, flattened buttocks, a short intergluteal cleft, a prominent iliac crest, absent coccyx/sacral elements, and impaired lower extremity motor function [34]. These clinical findings are linked by a common error in embryologic development, a malformed caudal eminence resulting in abnormal canalization of secondary neural tube, subsequently leading to a dysfunctional ventral spinal cord [35].

Lipomas

Lipomas can arise in numerous locations at the caudal end of the spinal cord. Presumably, lipomas arise after the completion of primary neurulation but before secondary neurulation and arise from embryonic mesodermal tissue that has infiltrated into an abnormal area [33]. Lipomas in the filum terminale were discussed earlier; the focus here is on lipomas affecting the conus medullaris. These lipomas most are commonly subpial, although a small number can be subdural. Subdural lipomas are infrequently associated with tethering and more commonly present like a mass lesion with cord compression [33].

More commonly, however, lipomas of the spinal cord occur in the lumbosacral region and have an associated dural defect. Chapman [36] classified such conus lipomas into three categories, those arising from (1) the terminal end of the conus, (2) the dorsal surface of the conus, or (3) both the terminal end and dorsal surface of the conus. The most important clinical distinction is whether the lipoma involves neural tissue (ie, conus/cauda) or not (eg, filum) [33]. Approximately 75% occur in the conus, approximately 15% to 20% in the filum, with the remainder involving both the conus and filum [37]. In addition, lipomatous tissue can infiltrate almost any caudal spinal defect to give rise to malformations including the atypical forms lipomyelocele, lipomyelomeningocele, and lipomyelocystocele.

In a large series by Pierre-Kahn and colleagues [37], 63% of lipomas were classified as atypical. These embryologically distinct entities have direct relevance to surgical planning. The exact embryologic mechanism underlying this pathogenesis has been debated, with alternative theories proposed by several groups [30,38]. Several of these models propose that traction on the spinal cord caused by the lipoma may be asymmetric. This theory has been supported by findings at surgery, where eccentric lipomas have been observed to cause the affected side of the cord to be directed more posterolaterally, stretching the ipsilateral nerve roots [23,33].

Histologic analysis of fat supports the concept of primary and secondary neurulation contributing to distinct pathophysiologic processes, because lipomas rostral to S2 often contain typical fat cells, whereas lipomas caudal to S2 often contain other mesenchymal cell derivatives including a thick fibrous stroma as well as tissue with characteristics suggestive of muscle or bone [23,33]. Another study by Pierre-Kahn and colleagues [37] has shown that lipomas in their series contain nonadipose tissue apparently derived from all three primary germ layers.

Dermoid/sinus tract

Whereas lipomas are thought to occur from premature disjunction, delayed disjunction is the proposed cause for both dermal sinus tracts and dermoid/epidermoid tumors [23]. At a certain point in normal neural tube fusion, the neural tube separates from the cutaneous ectoderm, allowing mesenchymal cells to invade and separate the neural tube from the surface ectoderm. If the surface tissue does not separate successfully from the central nervous system, residual tissue or sinus tracts can develop in association with the central nervous system.

Another theory proposes that a more general disorder of gastrulation in which two paired notochordal anlagen do not fuse properly results in the inappropriate deposition of ectodermal tissue between the notochords, engendering the development of dermoids, sinus tracts, and epidermoid tumors [39]. According to this theory, the separation of tissue layers is delayed, resulting in cutaneous ectodermal cells being carried in from the skin and subsequently residing at the site of neural tube closure. These cells can develop into a dermal sinus tract, an epidermoid, or a dermoid [23].

Complex spinal dysraphisms

Complex spinal dysraphisms are disorders affecting all three primary germ layers during embryogenesis, and they share a common embryologic basis. The common complex spinal dysraphisms that can lead to tethering are spina bifida, split cord malformations (ie, diastematomyelia and diplomyelia), and neurenteric cysts. They can occur as open neural tube defects but more often are closed defects [23]. (For a more detailed review, see Dias and McLone [23].)

One theory has been proposed by Dias and Walker [39], who believe that these malformations arise when the anlagen of all three germ layers are established in gastrulation. During the formation of the notochordal process, paired bilateral notochordal anlagen come together to form a single notochord with a narrow primitive streak. Should these bilateral anlagen become separated, two distinct spinal cords would develop. The space between the hemicords also could give rise to tissues from each of the three germ layers: endoderm (neurenteric cysts), mesoderm (bony spurs, muscle, fat), and ectoderm (dermoid/epidermoid tumors) [39]. This proposed mechanism of complex spinal dysraphisms also supports the unified theory of split cord malformation proposed by Pang [40,41], who posits a common embryologic basis for type I split cord malformations (diastematomyelia, two spinal cords with two dural sleeves) and type II malformations (diplomyelia, two spinal cords sharing one dural sleeve).

Split cord malformations (diastematomyelia and diplomyelia) often are associated with tethered cords, with the tethering often attributed to bony or fibrous spurs and/or thickened fila. In a series of 31 children, all split cord malformations below T7 were associated with a low-lying conus and a spinal lipoma or fatty filum [40,41].

Neurenteric cysts often are found on the ventral side of the spinal canal and consist of a fluid-filled cyst that may communicate with the gastrointestinal tract through a vertebral defect such as a hemivertebra or butterfly vertebra [34]. The neurenteric cyst itself can cause compression, but its adherent fibrous bands also can result in tethering [34]. They usually are intradural and extramedullary, and their origin is debated, although positive immunoreactivity for carcinoembryonic antigen suggests endodermal origins [42].

In all these cases, tethering can occur when improperly placed mesenchymal tissue creates various abnormal structures such as bony spurs, fat, and fibrous bands that impede the normal ascent of the conus or attach to tissue at inappropriate locations, causing a tethering effect.

Myelomeningocele, meningocele, meningocele manqué

Myelomeningocele, meningocele, and meningocele manqué reflect abnormal development during primary neurulation or immediately after during the formation of the meninges. In myelomeningocele, the spinal cord does not fuse dorsally, leaving neural tissue known as the "neural placode." The groove in the neural placode is the remnant of the central canal [43]. In meningocele, the neural tube fuses properly, but the dura does not fuse correctly, creating a cystic lesion that is often skin-covered. In both cases, tethering can occur as functional cord attaches itself dorsally either to dura or to surface ectoderm. An interesting case of meningocele known as the "meningocele manqué" (the "missing" meningocele) occurs when a meningocele has formed during embryogenesis but has healed spontaneously or scarred creating a dorsal band. These dorsal bands can extend from intrathecal structure into the dura or outside structures creating a significant tethering effect [34]. The dorsal band of meningocele manqué may reflect a fibroneurovascular stalk derived from the same endomesenchymal tract that is the basis for split cord malformations [41].

Clinical presentation and evaluation

In the original description of the tethered cord syndrome, Hoffman and colleagues [1] chose in their subtitle to refer to the syndrome's "protean manifestations," a term that comes from the Greek god Proteus who would change shape. "Protean" is an apt term for the tethered cord syndrome because its presentations are as varied as its causes. This section describes some common presentations and highlights some unique findings.

Cutaneous findings

Cutaneous findings are commonplace in closed spinal dysraphism. A retrospective study by Guggisberg and colleagues [44] examined the diagnostic value of midline cutaneous lesions in the lumbosacral region for closed spinal dysraphism. A large number of cutaneous lesions were reviewed, including cutaneous lipoma, tail, dermal sinus, atypical dimple, deviation of gluteal crease, hamartoma, hemangioma, port-wine stain, hypertrichosis, and pigmentary nevus, among others, with the recommendation of MRI testing if patients had two or more of the listed cutaneous lesions or one high-risk lesion such as a lipoma, tail, or dermal sinus [44]. Other lower-risk lesions such as an atypical dimple, a deviation of the gluteal crease, or an unclassified hamartoma suggest the need for ultrasound evaluation before 6 months of age or an MRI after 6 months. The rationale for the age difference is that the acoustic window to the spine closes at approximately 3 to 6 months. Other isolated findings such as hypertrichosis or vascular abnormalities have a lower likelihood of being associated with spinal cord tethering in the absence of any other signs or symptoms [44].

A common finding in closed spinal dysraphism is a palpable subcutaneous lipoma, often associated with a cutaneous hemangioma [33]. Dimples often are cited as a common finding, but it is important to distinguish a sacrococcygeal dimple as a marker for a dermal sinus tract or more dangerous abnormality from a more benign coccygeal dimple [23]. Sacrococcygeal dimples are almost always cranial to the intergluteal cleft, and the intergluteal cleft is often abnormal or deviated. Its distance from the anus is more than 2.5 cm, its diameter is larger (>5 mm), and cutaneous stigmata often are present [45]. Simple coccygeal dimples usually are intergluteal and smaller than sacrococcygeal dimples with no significant cutaneous abnormalities and are thought to be a remnant of the primitive pit with some cells from the caudal eminence [23,45]. There are rare reports associating low, coccygeal dimples and presacral masses that might warrant a conservative approach including ultrasound examination and digital rectal examination [33].

As a rule of thumb, a lesion rostral to the gluteal cleft often is associated with neurosurgical disease and should be considered for detailed imaging evaluation, whereas lesions within or caudal to the gluteal cleft are less likely to require neurosurgical attention.

Neurologic findings

A variety of neurologic findings can be present in patients who have tethered cord syndrome. Common findings change with age and depend on the underlying cause of the tethered cord [34]. A full neurologic examination is vital for initial diagnosis and for establishing a baseline for follow-up. In infants, one may find decreased spontaneous leg movement, abnormal reflexes, foot asymmetry, and leg atrophy (occasionally hidden by baby fat). Toddlers often show developmental delay in acquiring gait or have an abnormal gait. Older children have asymmetric motor and sensory dysfunction, painless foot burns (trophic ulcerations), hyperreflexia, and back and leg pain that often is worsened with flexion or vigorous physical activity. Young adults have similar pain and reflex changes but may present with predominantly sensory dysfunction. Generally, however, pain and motor dysfunction are more prominent, perhaps because the ventral aspect of the conus medullaris derives primarily from the secondary neural tube, whereas the primary neural tube extends slightly dorsally into the conus during development [34].

Orthopedic findings

Common deformities include clubfeet (often equinovarus), asymmetry in leg length, trophic ulcerations of the foot in advanced cases, atrophy of lower leg muscle occasionally masked by baby fat in an infant, hip subluxation, and scoliosis [33]. These conditions call for orthopedic consultation and mandate treatment of the underlying tethering by the neurosurgeon. In the older patient, severe scoliosis, gait change, leg weakness and atrophy, and pain can occur either as an exacerbation of a previously undiagnosed tethering or as a retethering of the cord [33]. Spinal radiographs, as discussed later, are useful in cases of scoliosis and are recommended when vertebral deformities are present.

Urologic function and assessment

Urologic decline is one of the most important indicators for early and definitive treatment. As a child grows older or as urologic function deteriorates, it often becomes more difficult to restore urologic function after untethering [33]. Common symptoms include frequent urinary tract infections, abnormal voiding, urinary incontinence, and fecal soiling. Incontinence and infections are more common in older children and young adults [34].

A careful history and physical examination are important screening tools for evaluating urologic function, especially in infants and young children. Particular attention should be given to histories that include a loss of previously attained milestones in continence that is progressive in nature. Treatment for any urinary tract infection and a full work-up for any hematuria should be performed [46].

Urodynamic assessment provides quantifiable evidence of neurologic dysfunction in the setting of tethered cord. Evaluation includes urodynamic measurements by simultaneous cystourethrography/cystometrography and sphincter electromyography. Sacral innervation can also be tested by examination of perianal sensation, anal sphincter tone, the bulbocavernosus reflex, and voluntary sphincter control [46].

Electromyographic measurements include a bulbocavernosus reflex latency time and an electromyographic examination of the perineal floor muscles. If the sympathetic pathways are damaged, incontinence results from lack of internal sphincter control. If parasympathetic pathways are damaged, an areflexic and either hypotonic or hypertonic bladder will result. Patients who have hypertonic bladders may be treated with anticholinergics and self-catheterization in addition to treatment of any underlying neurologic proximal cause, such as spinal cord tethering [46]. Detrusor dyssynergia, another common finding with hypotonic and hypertonic bladder, is caused by a lesion between the brainstem and the sacral spinal cord [33]. Both dyssynergia and hypertonic bladder with high intravesical filling pressures require treatment to prevent further upper urinary tract disease. High intravesical pressures have been shown to be predictive of future urinary tract problems in patients who have tethered cord syndrome [47].

As discussed later, urologic examination and assessment are vital in the follow-up after surgical treatment of a tethered cord, because new dysfunction or a postoperative progression of dysfunction may herald retethering of the cord. Successful treatment of a tethered cord may lead to stabilization or even reversal of urologic dysfunction. In addition, preoperative urodynamics can document pre-existing problems that may not be clinically evident immediately but may present later in life (for example, in younger children who later may have difficulty in toilet training). These preoperative tests may provide evidence that problems discovered later in life are not a result of the surgical intervention or necessitate additional treatment. Nevertheless, the consensus view is that early, aggressive treatment, particularly in the infant and young child, can help significantly with urologic function in the context of a tethered cord [48,49].

Imaging

Ultrasonography

Ultrasound imaging, although not very useful for surgical planning or proper spinal anomaly evaluation, can have a role as a relatively quick and easy screening tool in young children. The acoustic window into the lumbar spine in the infant closes in the first months of life. Ultrasound is best able to detect the position of the conus, the presence of any fat, and decreased spinal cord motion, any of which might indicate tethering [34]. Should ultrasonography be performed, it can be useful to image with the patient's head elevated to distend any potential meningocele or closed spinal dysraphism [50].

Plain-film radiography

When a congenital defect with a vertebral or bony component (such as midline bony spurs in split cord malformation type I) is suspected, plain-film radiographs may be useful but in most cases have been largely supplanted by MRI and CT. In complex spinal dysraphisms, one should look for anomalies in the laminae, vertebral bodies, disc spaces, or pedicles [34]. Widening of the spinal canal, as evidenced by an increased interpedicular distance or scalloping of the posterior of the vertebrae, is particularly evident on plain-film radiographs [34]. More global assessments, including any change in the number of vertebra or obvious malformation of an individual vertebra, should be made also. In cases of caudal agenesis, radiographic evidence of absence or splitting of the sacrum should be noted.

The one particularly helpful role of plain-film radiography is in assessment of spinal curvature. Radiographs can be measured to evaluate the degree of kyphosis, lordosis, or scoliosis.

CT and MRI

Previously, the standard of diagnosis for tethered cord was lumbar myelography. CT

myelography (CTM) later became accepted, and criteria were established for the diagnosis of a tethered cord: a low-lying conus (below L2-L3), a thickened filum (>2 mm), or fat in the filum. CTM has proven useful when examining the axial plane to see the relationship between lipomas, subarachnoid space, nerve roots, and neural placode, if there is one. Pang [40] also has suggested that CTM with iohexol is superior to MRI in the diagnosis of split cord malformations. Through varying window settings, CTM can elaborate on bony spurs and other midline structures more clearly, and in the case of a bony spur without a marrow cavity, it is more sensitive than T1-weighted MRI, which loses the signal void of the bone marrow. MRI, however, better delineates intramedullary syrinxes and is comparable to CTM for tethering lesions such as thickened fila, lipomas, and dural adhesions [40].

More recently, however, MRI has replaced CTM myelography as the reference standard for the diagnosis of various causes of the tethered cord syndrome. MRI is particularly good at highlighting fat on T1-weighted imaging (Fig. 1). Nevertheless, a small number of reports have described patients who have tethered cord syndrome without a low-lying conus or other clues from imaging [4,6]. MRI is well suited to identifying the level of the conus relative to vertebral bodies, the presence of a syrinx, or visualization of other pathologic processes. MRI also is able to define the anatomy of other causes of tethered cord, such as the anatomy of terminal or multiple lipomas (Fig. 2), the presence of congenital lesions (such as dermoids), and the presence of myelomeningocele.

Pathophysiology

The mechanism by which tethering produces its effect on the spinal cord has long been the subject of debate [17]. Yamada and colleagues [51] performed the first scientific experiments to investigate the pathophysiologic basis of tethered cord. Using spectrophotometry on human and animal spinal cords to measure reduction/oxidation changes in cytochrome c, they demonstrated decreased mitochondrial oxidative metabolism with constant or intermittent cord stretching, particularly at higher forces of traction. Furthermore, they proposed that local hypoxia might contribute to the pathogenesis of symptoms in patients who have tethered cords. The hypothesis that the spinal cord may undergo ischemic changes in

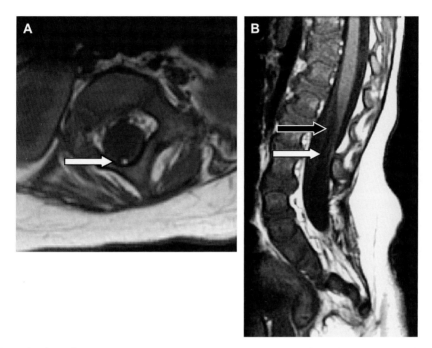

Fig. 1. MRI showing a fatty filum (*white arrow*), bright on T1 image (*A*), with low-lying conus (*black arrow*) (*B*).

response to tension was bolstered by the findings of experiments using laser Doppler to monitor the microcirculation of human spinal cords during untethering operations [52]. Using this approach, the authors demonstrated increased blood flow after surgical release of the spinal cord by untethering.

Sarwar and colleagues [3] and Tani and colleagues [53] provided evidence that helps explain why symptoms of tethered cord are referable predominantly to the caudal spinal cord and roots. Their work revealed that caudal cord traction produces primarily local elongation in the lumbar cord and that the filum acts as a distensible buffer to prevent cord stretching [3,53].Thus, any process that reduces the filum's distensibility and role as a buffer leaves the cord more susceptible to stretching forces. A shortened, thickened, or fatty filum may exert this effect and produce injury to the distal spinal cord.

It also has been demonstrated that flexion of the torso increases longitudinal tension if the cord is tethered and increases local compression of the spinal cord if a mass is present [54]. This finding suggests a dual mechanism of injury in the setting of a large spinal lipoma, because a terminal lipoma can tether the cord and, when the lipoma is large, can compress it [55]. Taken together,

these findings indicating that that forces on the spinal cord are exacerbated by flexion may help explain the development of symptoms during or after repetitive activity involving flexion (eg, Spiller's adolescent patients who were rowing and cycling [15]).

Traction on the spinal cord can occur from a variety of directions depending on the underlying cause of the tethered cord. Thickened filum terminale and some lipomyelomeningoceles produce caudal traction, as can dorsal bands, meningocele manqué, dorsal lipomas, and dermal sinus tracts. Split cord malformations and neurenteric cysts may cause ventral traction [34]. The tethered cord syndrome can occur without any obvious lowering of the conus [4,6,8–11]. In support of tethered cord syndrome with a normally positioned conus, Selcuki and colleagues [9] have postulated that an increase in abnormal dense connective tissue around the ependymal canal of the conus can reduce the elasticity of the normal-lying conus and its ability to act as a buffer against tethering.

In aggregate, this evidence supports the premise that entities that produce excessive tethering or compression of the spinal cord can produce neurologic dysfunction, presumably through a combination of local ischemia and direct

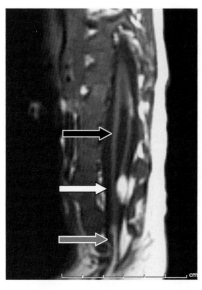

Fig. 2. MRI showing dorsal (*white arrow*) and terminal (*gray arrow*) lipomas with an associated syrinx (*black arrow*).

mechanical dysfunction. Limitation of injurious activity (such as excessive flexion) may minimize cord injury. Furthermore, relief of this tension and/or compression (as seen with surgical untethering) may result in improved circulation and abrogation of further damage.

Indications and rationale for treatment

Children who present with tethered cord syndrome fall into one of two groups, symptomatic or asymptomatic. In general, treatment of symptomatic children found to have tethered cord by imaging is indicated. It is important, however, to note two potential confounding conditions related to specific disease entities.

Confounding conditions

One group that merits special mention is the population of patients who have large spinal lipomas that exhibit mass effect on the spinal cord. A limited subpopulation of this group can develop worsening in symptoms in association with rapid weight gain. It has been hypothesized that the spinal lipoma increases in size, and thus in mass effect, as the patient gains weight. Some have proposed that weight loss may be a helpful adjunct in the treatment of this patient population. Although it may be difficult to justify

delaying treatment of patients who have neurologic deficits, those presenting only with pain may be considered for a trial of weight loss before committing to surgical intervention.

A second population that is important to discuss is the group of myelomeningocele patients who have symptoms suggestive of tethered cord syndrome and who also have ventricular shunts. A malfunctioning shunt sometimes can cause signs and symptoms that may mimic a tethered cord. In these patients, even with radiographic evidence of findings suggestive of a tethered cord (eg, progressive scoliosis or a syrinx), it is important to confirm that the shunt is working before committing to an untethering operation.

General principles

Outside these two specific scenarios, the development or progression of symptoms in patients who have a tethered cord often calls for an untethering operation [56]. Symptoms may develop early in life but can occur later, as exemplified by one case report of the development of symptomatic diastematomyelia in a 78-year-old woman [57]. In general, these more complicated cases should be referred to neurosurgeons who have extensive experience in the treatment of this condition and only after a discussion with the child's family and caregivers outlining the risks and benefits of the procedure.

Chronicling a decline in neurologic, orthopedic, or urologic status may be difficult across multiple health care providers. As discussed previously, neurologic symptoms include lower extremity weakness, gait impairment, and pain. A detailed neurologic examination can provide clues to the causes of sensory/motor disturbances and progression of lower back and leg pains. Obvious deficits on initial examination may be fixed, but progression of any of these symptoms as documented by serial neurologic examinations further supports the indication for surgery. Surgery can arrest the progression of symptoms in the majority of patients; a smaller percentage of patients show improvement after untethering [34]. Improvement is more likely to be seen in patients whose primary symptom is pain, although these patients tend to be an older population including young adults and adults [34].

Orthopedic symptoms may be present also and should be considered in deciding on indications for treatment. Patients sometimes are seen first by an orthopedic surgeon for progressive scoliosis, gait problems, or for consideration of heel cord release because of toe walking. These symptoms in the setting of a tethered cord should prompt consideration of surgical release of the cord. It also is crucial to be aware of the population of children who have the concomitant presentation of severe scoliosis and a tethered cord. Untethering often arrests symptoms, but orthopedic intervention still may be required in cases of more severe scoliosis. If these children are scheduled for correction of the curvature of the spine, the cord should be untethered first to avoid excessive traction on the cord when subsequent bony realignment and lengthening occurs.

Pang's [40] study of split cord malformation in patients who had scoliosis reveals that in the majority of patients the scoliosis was stabilized after untethering, although subsequent correction of the deformity was limited. Similarly, Pierz and colleagues [58] studied 19 children who had myelomeningocele, scoliosis, and a tethered cord. They found that for curves of less than 40° there was subsequent improvement in the correction of the deformity, but there was no improvement for curves greater than 40°. These data suggest that the neurosurgeon should recommend untethering as treatment of the root cause of scoliosis in selected cases, but that correction of the deformity may be limited, and orthopedic involvement may be necessary.

Urologic symptoms can be stabilized or improved in many cases following successful untethering operations. Metcalfe and colleagues [59] demonstrated marked improvement of medically managed neuropathic bladders after sectioning of the filum terminale in 36 pediatric patients (age range, 1.2–15 years). Other studies also have shown marked improvement in urologic function after untethering, even in patients who have a normally positioned conus and a normal thickness filum [6,10,60–62]. When retethering occurs in patients who have myelomeningocele, Tarcan and colleagues [63] have shown that a second untethering surgery can improve urologic outcome markedly.

Controversy, however, still surrounds treatment options for the asymptomatic patient who has signs of a spinal anomaly, particularly a milder anomaly such as a thickened filum or an asymptomatic lipoma. (For a thorough review, see McLone and Thompson [33].) The risks must be weighed, because lipomas of the filum (or a thickened filum) have much better surgical outcomes than those of the conus, which can be significantly more difficult to remove. Some patients can lead fully active lives with a fatty filum and remain symptom-free throughout their lifetimes. In this setting, surgery may not be necessary and may not justify the risk of complications such as cerebrospinal fluid (CSF) leak.

Conversely, some believe that evidence supports a role for prophylactic surgery, noting that surgery does not always provide a reversal of dysfunction or abnormality in symptomatic patients. Studies of patients who had delayed diagnosis and treatment of occult spinal dysraphisms reveal that they are more likely to present with irreversible urologic and neurologic deficits that might have been prevented with an earlier diagnosis and surgical treatment [64]. Thus, proponents of early surgery argue that there is value in attempted prevention of irreversible defects, particularly in avoiding urologic dysfunction. Improvements in surgical technique with reductions in perioperative complications have added to the enthusiasm for early treatment and treatment of asymptomatic patients. Amid this controversy, however, many agree about the need for well-designed, randomized, controlled trials involving patients who have asymptomatic closed spinal defects [5,56,65].

Treatment options

General principles

Latex precautions

Full latex allergy precautions should be considered. The incidence of latex allergy in children who have spinal dysraphism is high because of the likelihood of exposure to latex antigens from repeated bladder catheterization [66].

Intraoperative monitoring

The differentiation of nerve roots from other structures such as a lipoma, dorsal band, or filum terminale is a critical element of any detethering procedure and is facilitated by the use of intraoperative neurophysiologic monitoring with combinations of motor-evoked potentials and sensory-evoked potentials. Monopolar nerve stimulators can be used to stimulate nerves so that they can be identified and preserved. Stimulation of S2, S3, and S4 can be monitored through anal manometry or electromyographic recordings [67]. The external anal sphincter is innervated by the anterior roots of S2 and S3 and by both roots of S4 through the proximal branch of the pudendal nerve. Because the distal branch of the pudendal nerve, the perineal nerve, supplies the external urethral sphincter, rectal manometry usually reflects activity of the external urethral sphincter as well [67]. The integrity of the conus medullaris and the cauda equina can be monitored by motor root mapping, motor-evoked potentials, sensory-evoked potentials, and electromyography.

Avoiding cerebrospinal fluid leak

Measures should be taken to decrease the risk of CSF leak. These measures include careful attention to a watertight dural closure, with graft if necessary. The integrity of the closure can be tested by a Valsalva maneuver under direct observation. Adjuvant sealants, such as fibrin glue or other commercially available products, may be used to enhance closure of the dura. In addition to the dural closure, careful attention also is paid to the superficial soft tissue closure as a further means of minimizing CSF leak. Consultation with plastic surgery colleagues may be helpful in complex cases to assist in possible planning of alternative closure strategies, such as rotational flaps. Postoperatively, the child often is kept flat for 1 to 5 days (depending on the complexity of the repair) and gradually is elevated in bed to minimize pressure from a standing column of fluid on the repair site.

Avoiding retethering

Many spinal anomalies with tethered cord have a tendency to retether postoperatively. To avoid retethering, meticulous attention is needed in hemostasis and closure. Dural closure with 4-0 Nurolon is adequate for many straightforward detethering operations. With more complex spinal dysraphisms, a running monofilament suture can be used with good results [68]. In complex lesions, such as extensive lipomas, resection of the maximal amount of pathologic tissue should be performed, followed by imbrication of the pial surface to create a smooth surface apposed to the dura [69,70].

Sometimes the dural sac is developmentally deficient or becomes compromised during the operation so that a significant portion of the dural sac must be reconstituted. Various materials have been used as grafts with varying degrees of success including autologous fascia, Gore-Tex (W. L. Gore & Associates, Baltimore, Maryland), biological collagen, and cadaveric tissue such as Alloderm (Lifecell, Branchburg, New Jersey) [71,72]. Silastic sheeting (Dow Corning, Midland,

Missouri) has been used in the past, but it can cause the formation of a fibrous envelope to which neural structures may attach [68]. Finally, in severe cases of retethering in patients who have myelomeningocele and compromised neural function, transaction of the spinal cord above the neural placode can be performed to prevent the placode from scarring and forming adhesions [73].

In the immediate postoperative period, some have reported keeping patients prone to minimize adhesions of the cord to the dural suture line. The patients are turned supine and slowly elevated in bed over several days.

General strategies

Many untethering operations are associated with markedly abnormal anatomy resulting from primary development and also secondary postoperative scarring. A general strategy of starting the dissection from normal tissue (usually rostrally) is often helpful. The finding of a normal bony lamina may allow identification of the dura and subsequent improved understanding of abnormal tissue planes. This principle holds true intradurally as well, where rostral exposure of normal spinal cord may facilitate safer dissection of more caudal abnormalities.

For many cases involving lipomatous tissue or scar, the use of the laser can greatly enhance the ease and safety of surgery. Excellent results have been reported with both the carbon dioxide laser and the yttrium-aluminum-garnet contact laser. Lipomatous masses in the conus and spinal cord can cause significant tethering and can be difficult to remove completely, but marked debulking often can be achieved, despite the occasional need to leave a rim of residual lipoma. At closure, a pial imbricating sutures to reconstitute more normal spinal anatomy may help reduce retethering [69].

Specific entities

Filum terminale

In filum terminale, only the distal filum terminale needs to be exposed. The filum is recognizable by its fatty appearance, by its straight midline location, and by its vasculature (Fig. 3). It is important to visualize the underside of the filum before sectioning, because nerve roots can travel along with the filum (Fig. 4). The intraoperative microscope can be invaluable in this exercise. Intraoperative nerve monitoring can be helpful in improving discrimination of nerve root from

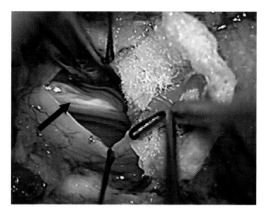

Fig. 3. A fatty filum (*arrow*).

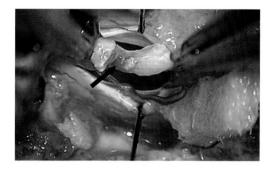

Fig. 5. Sectioning of the fatty filum (*arrow*). Note the fatty appearance and the absence of bleeding after coagulation.

filum. Once the filum is sectioned, care should be taken that there is no bleeding at the site of section before the proximal stump is released, because it may retract out of reach (Fig. 5). A watertight dural closure should be performed (Fig. 6).

Split cord malformations including meningocele manqué

Hemicords tether at the median septum, and therefore it is imperative to remove the septum. During the approach, care must be taken to avoid damaging to the spinal cord through inadvertent traction, because the cord often is tethered strongly to the bony septum or bony structures with dorsal bands. For a type I split cord malformation, the bony spur is removed subperiosteally from the dura and resected with either rongeurs or a drill. Then the dural sleeves of both hemicords are opened, and the median dura is resected along with the ventral dura with no ventral repair. A similar and easier approach to

the median fibrous band is applicable to type II split cord malformations.

Meningocele manqué should be treated similarly to a split cord malformation or a lipomyelomeningocele. The primary finding is dorsal bands tethering the cord. These bands can extend extradurally to attach to the laminae, and adherent nerve roots may be found also.

Other entities

Dermal sinus tracts identified radiographically as being in continuity with the central nervous system also may lead to tethering and should be explored intradurally. Simple excision of the extradural component of the tract may not alleviate intradural tethering. The child who presents with a patent sinus tract (as evidenced by obvious leaking of CSF or recurrent bouts of meningitis) should be treated in an expeditious fashion to minimize the risk of further infection. Preoperative imaging should be reviewed carefully for evidence of an intradural or intramedullary dermoid, which must be completely excised to avoid recurrence.

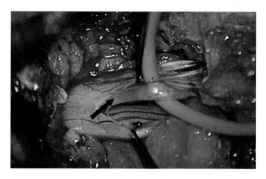

Fig. 4. Isolation of the fatty filum (*arrow*) with normal nerves below.

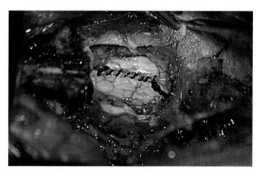

Fig. 6. Watertight dural closure using a running stitch.

Neurenteric cysts often are extremely adherent to the spinal cord and, because of the risk of recurrence, should be resected completely if possible. The surgeon must weigh the risks and benefits of total resection against the possibility of creating unacceptable neurologic deficits, paying particular attention to vital ventral spinal cord vasculature to avoid inadvertent cord ischemia. Finally, in some neurenteric cysts it may be useful to consider a ventral approach for improved exposure [42].

Surgical complications

Complications

Cerebrospinal fluid leak

CSF leak is a worrisome complication of surgeries in children who have a tethered cord because the dural anatomy may be abnormal before surgery and may be compromised further by the operative procedure. A meticulous, watertight dural closure is critical to avoid this potential complication, with dural substitutes and sealants used when necessary [68]. Several centers, including Children's Hospital of Boston, routinely keep patients who have complex untethering operations (but not an uncomplicated fatty filum) prone for several days following durotomy to facilitate dural apposition, with slow incremental elevation of the patient's head over subsequent days. Re-exploration may be warranted should CSF leak be observed, and the inclusion of plastic surgery staff for patients who have had extensive surgery or multiple operations may be helpful in planning alternative methods of closure, such as transposition flaps.

Retethering

Retethering of the cord is common, particularly in complex cases when not all of the adherent, tethering tissue can be removed, such as in a deep-seated transitional lipoma. At Children's Hospital of Boston children who have complex lesions may be kept prone to minimize adhesions to the dural suture line in the immediate postoperative period. In addition, this positioning helps minimize potential contamination of the wound by urine and feces.

Patients who have transitional lipomas have a significantly higher frequency of symptomatic retethering than patients who have either caudal or dorsal lipomas [36,74]. In a retrospective study by Colak and colleagues [74] with a median follow-up of 58 months after lipomyelomeningocele repair, 20.2% of patients had symptomatic retethering.

No dural graft material is completely free from the complication of retethering, including Gore-Tex, pericardial grafts, Silastic, and allograft dura.

In general, the diagnosis of retethering often is based on clinical examination and history. Any new or significantly progressive orthopedic, urologic, or neurologic symptom should be evaluated for the possibility of retethering. Unfortunately, although a large number of diagnostic tools are available to the clinician, few have reliably predicted retethering.

Worsening scoliosis may be part of the clinical picture of retethering and may be identified objectively by serial plain-film radiographs. Urodynamics has been shown to be a useful tool in the evaluation of the patient suspected of having symptomatic retethering. Creating a urodynamic score (based on bladder volume, compliance, detrusor activity, and vesico-sphincteric synergy) both preoperatively and postoperatively has been shown to be a reliable method for detecting retethering [75]. MRI has not proven particularly effective in evaluating retethering because the postoperative conus position often is similar to preoperative images, although evidence of an enlarging syrinx often is considered worrisome for retethering. Serial somatosensory-evoked potential testing for retethering has high false-positive (71%) and false-negative (43%) rates and has not proven to be particularly useful in supporting the clinical diagnosis of retethering [74,76].

Follow-up

Strategies for following patients who have been diagnosed as having a tethered cord often vary based on the underlying cause, treatment, and outcome. Patients who have been treated for a fatty filum with a straightforward sectioning operation and who are neurologically well may not need much in the way of long-term follow-up. In contrast, children who have more anatomically complex lesions, such as large lipomas or myelomeningocele, may need long-term, regular follow-up, involving multidisciplinary medical and social services, to monitor for potential retethering [66]. Interdisciplinary care, often including neurosurgery, orthopedics, urology, psychiatry, medicine, and social work, may be required to minimize potential further medical complications while maintaining the child's educational and social developmental trajectory as much as possible. In addition, some patients may suffer from complex pain syndromes, and consultation with a pain service team may be helpful.

From practical standpoint, the role of the neurosurgeon in the follow-up of patients who have complex tethered cords often involves annual neurologic examinations, periodic imaging studies (to evaluate for scoliosis, syrinx development or—in shunted patients—shunt failure), and review of periodic urodynamic studies.

Although retethering can occur at any time, the risk often decreases once adult stature is reached and growth has stopped. Nonetheless, in children who have complex tethering lesions delayed retethering can occur, sometimes decades later. A current problem faced by many pediatric neurosurgeons is managing the transition of patients treated initially as children into adulthood. Although debate regarding the best strategy to manage this transition is ongoing, it is accepted that a continued relationship with neurosurgery is mandatory for the treatment of this challenging population.

Summary

Tethered cord syndrome is a clinical phenomenon resulting from anatomic restriction of the normal movement of the spinal cord or vascular compromise leading to hypoxia of its distal structures. Causes of tethering can be acquired (secondary) or congenital (primary). A detailed understanding of the embryologic causes of primary tethered cord can aid in the diagnosis and treatment of patients who have these conditions. Surgical intervention, when indicated, is directed at releasing the tethered cord; intraoperative neurophysiologic monitoring in certain patients and meticulous dural closure whenever possible are important adjuncts to the operative procedure, regardless of the mechanism of cord restriction. Retethering of the released spinal cord may occur over time in certain subgroups of patients who should be regularly followed over time to monitor their neurologic, orthopedic, and urologic stability.

References

[1] Hoffman HJ, Hendrick EB, Humphreys RP. The tethered spinal cord: its protean manifestations, diagnosis and surgical correction. Childs Brain 1976; 2(3):145–55.

[2] Yamada S, Iacono RP. Tethered cord syndrome. In: Pang D, editor. Disorders of the pediatric spine. New York: Raven Press; 1995. p. 159–73.

[3] Sarwar M, Crelin ES, Kier EL, et al. Experimental cord stretchability and the tethered cord syndrome. AJNR Am J Neuroradiol 1983;4(3):641–3.

[4] Warder DE, Oakes WJ. Tethered cord syndrome and the conus in a normal position. Neurosurgery 1993;33(3):374–8.

[5] Selden NR. Occult tethered cord syndrome: the case for surgery. J Neurosurg 2006;104(Suppl 5):302–4.

[6] Nazar GB, Casale AJ, Roberts JG, et al. Occult filum terminale syndrome. Pediatr Neurosurg 1995; 23(5):228–35.

[7] Tubbs RS, Oakes WJ. Can the conus medullaris in normal position be tethered? Neurol Res 2004; 26(7):727–31.

[8] Selcuki M, Coskun K. Management of tight filum terminale syndrome with special emphasis on normal level conus medullaris (NLCM). Surg Neurol 1998;50(4):318–22 [discussion: 322].

[9] Selcuki M, Vatansever S, Inan S, et al. Is a filum terminale with a normal appearance really normal? Childs Nerv Syst 2003;19(1):3–10.

[10] Khoury AE, Hendrick EB, McLorie GA, et al. Occult spinal dysraphism: clinical and urodynamic outcome after division of the filum terminale. J Urol 1990;144(2 Pt 2):426–8 [discussion: 428–9, 443–4].

[11] Wehby MC, O'Hollaren PS, Abtin K, et al. Occult tight filum terminale syndrome: results of surgical untethering. Pediatr Neurosurg 2004;40(2):51–7 [discussion: 58].

[12] Hoffman HJ. The tethered spinal cord. In: Holtzman RNN, Stein BM, editors. The tethered spinal cord. New York: Theime-Stratton; 1985. p. 91–8.

[13] Johnson A. Fatty tumour from the sacrum of a child, connected with the spinal membranes. Transactions of the Pathological Society of London 1857; 8:16–8.

[14] Jones WL. Spina bifida occulta: no paralytic symptoms until seventeen years of age: spine trephined to relieve pressure on the cauda equina: recovery. Br Med J 1891;1:173–4.

[15] Spiller WG. Congenital and acquired enuresis from spinal lesion: a) myelodysplasia; b) stretching of the cauda equina. Am J Med Sci 1916;151: 469–75.

[16] Brickner WM. Spina bifida occulta: (1) with external signs, with symptoms; (2) with external signs, without symptoms; (3) without external signs, with symptoms; (4) without external signs; without symptoms. Am J Med Sci 1918;155(4):473–502.

[17] Warf BC. Pathophysiology of tethered cord syndrome. In: McLone DG, editor. Pediatric neurosurgery: surgery of the developing nervous system. 4th edition. Philadelphia: Saunders; 2001. p. 282–8.

[18] Fuchs A. Über den klinischen Nachweis kongenitaler Defektbildungen in den unteren Rückenmarksabschnitten ("Myelodysplasia"). Wien Med Wochenschr 1909;37:2141–7.

[19] Ingraham FD, Lowrey JJ. Spina bifida and cranium bifidum. N Engl J Med 1943;228(23):745–50.

[20] Lichtenstein BW. "Spinal dysraphism": spina bifida and myelodysplasia. Arch Neurol Psychiatry 1904; 44:792–890.

[21] Garceau GJ. The filum terminale syndrome (the cord-traction syndrome). J Bone Joint Surg Am 1953;35A(3):711–6.

[22] Hendrick EB, Hoffman HJ, Humphreys RP. The tethered spinal cord. Clin Neurosurg 1983;30: 457–63.

[23] Dias MS, McLone DG. Normal and abnormal early development of the nervous system. In: McLone DG, editor. Pediatric neurosurgery: surgery of the developing nervous system. 4th edition. Philadelphia: Saunders; 2001. p. 31–71.

[24] Muller F, O'Rahilly R. The development of the human brain, the closure of the caudal neuropore, and the beginning of secondary neurulation at stage 12. Anat Embryol (Berl) 1987;176(4):413–30.

[25] Muller F, O'Rahilly R. The primitive streak, the caudal eminence and related structures in staged human embryos. Cells Tissues Organs 2004;177(1):2–20.

[26] O'Rahilly R, Muller F. Neurulation in the normal human embryo. Ciba Found Symp 1994;181:70–82 [discussion: 82–79].

[27] Van Allen MI, Kalousek DK, Chernoff GF, et al. Evidence for multi-site closure of the neural tube in humans. Am J Med Genet 1993;47(5):723–43.

[28] Wilson DA, Prince JR. John Caffey award. MR imaging determination of the location of the normal conus medullaris throughout childhood. AJR Am J Roentgenol 1989;152(5):1029–32.

[29] Wolf S, Schneble F, Troger J. The conus medullaris: time of ascendence to normal level. Pediatr Radiol 1992;22(8):590–2.

[30] Catala M. Embryogenesis. Why do we need a new explanation for the emergence of spina bifida with lipoma? Childs Nerv Syst 1997;13(6):336–40.

[31] Catala M. Embryonic and fetal development of structures associated with the cerebro-spinal fluid in man and other species. Part I: the ventricular system, meninges and choroid plexuses. Arch Anat Cytol Pathol 1998;46(3):153–69.

[32] O'Rahilly R, Muller F. The meninges in human development. J Neuropathol Exp Neurol 1986;45(5): 588–608.

[33] McLone DG, Thompson DNP. Lipomas of the spine. In: McLone DG, editor. Pediatric neurosurgery: surgery of the developing nervous system. 4th edition. Philadelphia: Saunders; 2001. p. 289–301.

[34] Iskander BJ, Oakes WJ. Anomalies of the spine and spinal cord. In: McLone DG, editor. Pediatric neurosurgery: surgery of the developing nervous system. 4th edition. Philadelphia: Saunders; 2001. p. 307–23.

[35] Emans PJ, van Aalst J, van Heurn EL, et al. The Currarino triad: neurosurgical considerations. Neurosurgery 2006;58(5):924–9.

[36] Chapman PH. Congenital intraspinal lipomas: anatomic considerations and surgical treatment. Childs Brain 1982;9(1):37–47.

[37] Pierre-Kahn A, Zerah M, Renier D, et al. Congenital lumbosacral lipomas. Childs Nerv Syst 1997;13(6): 298–334 [discussion: 335].

[38] McLone DG, Naidich TP. Terminal myelocystocele. Neurosurgery 1985;16(1):36–43.

[39] Dias MS, Walker ML. The embryogenesis of complex dysraphic malformations: a disorder of gastrulation? Pediatr Neurosurg 1992;18(5–6):229–53.

[40] Pang D. Split cord malformation: part II: clinical syndrome. Neurosurgery 1992;31(3):481–500.

[41] Pang D, Dias MS, Ahab-Barmada M. Split cord malformation: part I: a unified theory of embryogenesis for double spinal cord malformations. Neurosurgery 1992;31(3):451–80.

[42] Menezes AH, Traynelis VC. Spinal neurenteric cysts in the magnetic resonance imaging era. Neurosurgery 2006;58(1):97–105 [discussion: 197–105].

[43] Cohen AR, Robinson S. Early management of myelomeningocele. In: McLone DG, editor. Pediatric neurosurgery: surgery of the developing nervous system. 4th edition. Philadelphia: Saunders; 2001. p. 241–59.

[44] Guggisberg D, Hadj-Rabia S, Viney C, et al. Skin markers of occult spinal dysraphism in children: a review of 54 cases. Arch Dermatol 2004;140(9): 1109–15.

[45] Schenk JP, Herweh C, Gunther P, et al. Imaging of congenital anomalies and variations of the caudal spine and back in neonates and small infants. Eur J Radiol 2006;58(1):3–14.

[46] Blaivas JG. Urologic abnormalities in the tethered spinal cord. In: Holtzman RNN, Stein BM, editors. The tethered spinal cord. New York: Theime-Stratton; 1985. p. 59–73.

[47] McGuire EJ, Woodside JR, Borden TA, et al. Prognostic value of urodynamic testing in myelodysplastic patients. J Urol 1981;126(2):205–9.

[48] Scott RM. Delayed deterioration in patients with spinal tethering syndromes. In: Holtzman RNN, Stein BM, editors. The tethered spinal cord. New York: Theime-Stratton; 1985. p. 116–24.

[49] Tarcan T, Onol FF, Ilker Y, et al. The timing of primary neurosurgical repair significantly affects neurogenic bladder prognosis in children with myelomeningocele. J Urol 2006;176(3):1161–5.

[50] Naidich TP, McLone DG. Neuroradiology: ultrasonography versus computed tomography. In: Holtzman RNN, Stein BM, editors. The tethered spinal cord. New York: Theime-Stratton; 1985. p. 47–58.

[51] Yamada S, Zinke DE, Sanders D. Pathophysiology of "tethered cord syndrome". J Neurosurg 1981; 54(4):494–503.

[52] Schneider SJ, Rosenthal AD, Greenberg BM, et al. A preliminary report on the use of laser-Doppler flowmetry during tethered spinal cord release. Neurosurgery 1993;32(2):214–7 [discussion: 217–8].

[53] Tani S, Yamada S, Knighton RS. Extensibility of the lumbar and sacral cord. Pathophysiology of the tethered spinal cord in cats. J Neurosurg 1987;66(1): 116–23.

[54] Breig A. Overstretching of and circumscribed pathological tension in the spinal cord—a basic cause of symptoms in cord disorders. J Biomech 1970;3(1): 7–9.

[55] Fujita Y, Yamamoto H. An experimental study on spinal cord traction effect. Spine 1989;14(7): 698–705.

[56] Steinbok P, Garton HJ, Gupta N. Occult tethered cord syndrome: a survey of practice patterns. J Neurosurg 2006;104(5 Suppl):309–13.

[57] Pallatroni HF, Ball PA, Duhaime AC. Split cord malformation as a cause of tethered cord syndrome in a 78-Year-old female. Pediatr Neurosurg 2004; 40(2):80–3.

[58] Pierz K, Banta J, Thomson J, et al. The effect of tethered cord release on scoliosis in myelomeningocele. J Pediatr Orthop 2000;20(3):362–5.

[59] Metcalfe PD, Luerssen TG, King SJ, et al. Treatment of the occult tethered spinal cord for neuropathic bladder: results of sectioning the filum terminale. J Urol 2006;176(4 Pt 2):1826–9 [discussion: 1830].

[60] Nogueira M, Greenfield SP, Wan J, et al. Tethered cord in children: a clinical classification with urodynamic correlation. J Urol 2004;172(4 Pt 2):1677–80 [discussion: 1680].

[61] Selcuki M, Unlu A, Ugur HC, et al. Patients with urinary incontinence often benefit from surgical detethering of tight filum terminale. Childs Nerv Syst 2000;16(3):150–4 [discussion: 155].

[62] Tarcan T, Bauer S, Olmedo E, et al. Long-term followup of newborns with myelodysplasia and normal urodynamic findings: is followup necessary? J Urol 2001;165(2):564–7.

[63] Tarcan T, Onol FF, Ilker Y, et al. Does surgical release of secondary spinal cord tethering improve the prognosis of neurogenic bladder in children with myelomeningocele? J Urol 2006;176(4 Pt 1):1601–6 [discussion: 1606].

[64] Satar N, Bauer SB, Shefner J, et al. The effects of delayed diagnosis and treatment in patients with an occult spinal dysraphism. J Urol 1995;154(2 Pt 2): 754–8.

[65] Drake JM. Occult tethered cord syndrome: not an indication for surgery. J Neurosurg 2006;104(5 Suppl): 305–8.

[66] McDonald CM. Rehabilitation of children with spinal dysraphism. Neurosurg Clin N Am 1995;6(2): 393–412.

[67] Pang D. Use of an anal sphincter pressure monitor for identification of sacral nerve roots and conus. In: Holtzman RNN, Stein BM, editors. The tethered spinal cord. New York: Theime-Stratton; 1985. p. 74–84.

[68] Pang D. Surgical complications of open spinal dysraphism. Neurosurg Clin N Am 1995;6(2): 243–57.

[69] McLone DG. Lipomeylomeningocele repair. In: McLone DG, editor. Pediatric neurosurgery: surgery of the developing nervous system. 4th edition. Philadelphia: Saunders; 2001. p. 302–6.

[70] McLone DG, Naidich TP. Spinal dysraphism: experimental and clinical. In: Holtzman RNN, Stein BM, editors. The tethered spinal cord. New York: Theime-Stratton; 1985. p. 14–28.

[71] Aliredjo RP, de Vries J, Menovsky T, et al. The use of Gore-Tex membrane for adhesion prevention in tethered spinal cord surgery: technical case reports. Neurosurgery 1999;44(3):674–7 [discussion: 677–8].

[72] Inoue HK, Kobayashi S, Ohbayashi K, et al. Treatment and prevention of tethered and retethered spinal cord using a Gore-Tex surgical membrane. J Neurosurg 1994;80(4):689–93.

[73] Blount JP, Tubbs RS, Okor M, et al. Supraplacode spinal cord transection in paraplegic patients with myelodysplasia and repetitive symptomatic tethered spinal cord. J Neurosurg 2005;103(1 Suppl): 36–9.

[74] Colak A, Pollack IF, Albright AL. Recurrent tethering: a common long-term problem after lipomyelomeningocele repair. Pediatr Neurosurg 1998;29(4): 184–90.

[75] Meyrat BJ, Tercier S, Lutz N, et al. Introduction of a urodynamic score to detect pre- and postoperative neurological deficits in children with a primary tethered cord. Childs Nerv Syst 2003;19(10–11): 716–21.

[76] Li V, Albright AL, Sclabassi R, et al. The role of somatosensory evoked potentials in the evaluation of spinal cord retethering. Pediatr Neurosurg 1996; 24(3):126–33.

NEUROSURGERY
CLINICS
OF NORTH AMERICA

Neurosurg Clin N Am 18 (2007) 549–568

ELSEVIER
SAUNDERS

Chiari Malformations, Syringohydromyelia and Scoliosis

Todd C. Hankinson, MD[a],*, Paul Klimo, Jr, MD, MPH, Maj, USAF[b],
Neil A. Feldstein, MD[a], Richard C.E. Anderson, MD[a],
Douglas Brockmeyer, MD[c]

[a]Department of Neurosurgery, Columbia University, College of Physicians and Surgeons,
710 West 168th Street, New York, NY 10032, USA
[b]88th Medical Group SGOS/SGCXN, 4881 Sugar Maple Drive, WPAFB, OH 45433, USA
[c]Department of Neurosurgery, University of Utah, Division of Pediatric Neurosurgery,
Primary Children's Medical Center, 100 North Medical Drive, Salt Lake City, UT 84113, USA

This article addresses the key features, presentation, and current management of pediatric patients who have Chiari I and Chiari II malformations. It further discusses syringohydromyelia and scoliosis as they relate to pediatric Chiari malformations. Because of the focus on pediatric patients, acquired Chiari malformations are not discussed. Current management algorithms for the more recently described Chiari 0 (syringohydromyelia in the absence of cerebellar tonsillar herniation) and Chiari 1.5 (tonsillar herniation with associated brain stem herniation) malformations are based on the principles developed for the treatment of the more common Chiari I and Chiari II malformations. As such, Chiari 0 and 1.5 are not discussed.

Chiari I malformation

Key features

The key feature of Chiari I malformation (CMI) is downward hindbrain herniation through the foramen magnum. Herniation always includes the cerebellar tonsils, and, in more severe cases, it can include portions of the medulla and fourth ventricle. The presentation of CMI is influenced

by the age of the patient and the specific site of compression. Syringohydromyelia and scoliosis are present in 10% to 20% of patients who have CMI and often contribute to the clinical findings. There is no effective medical treatment for the neurological symptoms of CMI. Surgical therapy through posterior fossa decompression is the most common treatment for symptomatic pediatric patients who have CMI.

Imaging

The introduction of MRI technology resulted in a dramatic increase in the diagnosis of tonsillar herniation and demonstrated that prevalence is likely greater than previous estimates of 1 in 1000. Although often debated, most clinicians will give a diagnosis of CMI if the cerebellar tonsils descend 5 mm below the foramen magnum and demonstrate a peg-like morphology, rather than the normal rounded shape. (Fig. 1) Using MRI data from 221 patients without hindbrain pathology, Mikulis and colleagues [1] proposed criteria defining tonsillar ectopia. During the first decade of life, ectopia would be present in cases of herniation greater than 6 mm below the foramen magnum. During the second and third decades, herniation of greater than 5 mm would constitute ectopia. Although herniation of greater than 5 mm generally is associated with symptoms, patients who have as much as 12 mm of tonsillar herniation may be asymptomatic [2]. Therefore,

* Corresponding author.
 E-mail address: tch12@columbia.edu
(T.C. Hankinson).

1042-3680/07/$ - see front matter © 2007 Elsevier Inc. All rights reserved.
doi:10.1016/j.nec.2007.04.002

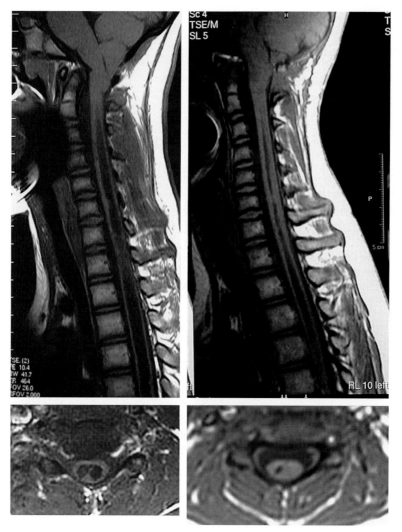

Fig. 1. Preoperative (*left*) and 4-month postoperative (*right*) sagittal and axial T1 weighted MRI scans of a patient who underwent bony decompression without duraplasty for Chiari I malformation with syringomyelia The postoperative images demonstrate a significant reduction in hindbrain compression and syrinx size. The patient's symptoms completely resolved postoperatively.

radiological findings must be judged within the clinical context [3–6].

Pathophysiology

Current research indicates that noniatrogenic hindbrain herniation usually results from a volume discrepancy between the posterior fossa cranium and the neural tissue residing within it. In adult patients who have CMI, Stovner and colleagues [7] identified a significantly smaller posterior fossa in patients who had CMI, and Milhorat and colleagues [8] recorded a 40% reduction in posterior fossa cerebrospinal fluid (CSF) volume with normal brain volume. Some work in children has suggested that those who have syringohydromyelia have disproportionately small posterior fossa volumes, whereas those without a syrinx may have normal posterior volumes [9]. In the 1960s, Gardner proposed that CSF pulsations from the choroid plexus play a significant role in the expansion of the neural tube [10]. He suggested that the balance between the pulsatile flow in the supratentorial and fourth ventricular choroids plexi directed brain growth differentially. If the fourth ventricular pulsations were overactive, the tentorium would be pushed upward, and a Dandy Walker malformation could develop; conversely, if the supratentorial pulsations were overactive, tentorial migration became such that the posterior fossa was small, thus creating the Chiari malformation. Propagation of the Chiari malformation by repeated Valsalva's maneuvers was suggested by Williams [11,12]. He believed that with Valsalva's maneuvers, there is an increase in the intracranial and intraspinal compartments causing fluid to flow cranially and caudally. There is no resistance to cranial flow; however, caudal flow is delayed by hindbrain adhesions and outlet obstruction, creating a pressure differential that then leads to worsening hindbrain impaction and syringohydromyelia. Modern theories suggest that maldevelopment of the para-axial mesoderm of the fourth occipital sclerotome produces subnormal posterior fossa volume, while there is no reduction in infratentorial brain volume, precipitating hindbrain herniation through the foramen magnum [13–18].

Although no gene or gene combination has been correlated with CMI, familial clustering and an association with genetic syndromes such as achondroplasia, hypophosphatemic rickets, Albright's hereditary osteodystrophy, and William's syndrome provide evidence for a genetic contribution to some cases [19–22]. Many children who have CMI are not symptomatic with other illnesses. In children who have symptomatic and asymptomatic CMI, however, Genitori and colleagues [23] described concomitant conditions including hydrocephalus, cranio–facial syndromes, epilepsy, occult spinal dysraphism, and precocious puberty. Other cranio–vertebral abnormalities associated with CMI include syringohydromyelia, proatlantal remnants, basilar invagination, atlanto–occipital assimilation, and Klippel-Feil malformation [15,23–25].

Signs and symptoms

In children who have CMI, the most common presenting symptom is headache, with or without posterior cervical pain, which occurs in 28% to 63% of patients (Table 1) [13,16,23,24,26–30]. Classically, the pain is severe and paroxysmal, often related to Valsalva's maneuvers; less frequently it is dull and persistent [13,14,25,26, 29,31]. In nonverbal children, pain may manifest as persistent crying or irritability and sometimes with hyperextension of the neck or opisthotonos [25,30,32]. In adults and older children, symptoms have been correlated with the site of compression. Cerebellar compression may cause ataxia and nystagmus; brain stem compression may produce pain, dysphagia and facial numbness. Spinal cord compression, often caused by a syrinx, may cause pain, weakness and/or sensory changes [13,24]. Lower cranial nerve dysfunction is present in approximately 20% of patients and can manifest as sleep apnea, dysarthria, hoarseness, recurrent aspiration, and tongue atrophy [25,26,33–36].

In series of children presenting with CMI, numbness or sensory loss has been reported in 26% to 50% of patients [23,26–28]. Motor loss is present in 12% to 19% of patients, and it is considerably more common in patients who harbor a syrinx [26,28]. Genitori reported vertigo in 31% of patients without a syrinx and 40% of patients who have syringohydromyelia [23].

Clinical evaluation

As stated previously, MRI has allowed many children who have CMI to be diagnosed before significant symptoms develop [4,16,25,26]. Workup of a child who presents with CMI should include supratentorial imaging to rule out an acquired Chiari caused by a mass lesion or hydrocephalus, and total spine imaging to assess for the presence of a syrinx, scoliosis, or other less common abnormality such as a tethered cord. If a shunt is present, evaluation of shunt function also should be completed [13]. In cases where symptoms have not yet developed, some authors have advocated CSF flow studies such as phase-contrast MRI to help the clinician determine if CSF flow is impaired at the cranio–cervical junction [13,37]. Thin-cut CT scan with two-dimensional reconstructions, although less sensitive than MRI for the diagnosis of tonsillar herniation or syringohydromyelia, may aid in the identification of bony abnormalities at the cranio–cervical junction. Upright total spine radiographs are best to assess for scoliosis, and flexion/extension radiographs may be needed to rule out instability.

Treatment and outcomes

The primary goal of surgical treatment of CMI is to restore normal physiologic CSF flow at the cranio–cervical junction. Posterior fossa decompression accomplishes this by restoring the posterior fossa subarachnoid space. This decompresses

Table 1
Presenting symptoms in pediatric Chiari I malformation

Author (year)	N	HA/neck pain	Sensory loss	Motor loss	CN/BS/cerebellar	Ataxia	Scoliosis
Navarro [16] (2004)	96	53 (55.2%)	NS	NS	19 (19.8%)	NS	14 (14.6%)
Tubbs, et al [30] (2003)	130	55 (42.3%)	NS	NS	NS	12 (9.2%)	23 (17.7%)
Alzate [26] (2001)[a]	66	36 (54.5%)	20 (30.3%)	8 (12.1%)	14 (21.2%)	4 (6.1%)	11 (16.7%)
Park [28] (1997)	68	43 (63.2%)	18 (26.5%)	13 (19.1%)	NS	NS	19 (27.9%)
Ellenbogen, et al [14] (2000)	36	27 (75.0%)	20 (55.6%)	17 (47.2%)	NS	9 (25.0%)	19 (52.8%)
Kreiger (1999)	31	16 (51.6%)	9 (29.0%)	12 (38.7%)	NS	7 (22.6%)	20 (64.5%)

Abbreviations: CN/BS, cranial nerve/brain stem; HA, headache; NS, not stated.
[a] 52 of 66 patients were <20 years of age.

the cerebellar tonsils and brain stem and also may eliminate the cranial–spinal CSF pressure differential that likely contributes to syrinx formation [38,39].

The first step in surgical planning is the decision whether to open the dura (Figs. 1 and 2). There is evidence to support preservation of the dura and dural opening [30,40], and this decision is based upon the surgeon's experience and preference. If the dura is opened, intradural maneuvers may be completed (Fig. 3). Although recent literature indicates a decrease in the use of shunting and tonsillar reduction [4,16,24,26,27,39,41–43], there is no consensus regarding the application of intradural

maneuvers to improve CSF flow following bony decompression [4,16,24,26,28,34,39]. Two recent surveys of pediatric neurosurgeons reflect this variability [4,39]. In the treatment of symptomatic patients without a syrinx, Haroun received an almost even distribution of respondents (between 20% and 30% each) recommending bony decompression alone, duraplasty, intradural dissection, or tonsillar manipulation. Schijman and Steinbok [39] found that 76% of surgeons always open the dura, and 20% sometimes do so. Using intraoperative brain stem auditory-evoked responses (BAERs) during CMI decompression, Anderson and colleagues [44] have offered evidence that

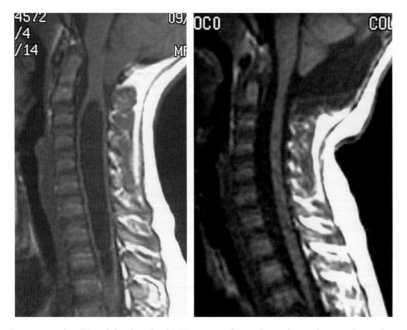

Fig. 2. Pre- and postoperative T1 weighted sagittal MRI scans of a patient who underwent bony decompression with duraplasty for Chiari I malformation with syringomyelia. Postoperative images demonstrate a significant retrocerebellar cisternal space and resolution of hindbrain compression and syringomyelia. The patient's symptoms completely resolved postoperatively.

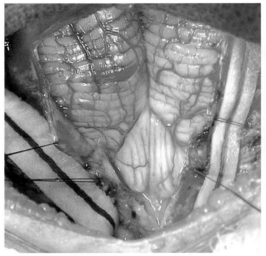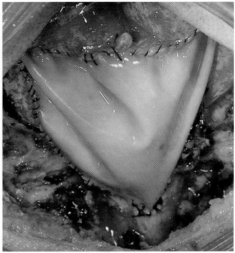

Fig. 3. Intraoperative photographs of the patient in Fig. 2. The left panel demonstrates the peg-like appearance of the herniated cerebellar tonsils following dural opening. The right panel demonstrates the relaxed appearance of the duraplasty before closure. No tonsillar reduction was undertaken.

improved conduction of nerve impulses through the brain stem occurs after the bony decompression rather than the dural opening.

In a recent study by Yeh and colleagues [45], the authors used intraoperative ultrasound to determine whether bony decompression alone was adequate. Following a standard suboccipital craniectomy and one or more laminectomies, ultrasound was used to evaluate the decompression. Decompression was considered adequate if there was a CSF space anterior to the brainstem and dorsal to the tonsils without evidence of abnormal tonsillar piston activity. If the decompression was inadequate, the dura was opened with inspection of the fourth ventricle, tonsillar reduction, and stent placement in some cases. In their series of 130 patients, 91 underwent a bony decompression and duraplasty, and 39 underwent bony decompression alone. There were four surgical failures in the bone decompression group and two in the duraplasty group, but 12 patients in the duraplasty group had complications, whereas no patients in the bone decompression group had complications.

Despite significant literature describing the treatment of CMI, a lack of standard treatment regimens and outcome measures, along with an absence of randomized trials, makes results somewhat difficult to assess. Most authors report clinical improvement in 65% to 90% of cases (Table 2).

The largest series of pediatric decompression for Chiari I includes 130 patients who underwent posterior fossa decompression and duraplasty by

a single surgeon [30]. Stent placement was used early in the series but later abandoned. Tonsillar coagulation was used in 22 patients (17%), eight of whom had subsequent procedures to treat syringohydromyelia. Relief of preoperative pathology was accomplished in 83% of patients. Headache did not resolve in 12% of patients, and complications occurred in 2.3%.

Navarro and colleagues [16] compared outcomes between surgical regimens in 96 children who had CMI. Posterior fossa decompression without dural opening led to improved symptoms in 72.2% of patients. Dural opening without tonsillar manipulation improved symptoms in 68.4% of patients, and symptoms improved in 60.8% of those who underwent tonsillar manipulation. Although rates of clinical improvement were similar, complications were significantly more frequent in the groups who underwent dural opening. There was a 5.6% complication rate in those who did not undergo dural opening, while the rate with duraplasty alone was 42.1%, and with tonsillar manipulation it was 21.7%. Most complications were related to CSF flow. As a result, patients later in the series were treated without dural opening unless intraoperative ultrasound failed to demonstrate adequate decompression. Neither the presence of syringohydromyelia nor any other specific presenting symptom was predictive of clinical outcome. The only variable predictive of a positive clinical outcome was age at diagnosis younger than 8 years.

Table 2
Outcomes following surgical intervention for Chiari I malformation

Author (year)	N	Syrinx (%)	Intervention	N	Clinical improvement	Syrinx improvement	Complications	Reoperation
Navarro [16] (2004)	96#	41 (42.7)	PFD	71	72%	25/38´ (65.7%)	5.6%	11.3%
			PFD+D	24	68%		42.1%	4.2%
			PFD+D+IM	14	61%		21.7%	28.6%
Tubbs [30] (2003)	130	75 (57.7)	PFD+D+IM		107 (82.3%)	67 (89.3%)	2.3%	6.9%
Alzate [26] (2001)	66	34 (51.5)	PFD+D+IM		66 (100%)	30 (88.2%)	11 (16.7%)	7.5%
Park [28] (1997)	68	40 (58.9)	PFD+D+IM		100%*	32 (80.0%)	7 (10.3%)	4.4%
Kreiger (1999)	31	26 (83.9)	PFD+D+IM		94%**	23 (88.5%)	3 (9.7%)	9.7%
Ellenbogen [14] (2000)	36	28 (80.6)	PFD+D+IM		35 (97.2%)	27 (96.4%)	NS	NS
Genitori et al [23] (2000)	26	10 (38.4)	PFD		100% (no syrinx)	—	0.0%	0.0%
			PFD		94% (syrinx)	8 (80.0%)	7.7%	7.7%
Anderson [40] (2003)	11	6 (54.6)	PFD+D		11 (100%)	6 (100%)	1 (9.1%)	0.0%
Feldstein and Choudhri [86] (1999)	7	7 (100)	PFD+D		7 (100%)	7 (100%)	0 (0.0%)	0.0%˝

Abbreviations: D, duraplasty; IM, intradural maneuvers; NS, not stated; PFD, posterior fossa decompression.
109 total operations
´ Includes all surgical techniques. No difference between techniques was identified
* % of symptoms improved.
** % of total signs and symptoms improved.
˝ 1 child required spinal fusion for 46-degree scoliosis.

Genitori and colleagues [23] studied the effectiveness of posterior fossa decompression with removal of the outer layer of dura in 26 children who had symptomatic CMI. Overall 97.2% of symptoms improved, and MRI demonstrated syrinx resolution in 8 of 10 patients. Complications were limited to two superficial wound infections.

In series that describe the use of variable operative plans, no strategy has emerged as superior under all circumstances. Recent trends in first-line management have been away from invasive intradural maneuvers such as stenting or syrinx shunting. Obex plugging largely has been abandoned. The roles of tonsillar reduction and duraplasty remain to be determined. In general, headache, sleep apnea, and other posterior fossa compression syndromes improve in 70% to 100% of cases [16,23,28,41]. In patients presenting with sensory symptoms, improvement also is seen in 70% to 100% of patients, although many do not experience complete resolution [23,26,27,46]. Rates of syrinx improvement or resolution range from 80% to 88% [13,27,28]. Following dural opening, CSF-related complications can be expected in approximately 10% [13,27]. Despite encouraging initial results, a significant number of patients may experience recurrent symptoms 6 to 12 months postoperatively; therefore close clinical follow-up should be maintained [16].

Summary

Current theories regarding CMI assert that mesodermal maldevelopment results in a posterior fossa that lacks the volume to contain the entirety of the neuroectodermal structures that grow within it. Posterior fossa decompression has become the accepted first step in surgical treatment. Whether to open the dura and what intradural maneuvers to perform both remain subjects of significant debate, although there is evidence that the pediatric population responds well to simple bony decompression without dural opening. This may be because of an increased distensibility of the dura itself, or it may be because the disease process is addressed earlier in its course. At this point, there are no standard outcome measures, nor has there been a randomized trial comparing different surgical strategies. Despite good initial results, some patients likely will present with recurrent symptoms. Factors that may contribute to a good outcome include early intervention and surgical technique that minimizes complications.

Chiari II malformation

Key features

The Chiari II malformation (CMII) is more complex and generally more severe than CMI. CMII always is paired with myelomeningocele, which occurs in 0.6 of 1000 live births [47]. In neonatal patients, brain stem compression caused by CM II can cause rapid irreversible neurological deterioration; therefore these patients require a high degree of clinical vigilance. All patients born with Chiari II and myelomeningocele require closure of the myelomeningocele within 72 hours of birth (Fig. 4). Most will require CSF diversion for hydrocephalus, and up to 20% ultimately will need cranio–cervical decompression for brain stem decompression [48,49]. The management of hindbrain compression and, to a lesser extent, hydrocephalus, form the focus of this section.

Imaging

The main features of Chiari II are caudal displacement of the pons, medulla, and fourth ventricle, often with elongation and kinking (Box 1). The cerebellar vermis herniates into the cervical spinal canal through an enlarged foramen magnum, and the superior aspect of the cerebellum sits above a dysplastic and low-lying tentorium cerebelli. Cerebellar heterotopias are also common. Supratentorial anomalies include collicular fusion, which gives the radiological impression of tectal plate beaking, and an enlarged massa intermedia. Partial or total agenesis of the corpus callosum is seen in 33% of cases (Fig. 5). Skull deformities include lückenschadel, scalloping of the petrous pyramids, clival shortening, and the previously mentioned enlargement of the foramen magnum [5,50–52]. Hydrocephalus will develop in more than 80% of infants born with CMII, and syringohydromyelia will develop in 48% to 88% [34,53]. Scoliosis will present in 50% to 90% of patients who have CMII, and this is particularly difficult to manage [54].

Pathophysiology

The origin of the myriad abnormalities associated with CMII remains elusive. Current theories suggest that effects from an open neural tube produce multiple independent developmental anomalies, which together generate the widespread abnormalities present in this patient population.

McLone and Knepper [48] posited that the open neural tube defect allows CSF drainage

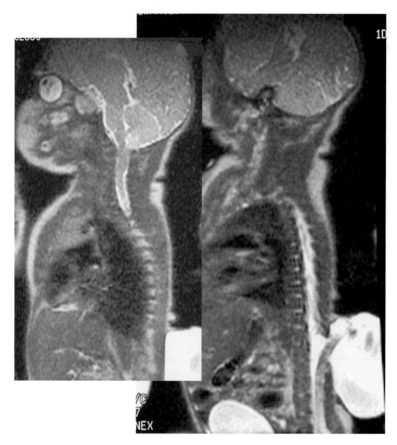

Fig. 4. Mid- and parasagittal T2 weighted MRI images of a neonate with Chiari II malformation and a large myelomeningocele. Note the fusion of the colliculi (tectal beaking), kinking of the medulla, and vermian herniation. The large, bulbous myelomeningocele is appreciated best on the right image.

from the developing ventricular system, reducing the stimulation for expansion upon the cranial vesicles. This produces a small posterior fossa and cerebral disorganization (supra- and infratentorial). The neural structures that reside in the posterior fossa, although below normal size, grow into a small vault, forcing the cerebellar vermis and parts of the brainstem to herniate into adjacent spaces. This theory explains many aspects of the clinical presentation in CMII, although rare cases of Chiari II with closed neural tube defects indicate that other mechanisms also may contribute [55].

Clinical experience in some number of cases supports the hypothesis that brain stem compression, rather than dysgenesis, is responsible for the signs and symptoms that manifest in the Chiari II population [56–59]. Some patients do not manifest symptoms of medullary dysfunction at birth, but instead develop progressive symptoms. Data demonstrating some recovery of function

following decompression further support the concept of a compressive, rather than developmental, etiology of medullary compromise and encourages the practice of rapid surgical decompression rather than palliative treatment in this small group of patients.

Signs and symptoms

The first sign that indicates a CMII malformation is the presence of an open neural tube defect, which invariably requires neonatal repair (Fig. 6). Greater than 80% of children who have myelomeningocele will develop hydrocephalus and require CSF diversion [53]. The signs of inadequate CSF absorption can be obvious (eg, increased occipitofrontal circumference, bulging anterior fontanelle, splaying of the sutures, increasing ventricular size) or subtle (eg, mild exacerbation of syringohydromyelia) [53]. Despite adequate CSF diversion,

Box 1. Anatomical features of Chiari II malformation

Anterior/middle fossa
  Lückenschadel
  Polygyria
  Cortical heterotopia
  Dysgenesis of the Corpus callosum
  Large Massa intermedia
  Tectal beak of the midbrain
  Quadrigeminal cysts
Posterior fossa
  Small bony vault
  Low-lying tentorium with large
    incisura
  Scalloping of the petrous bone
  Clival shortening
  Loss of pontine flexure
  Aqueductal stenosis or forking
  Caudal displacement of the pons,
    medulla, and posterior circulation
  Descent and elongation of the
    cerebellar vermis through the
    foramen magnum
  Descent and kinking of the brain stem
  Dorsal kink of the cervicomedullary
    junction
  Upward herniation of the superior
    cerebellum through the incisura
Spinal cord/canal
  Enlargement of the Foramen magnum
  Spina bifida aperta
  Stretching of the lower cranial nerves
  Caudal displacement of the upper
    cervical cord with horizontal or
    upward course of exiting nerve roots
  Syringohydromyelia

  Adapted from McLone DG, Naidich TP. Developmental morphology of the subarachnoid space, brain vasculature, and contiguous structures, and the cause of the Chiari II malformation. AJNR 1992;13:463–82. © by American Society of Neuroradiology.

8.7% to 21% of children born with myelomeningocele will go on to develop symptoms of hindbrain, cranial nerve, or spinal cord compression, most before the age of 3 months [48,49,56,57,59–61]. At this stage, the symptom complex and urgency of treatment differ between patients who present as neonates and those who present later in childhood.

In patients who present as neonates, mild signs and symptoms of respiratory or gastrointestinal (GI) dysfunction may be harbingers of severe cranial nerve and/or brain stem disease, and symptoms can progress over hours to days. Prompt diagnosis and possible intervention are important, as the preoperative neurological status of the patient is the most reliable predictor of outcome [56,57,60]. In older patients, symptoms are often more insidious, allowing time for proper diagnosis and treatment planning.

The most common source of mortality in the CMII population is respiratory dysfunction. Inspiratory stridor or apneic episodes signal significant lower cranial nerve or medullary dysfunction but may be confused with less severe maladies such as croup. Any symptoms consistent with upper respiratory illness should be investigated, and a low threshold for diagnosis using direct laryngoscopy should be maintained. The preoperative presence of bilateral vocal cord paralysis has been shown to predict poor outcome, which reinforces the current practice to aggressively treat infants with CMII and symptoms referable to hindbrain compression [56,57,60,62].

Neurogenic dysphagia also may represent life-threatening brain stem and lower cranial nerve dysfunction. Approximately 59% to 71% of children who have symptomatic CMII present with feeding or swallowing difficulties [59,60,62]. GI signs such as chronic aspiration, choking, nasal regurgitation, prolonged feeding time, and weight loss are often more subtle than respiratory symptoms, but they predispose to recurrent pneumonitis and may precede other brain stem syndromes [57,59,60]. Other signs of brainstem and spinal cord pathology associated with CMII in patients younger than 2 years of age include extremity weakness, hypotonia, nystagmus, opisthotonos, and a weak cry.

In patients who develop symptoms after the neonatal period, symptoms are more often chronic and rarely require emergent intervention. The most common presenting symptoms in this age group are related to cervical myelopathy and slowly progressive dysphagia. Ataxia and occipital or cranio–cervical pain are also common. As with younger patients, brain stem symptoms are generally progressive if left untreated [57].

Characterization of cervicomedullary and other structural neural abnormalities in patients who have CMII is best completed using MRI. The caudal extent of the brain stem herniation does not correlate with prognosis [63]. Neurophysiologic

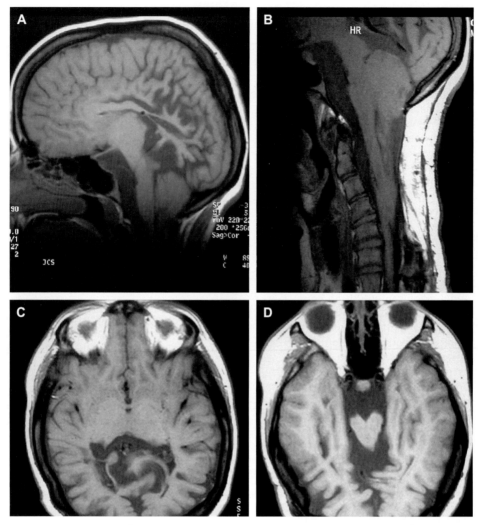

Fig. 5. MRI findings in Chiari II malformation sagittal (*A, B*) and axial (*C, D*). (*A*) Partial agenesis of the corpus callosum, tectal beaking, and low lying torcula. (*B*) Herniation of the cerebellar vermis and tonsils to the level of C5. (*C*) Fusion of the Thalami. (*D*) Tectal beaking and interdigitation of temporo–occipital gyri.

testing such as brainstem auditory evoked responses (BAERs) and somatosensory evoked potentials (SSEPs) may identify infants who are at risk to develop brainstem dysfunction, but it does not correlate with clinical outcome [62,64–66].

Treatment and outcomes

Early myelomeningocele repair is the first operative intervention for almost all infants born with CMII (see Fig. 6). Most patients also will require CSF diversion. If the patient subsequently becomes symptomatic because of hindbrain compression, neurosurgical intervention aims to prevent the progression of symptoms and hopes to reverse them. Current literature does not provide standards for the surgical management of symptomatic CMII; therefore multiple algorithms exist. As discussed previously, the natural history of the disease varies depending on the age of symptom onset [57,59,60,62]. In initially asymptomatic children who develop hindbrain compromise, a surgical strategy should be considered, as outcomes have been shown to correlate with preoperative neurological status [52,56,57]. Neonates who demonstrate significant respiratory distress and brainstem dysfunction from birth, however, are very unlikely to benefit from decompression.

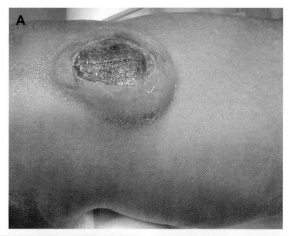

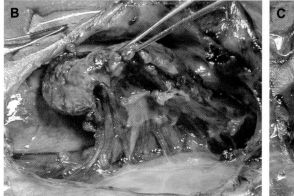
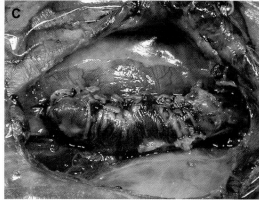

Fig. 6. Pre- and intraoperative photos of a myelomeningocele repair in a child with Chiari II malformation. (*A*) Exposed neural placode. (*B*) Lumbar nerve roots originating from the neural placode. (*C*) Surgically closed caudal neural tube.

Hydrocephalus must be treated adequately before cranio–cervical decompression. If a shunt is present, partial or complete obstruction must be ruled out before posterior fossa decompression. Successful treatment of hydrocephalus has been shown to improve symptoms in up to 23% of children who have Chiari II, and it reliably reduces syrinx size [62,67,68]. The optimal application of third ventriculostomy in this population requires further study, as failure rates of 20% to 30% have been described, and some authors feel that failure of third ventriculostomy is more difficult to diagnose than that of a ventricular shunt [69,70,122].

In successfully shunted patients presenting with significant respiratory dysfunction, preoperative tracheostomy is occasionally necessary. Patients presenting with severe GI dysfunction often stabilize with conservative measures such as metoclopramide and postural adjustment during feeding. Some, however, require preoperative nasogastric tubes or percutaneous gastrostomy to maintain nutrition and/or fundoplication to prevent aspiration [52,57,71].

Outcomes following decompression in patients with CMII vary based on the severity of the preoperative symptoms. Evidence of severe brain stem compromise, such as bilateral vocal cord paralysis or central hypoventilation or apnea, has been correlated with poor recovery and increased mortality [56,57,60,71]. Milder respiratory dysfunction and severe neurogenic dysphagia in the absence of other signs and symptoms from brain stem compromise, however, may respond well to decompression [56,57,59,71]. Age has not been shown to be independently predictive of outcome, but younger patients often present with rapidly progressive signs and symptoms. As such, up to 15% of young symptomatic patients will die before age 3, and a further one third will have permanent neurological deficits [52]. In older patients, mortality approaches 0%, and a good outcome can be expected in up to 60% to 80%

of these patients with aggressive surgical management, with 70% to 100% of patients presenting with cervical myelopathy enjoying an improvement in their symptoms [52,58].

As opposed to the surgical management of CMI, decompression of CMII rarely includes suboccipital craniectomy. Most authors feel adequate decompression is accomplished through cervical laminectomies, as the large foramen magnum that is frequently present in CMII rarely causes compression [59,60,62]. Cervical laminectomies should extend from C1 to the lowest involved cervical level, and, if the dura is opened, the exposure should reveal the caudal extent of the cerebellum. The use of dural opening and intradural exploration remains largely influenced by surgeon experience and preference [4]. When the dura is opened, adequate CSF outflow can be assessed through exploration of the fourth ventricle.

In both a retrospective and subsequent prospective series, Pollack and colleagues demonstrated excellent recovery rates in infants treated with urgent hindbrain decompression [56,57]. The authors used a limited suboccipital craniectomy, appropriate laminectomies, and duraplasty with or without CSF shunting. Sixty-eight percent to 76% of patients had complete or near complete resolution of all symptoms of cervicomedullary compression, while 20% to 23% showed no improvement. The authors found the most significant predictor of poor postoperative outcome to be the presence of bilateral vocal cord paralysis preoperatively. Age was not an independent predictor of outcome. In nine patients who had bilateral vocal cord paralysis, only one achieved notable improvement of symptoms postoperatively, and the five total deaths were all in patients from this group. Vandertop and colleagues [59] achieved complete symptom resolution is 15 of 17 (88%) neonates who were treated with prompt cranio–cervical decompression.

Bell and colleagues [72] treated 22 patients who had symptomatic brain stem compression and CMII. The authors used laminectomy with or without suboccipital decompression. Of the 17 patients who developed symptoms before 6 months of age, 14 underwent surgical intervention. Nine (52.3%) died because of progressive symptoms; three (17.6%) improved, and five (29.4%) became asymptomatic. Among the five patients who presented after 3 years of age, all had complete resolution of their symptoms.

In patients who have syringohydromyelia, posterior fossa decompression relieves symptoms in over 75% and is preferred over syrinx shunting [62,68]. If a syrinx persists or remains symptomatic postoperatively, the surgeon should consider why the decompression was unsuccessful. If the decompression remains adequate, some authors will consider syrinx shunting [62].

In a group of children older than 3 years who have symptomatic CMII, James and Brandt [73] used suboccipital craniectomy and laminectomy without dural opening. There were no perioperative complications, and 72.7% of symptoms improved, with no symptoms becoming worse after surgery. Another series of older patients (mean age at surgery 11.1 years) achieved complete resolution of symptoms in 80% at 1 year follow-up [58].

Postlaminectomy kyphosis is a concern in the pediatric population. A study involving 32 patients who had Chiari malformations (16 CMI and 16 CMII) demonstrated a 9% rate of cervical kyphosis following decompression, with only one patient requiring cervical stabilization. The authors concluded that facet preservation allows for safe cervical decompression in the juvenile population [74].

Summary

Chiari II represents a severe and complex constellation of abnormalities that generally requires multiple surgical interventions and vigilant supportive care through a multidisciplinary team of health care providers. Surgical management begins with closure of the open neural tube defect and also requires CSF diversion in the vast majority of patients. Up to 20% of patients also may require cranio–cervical decompression to prevent irreversible severe medullary compression [48,49]. Decompression should not be considered, however, until a properly functioning shunt is confirmed. When evidence of new-onset respiratory or GI dysfunction presents in the postnatal period, surgical intervention should be considered. Older patients may present with symptoms of hindbrain compression, syringohydromyelia and scoliosis. In this group, treatment is often difficult. The slower progression of symptoms in this group, however, affords clinicians more time to carefully choose the proper course of intervention.

Syringohydromyelia

Key features

Syringohydromyelia is defined by the presence of a cystic cavity in the spinal cord. Although many etiologies exist (eg, trauma and neoplasia), the most common cause of syringohydromyelia is posterior fossa malformation. CMI and CMII are the most common congenital posterior fossa malformations. Syringohydromyelia is present in approximately 20% to 85% of children who have CMI [13,14,16,18,23,27,28,30,31] and is present in 48% to 88% of children who have CMII [34,62]. For the purposes of this section, the term syringo-hydromyelia will be used in reference to all cystic cavities of the spinal cord.

Pathophysiology

Influential early theories explained syrinx formation and extension through a mechanism that depended upon open communication between the ventricular system and the syrinx through the obex [75,76]. The observation that many syringes did not directly communicate with the ventricular system, in addition to the disappointing efficacy of obex plugging [41,42,46] led to the proposal of further theories regarding the origin and physiology of syringohydromyelia [42,77,78]. A detailed discussion of previous theories is beyond the scope of this article, but is reviewed in Oldfield and colleagues [42]. In Oldfield's report, the authors propose that the impacted cerebellar tonsils act as a piston, compressing the cervical spinal cord and cranial aspect of the syrinx with each cardiac cycle [42,79]. This theory has been supported by phase contrast MRI findings demonstrating pathological obstruction of caudal CSF flow at the cranio–cervical junction during cardiac systole [14,42,80]. Likewise, recoil cranial flow during diastole is obstructed by cerebellar herniation. The obstruction to cranial CSF flow during cardiac diastole leads to trapping of CSF in the cervical subarachnoid space. CSF then tracks along peri-vascular spaces into the parenchyma of the spinal cord, creating a syrinx [14,77,81]. Two characteristics of syrinx formation not addressed by this theory are the mechanism underlying an isolated thoracic syrinx [14] and the observation that syringohydromyelia occurs more commonly with moderate degrees of tonsillar herniation as opposed to mild or severe herniation [5,82].

Signs and symptoms

Although children who have a Chiari malformation and no syrinx generally present with pain, those who have syringohydromyelia are more likely to present with motor or sensory changes or scoliosis. Adolescents more often present with motor and sensory disturbances, while younger patients commonly present with scoliosis [16,26,68,82,83]. Among series of children who have CMI and syringohydromyelia, 63% to 100% present with sensory deficits, and 76% to 85% present with scoliosis [83–85]. Genitori and colleagues found that children who presented with syringohydromyelia had an average symptom duration of 43.2 months rather than the 14.3 months observed in children without a syrinx [23]. This indicates a longer evolution of disease and may represent an opportunity for earlier treatment.

The most reliable test for the diagnosis and monitoring of a syrinx is MRI (see Figs. 1 and 2). Both sagittal and axial images should be reviewed to detect smaller syrinxes, although in up to 70% of cases, the syrinx will include the entire length of the cervicothoracic spinal cord [23,26]. Less reliable methods for the diagnosis and monitoring of syringohydromyelia include CT myelography and neurophysiologic testing (eg, BAERs and SSEPs) [23,26]. Children who have a syrinx also should undergo assessment for scoliosis with upright total spine radiographs.

Treatment and outcomes

The goal of treatment for syringohydromyelia in the context of Chiari malformation is to prevent syrinx progression and, if possible, to reduce or eliminate the syrinx. Although no single treatment algorithm is applied universally, experience suggests that decompression of the posterior fossa corrects the pathologic CSF flow dynamics associated with Chiari malformation, leading to syrinx collapse in many cases [38,86]. Current surgical options include posterior fossa decompression without or with dural opening, which then may be left opened or closed by means of duraplasty. Further optional intradural maneuvers include cerebellar tonsil reduction, lysis of adhesions, and exploration of the fourth ventricle. Obex plugging and fourth ventricular stenting largely have fallen out of favor [4,39]. The role of syrinx diversion is controversial, and it frequently is used to treat refractory syringohydromyelia.

The previously mentioned surveys by Haroun and Schijman demonstrate the considerable variation in the way syringohydromyelia is treated. In symptomatic patients, there is little clinical dilemma regarding the need for surgical intervention. There is considerable debate, however, regarding the treatment of patients who have an asymptomatic syrinx. In children who have a Chiari malformation and asymptomatic syringohydromyelia, 28% to 75% (depending upon syrinx diameter) of pediatric neurosurgeons in an international cohort chose surgical intervention. A survey of the pediatric section of the American Association of Neurological Surgeons (AANS) showed that only 9% would always operate on a similar patient. In the presence of occipital headaches, the percentage of surgeons who would operate on patients with an 8 mm syrinx increased to 90% in the international survey. In the AANS survey, 79% would operate under similar circumstances [4,39].

When syringohydromyelia persists or progresses following decompression, some authors choose to re-explore the posterior fossa, while others prefer to divert CSF by means of syringo- or ventricular shunting. Although international survey data indicate that 90% of pediatric neurosurgeons would shunt a refractory syrinx [39], rates of syrinx shunt success range from 30% to 75% and complication rates related primarily to failure or infection are 10% to 25%, with half of the initially successful shunts failing over a 1- to 3-year period [27].

Hida and colleagues [83] treated 16 children who had syringohydromyelia and CMI. Seven patients underwent foramen magnum decompression, and nine underwent syringosubarachnoid shunting. Motor function and sensory disturbance improved in 87.5% and 90% of patients, respectively. Radiographic reduction of syrinx size was achieved in all patients. In 13 patients who presented with scoliosis, five improved (38.5%); five were stable, and three (23.1%) deteriorated.

Feldstein and Choudhri [86] treated seven patients who had CMI and holocord syringomyelia. Using suboccipital decompression and duraplasty without further intradural exploration, six syrinxes were collapsed at 2 to 4 months, and one was reduced. One year following surgery, all collapsed syrinxes remained so, and the other syrinx was reduced by 50%. No patient required reoperation for treatment of a syrinx.

Other series employing posterior fossa decompression for the treatment of pediatric syringohydromyelia demonstrate that there is usually a stabilization of sensory and motor symptoms, but the return of lost tendon reflexes, muscle bulk, and lost sensation is less reliable [16,23,28,46]. Symptoms related to syringohydromyelia are improved in 50% to 75% of cases, and radiologic resolution has been recorded in 73% to 80% [23,27,28].

Nohria and Oakes [31] correlated an improvement in preoperative signs and symptoms with syrinx resolution in a group of 43 patients who had CMI, 31 of whom were younger than 19 years.

Current data do not demonstrate any specific surgical technique to be superior [16,28]. In a study examining surgical intervention with and without duraplasty for children with and without syringohydromyelia, Navarro and colleagues found the only significant predictor of improved outcome to be age less than 8 years at diagnosis. The authors concluded that first-line surgical intervention without dural opening is the safest intervention, given the lack of improved outcome and increased risk associated with dural opening. The superior outcome of younger patients and the possibility that prolonged syringohydromyelia may lead to glial scarring and irreparable spinal cord damage [43,87] indicate that early intervention for patients who have Chiari malformation with syringohydromyelia should be encouraged.

The expansion or appearance of syringohydromyelia following posterior fossa decompression merits a reassessment of the decompression rather than immediate shunting of the syrinx. The presence of hydrocephalus or subdural hygroma may indicate that CSF flow remains impaired. In the case of worsening or a newly appearing syrinx with hydrocephalus, the hydrocephalus should be addressed as the first step.

Summary

Although the pathogenesis of pediatric syringohydromyelia is not understood completely, the close relationship to posterior fossa herniation syndromes such as Chiari malformations indicates that dysfunctional cranio–cervical CSF flow dynamics play an integral role. Clinical and radiological responses following posterior fossa decompression are encouraging, but the optimal management of refractory syringohydromyelia remains controversial. Early intervention to halt or reverse symptoms and prevent irreversible spinal cord damage should be encouraged.

Syringohydromyelia and scoliosis

Although the association between syringohydromyelia and the development of scoliosis was established in the 1940s, it was not until the widespread use of MRI in the early 1990s that it was revealed just how common a neurologic etiology existed for patients diagnosed as having idiopathic scoliosis [88–90]. The mechanism by which the syrinx causes scoliosis has not been determined, but some believe that the syrinx injures either the lower motor neurons or the dorsomedial and ventromedial aspects of the gray matter of the anterior horn of the spinal cord, causing an imbalance of trunk musculature and predisposing to scoliosis [91–95]. Scoliosis has been reported in 25% to 85% of all children who have a syrinx, whereas the incidence of MRI abnormalities in patients who have scoliosis ranges from 4% to 58%, with age and the presence of abnormal clinical findings being two of the most important variables [83,84,96–98].

The proposed indications in the literature to image the neural axis in a patient who has presumed idiopathic scoliosis include:

Neurologic deficits [99–101]
Juvenile onset (<10 years of age) [102–105]
Male gender [105]
Torticollis [106]
Cervical lordosis greater than 0 degrees [104]
Loss of apical lordosis [107]
Abnormal curve patterns (left-sided curve, double thoracic, triple, and a long right thoracic curve with end vertebrae caudal to T12) [97,99,105,108,109]
Rapid curve progression [100,108,110]
Thoracic kyphosis of at least 30 40 degrees [104,105,111]
Presence of pain [100,105,108]

The level of the syrinx also appears to influence the level of the curve. The lower the largest area of the syrinx and the more caudal the level of the syrinx, the more caudally the curve apex and lower-end vertebra were located [112].

As stated previously, the most common cause of syringohydromyelia is herniation of the posterior fossa contents, namely CMI and CMII, followed by tethered cord. Regardless of the cause, it is clear that treatment of the syrinx can halt or reverse the progression of scoliosis. Furthermore, after decompression of the syrinx, surgical correction of scoliosis can be performed with less neurologic risk [105–113]. There are few reports documenting the natural history of syringohydromyelia and the associated changes neurologically and with scoliosis. Tokunaga and colleagues [114] followed 27 patients who had CMI and scoliosis. After an average follow-up of almost 6 years, 14 patients showed a spontaneous decrease in the size of the syrinx by more than 50%, whereas 13 patients had no change

in their syrinx. In the reduction group, cerebellar tonsillar herniation decreased from a mean of 11.3 to 6 mm; 69% showed an improvement in dissociated sensory disturbance, and their scoliosis improved by 5 degrees or more in six patients. Despite the findings of this study, most neurosurgeons feel that the presence of a syrinx warrants treatment, especially if it is causing neurologic deficits.

A syrinx may be treated directly by placing a shunt, most commonly a syringosubarachnoid or syringopleural shunt, or indirectly, by decompressing the posterior fossa contents. The development of scoliosis in the spina bifida (Chiari type II and myelodysplasia) population has been known for many years. It is classified as a neuromuscular scoliosis and is one of the most difficult to treat of all spinal deformities in children. It occurs in 50% to 90% of these patients and in virtually all patients where the lesion is at T12 or higher [54]. It is thought to be caused by a combination of generalized paresis of the trunk musculature, congenital structural changes in the vertebrae. and syringomyelia. Scoliosis can be stabilized or improved with treatment of the syrinx, but the results are not nearly as good compared with patients with Chiari type I [98]. Despite various neurosurgical interventions such as posterior fossa decompressions, cord detetherings and direct shuntings, many patients continue to have progressive spinal deformity and eventually require a fusion [113].

It has only been since the use of MRI that the relations between patients who have CMI, syrinx and scoliosis have been analyzed. The scoliosis generally is thought to be directly caused by the presence of a syrinx, but there are reports of Chiari I patients and scoliosis without a syrinx [92,115,116]. Many Chiari I patients will have scoliosis as their presenting sign and symptom [106]. A review of the literature is shown in Table 3. One of the earliest reports was by Muhonen and colleagues [117]. Eleven patients under the age of 16 who had scoliosis of at least 15 degrees were studied. Surgical intervention consisted of a dorsal posterior fossa decompression in all patients and a transoral ventral decompression in five. The scoliosis improved in eight patients, stabilized in one, and progressed in two, with only one patient eventually needing surgery to correct the deformity. All patients younger than 10 had resolution of their scoliosis, despite preoperative curves of more than 40 degrees. Farley and colleagues [118] had 14 patients with CMI, 10 of whom underwent a syringosubarachnoid shunt for their

Table 3
Outcome of scoliosis in Chiari I patients with treatment of their syrinx

Paper	Year	N	M/F	Average age	Type of surgery	# Curve stabilization (%)	# Curve improvement (%)	# Curve progression (%)	# Spinal fusion (%)
Muhonen, et al [117]	1992	11	N/A	10.1	PFD + TOD	1 (9)	8 (73)	2 (18)	1 (9)
Isu [92]	1992	6	N/A	N/A	N/A	2 (33)	4 (67)	0	0
Charry [121]	1994	8	2/6	8.7	PFD	2 (25)	5 (63)	1 (12)	1 (12)
Farley [118]	1995	10	5/5	10.5	SSS	8 (80)	N/A	2 (20)	1 (10)
Ghanem [123]	1997	7	N/A	10.3	PFD	1 (14)	1 (14)	5 (72)	5 (72)
Hida [86]	1999	13	6/7	10.2	PFD + SSS	5 (38)	5 (38)	3 (23)	3 (23)
Sengupta [124]	2000	16	10/6	11	PFD	1 (6)	5 (31)	10 (63)	8 (50)
Kontio [96]	2002	4	2/2	11.7	PFD	2 (50)	0	2 (50)	1 (25)
Eule [84]	2002	8	N/A	N/A	PFD	1 (13)	4 (50)	3 (37)	0
Farley [125]	2002	9	2/7	8	PFD + SSS	3 (33)	0	6 (67)	5 (56)
Özerdemoglu [113]	2003	18	9/9	16.9	PFD + SSS	3 (17)	7 (39)	8 (44)	3 (17)
Brockmeyer [116]	2003	21	7/14	8.7	PFD	4 (19)	9 (43)	8 (38)	4 (19)
Flynn [119]	2004	15	6/9	9.0	PFD + SSS	4 (27)	2 (13)	9 (60)	7 (47)

Abbreviations: PFD, posterior fossa decompression; SSS, syringosubarachnoid shunt; TO, transoral decompression.

syrinx. Although the number of patients whose deformity improved could not be ascertained, eight patients had no progression, and only one patient eventually required a fusion. Özerdemoglu and colleagues [113] demonstrated that patients who underwent a suboccipital craniectomy had a superior outcome in terms of improving their scoliosis compared with patients who had direct syrinx shunting and required fewer reoperations for recurrent syrinx. In the study by Brockmeyer and colleagues [116], 13 of 21 (62%) patients had their curves improve or stay the same during the follow-up period after suboccipital decompression. Patients who were male, less than 10 years of age and with curves less than 40 degrees at the time of their decompression were more likely to have their curves improve over time. Similarly, Flynn and colleagues [119] found that those children who had progression of their scoliosis tended to have a larger curve at presentation, later age at hindbrain decompression, double curves, kyphosis, and rotation. One of the most dramatic curve corrections was presented by Mollano and colleagues in a 5-year-old boy whose 54-degree curve improved to only 4 degrees after a posterior fossa decompression [120].

Summary

Chiari I and II are the most common hindbrain malformations in the pediatric population. Despite their prevalence, the complex nature of their presentation, often including hydrocephalus, syringohydromyelia, and scoliosis, has prevented clinicians from establishing universal treatment protocols.

The increased use of MRI has facilitated the early diagnosis of CMI and has helped clarify the relationship between pediatric scoliosis, syringohydromyelia, and the Chiari malformations.

The most common symptom in patients who have CMI is occipital headache/neck pain, which can be expected in 40% to 75% of patients. Syringomyelia is present in 20% to 85% of patients who have Chiari I and scoliosis is present in 14% to 50%. Patients who have CMII invariably have a myelomeningocele. Approximately 80% of these children will develop hydrocephalus, and 48% to 88% will develop syringohydromyelia. Scoliosis is detected in 50% to 90% of patients. The presentation of brain stem compression occurs in roughly 20% of patients who have Chiari II and generally takes on one of two patterns. In younger patients, respiratory and GI symptoms can be rapidly progressive, often requiring urgent surgical intervention. In older children, symptoms develop more slowly and rarely merit urgent intervention.

The mainstay for the surgical treatment of Chiari malformations is posterior fossa decompression. In children who have CMI, dural opening and exploration of intradural structures is favored by some surgeons, while others limit the procedure to extradural decompression. Posterior fossa decompression also indirectly treats syringohydromyelia and, along with syrinx shunting, represents the main surgical treatment modality for syringes associated with Chiari malformation. In many cases, syrinx treatment has been demonstrated to stabilize or improve pediatric scoliosis, and surgical fusion is reserved for children who progress despite posterior fossa decompression and syrinx treatment.

Future clinical research for patients who have Chiari malformation looks to identify which patients will benefit from dural opening at surgery, and which, if any, should have syrinx shunting or other intradural maneuvers performed as part of first-line surgical therapy.

References

[1] Mikulis DJ, et al. Variance of the position of the cerebellar tonsils with age: preliminary report. Radiology 1992;183(3):725–8.
[2] Armonda RA, et al. Quantitative cine-mode magnetic resonance imaging of Chiari I malformations: an analysis of cerebrospinal fluid dynamics. Neurosurgery 1994;35(2):214–23; discussion 223–4.
[3] Bejjani GK. Definition of the adult Chiari malformation: a brief historical overview. Neurosurg Focus 2001;11(1):E1.
[4] Haroun RI, et al. Current opinions for the treatment of syringomyelia and chiari malformations: survey of the Pediatric Section of the American Association of Neurological Surgeons. Pediatr Neurosurg 2000;33(6):311–7.
[5] Meadows J, et al. Asymptomatic Chiari Type I malformations identified on magnetic resonance imaging. J Neurosurg 2000;92(6):920–6.
[6] Nishizawa S, et al. Incidentally identified syringomyelia associated with Chiari I malformations: is early interventional surgery necessary? Neurosurgery 2001;49(3):637–40; discussion 640–1.
[7] Stovner LJ, et al. Posterior cranial fossa dimensions in the Chiari I malformation: relation to pathogenesis and clinical presentation. Neuroradiology 1993;35(2):113–8.
[8] Milhorat TH, et al. Chiari I malformation redefined: clinical and radiographic findings for 364 symptomatic patients. Neurosurgery 1999;44(5):1005–17.
[9] Sgouros S, Kountouri M, Natarajan K. Posterior fossa volume in children with Chiari malformation Type I. J Neurosurg 2006;105(2 Suppl):101–6.
[10] Gardner WJ. Hydrodynamic mechanism of syringomyelia: Its relationship to myelocele. J Neurol Neurosurg Psychiatry 1965;28:247–59.
[11] Williams B. On the pathogenesis of syringomyelia: a review. J R Soc Med 1980;73(11):798–806.
[12] Williams B. Pathogenesis of syringomyelia. Acta Neurochir (Wien) 1993;123(3-4):159–65.
[13] Alden TD, Ojemann JG, Park TS. Surgical treatment of Chiari I malformation: indications and approaches. Neurosurg Focus 2001;11(1):E2.
[14] Ellenbogen RG, et al. Toward a rational treatment of Chiari I malformation and syringomyelia. Neurosurg Focus 2000;8(3):E6.
[15] Menezes AH. Primary craniovertebral anomalies and the hindbrain herniation syndrome (Chiari I): data base analysis. Pediatr Neurosurg 1995;23(5):260–9.
[16] Navarro R, et al. Surgical results of posterior fossa decompression for patients with Chiari I malformation. Childs Nerv Syst 2004;20(5):349–56.
[17] Nishikawa M, et al. Pathogenesis of Chiari malformation: a morphometric study of the posterior cranial fossa. J Neurosurg 1997;86(1):40–7.
[18] Schijman E. History, anatomic forms, and pathogenesis of Chiari I malformations. Childs Nerv Syst 2004;20(5):323–8.
[19] Cavender RK, Schmidt JH 3rd. Tonsillar ectopia and Chiari malformations: monozygotic triplets. Case report. J Neurosurg 1995;82(3):497–500.
[20] Mavinkurve GG, et al. Familial Chiari type I malformation with syringomyelia in two siblings: case report and review of the literature. Childs Nerv Syst 2005;21(11):955–9.
[21] Speer MC, et al. A genetic hypothesis for Chiari I malformation with or without syringomyelia. Neurosurg Focus 2000;8(3):E12.
[22] Szewka AJ, et al. Chiari in the family: inheritance of the Chiari I malformation. Pediatr Neurol 2006;34(6):481–5.
[23] Genitori L, et al. Chiari type I anomalies in children and adolescents: minimally invasive management in a series of 53 cases. Childs Nerv Syst 2000;16(10–11):707–18.
[24] Cheng JS, Nash J, Meyer GA. Chiari type I malformation revisited: diagnosis and treatment. Neurologist 2002;8(6):357–62.
[25] Steinbok P. Clinical features of Chiari I malformations. Childs Nerv Syst 2004;20(5):329–31.
[26] Alzate JC, et al. Treatment of Chiari I malformation in patients with and without syringomyelia: a consecutive series of 66 cases. Neurosurg Focus 2001;11(1):E3.

[27] Krieger MD, McComb JG, Levy ML. Toward a simpler surgical management of Chiari I malformation in a pediatric population. Pediatr Neurosurg 1999;30(3):113–21.

[28] Park JK, et al. Presentation and management of Chiari I malformation in children. Pediatr Neurosurg 1997;26(4):190–6.

[29] Pascual J, Oterino A, Berciano J. Headache in type I Chiari malformation. Neurology 1992;42(8):1519–21.

[30] Tubbs RS, McGirt MJ, Oakes WJ. Surgical experience in 130 pediatric patients with Chiari I malformations. J Neurosurg 2003;99(2):291–6.

[31] Nohria V, Oakes WJ. Chiari I malformation: a review of 43 patients. Pediatr Neurosurg 1990;16(4–5):222–7.

[32] Listernick R, Tomita T. Persistent crying in infancy as a presentation of Chiari type I malformation. J Pediatr 1991;118(4 (Pt 1)):567–9.

[33] Combarros O, Alvarez de Arcaya A, Berciano J. Isolated unilateral hypoglossal nerve palsy: nine cases. J Neurol 1998;245(2):98–100.

[34] Dyste GN, Menezes AH, VanGilder JC. Symptomatic Chiari malformations. An analysis of presentation, management, and long-term outcome. J Neurosurg 1989;71(2):159–68.

[35] Ruff ME, et al. Sleep apnea and vocal cord paralysis secondary to type I Chiari malformation. Pediatrics 1987;80(2):231–4.

[36] Yoshimi A, Nomura K, Furune S. Sleep apnea syndrome associated with a type I Chiari malformation. Brain Dev 2002;24(1):49–51.

[37] Menick BJ. Phase-contrast magnetic resonance imaging of cerebrospinal fluid flow in the evaluation of patients with Chiari I malformation. Neurosurg Focus 2001;11(1):E5.

[38] Gambardella G, et al. Transverse microincisions of the outer layer of the dura mater combined with foramen magnum decompression as treatment for syringomyelia with Chiari I malformation. Acta Neurochir (Wien) 1998;140(2):134–9.

[39] Schijman E, Steinbok P. International survey on the management of Chiari I malformation and syringomyelia. Childs Nerv Syst 2004;20(5):341–8.

[40] Anderson RC, et al. Chiari I malformation: potential role for intraoperative electrophysiologic monitoring. J Clin Neurophysiol 2003;20(1):65–72.

[41] Klekamp J, et al. The surgical treatment of Chiari I malformation. Acta Neurochir (Wien) 1996;138(7):788–801.

[42] Oldfield EH, et al. Pathophysiology of syringomyelia associated with Chiari I malformation of the cerebellar tonsils. Implications for diagnosis and treatment. J Neurosurg 1994;80(1):3–15.

[43] Blagodatsky MD, et al. Surgical treatment of Chiari I malformation with or without syringomyelia. Acta Neurochir (Wien) 1999;141(9):963–8.

[44] Anderson RC, et al. Improvement in brainstem auditory evoked potentials after suboccipital decompression in patients with chiari I malformations. J Neurosurg 2003;98(3):459–64.

[45] Yeh DD, Koch B, Crone KR. Intraoperative ultrasonography used to determine the extent of surgery necessary during posterior fossa decompression in children with Chiari malformation type I. J Neurosurg 2006;105(1 Suppl):26–32.

[46] Munshi I, et al. Effects of posterior fossa decompression with and without duraplasty on Chiari malformation-associated hydromyelia. Neurosurgery 2000;46(6):1384–9; discussion 1389–90.

[47] Osborn A. Diagnostic Neuroradiology, Vol. 1. St. Louis: Mosby, Inc.; 1994. p. 802.

[48] McLone DG, Knepper PA. The cause of Chiari II malformation: a unified theory. Pediatr Neurosci 1989;15(1):1–12.

[49] McLone DG, Naidich TP. Developmental morphology of the subarachnoid space, brain vasculature, and contiguous structures, and the cause of the Chiari II malformation. AJNR Am J Neuroradiol 1992;13(2):463–82.

[50] Jacob R, Rhoton A. The Chiari I Malformation, in Neurosurgical Topics: Syringomyelia and the Chiari Malformations, JA A, Benzel E, Awad I. editors. Park Ridge, Ill: AANS; 1997.

[51] McLone DG. The Chiari II Malformation of the Hindbrain and the Associated Hydromyelia. In: Anson J, Benzel E, Awad I, editors. Neurosurgical Topics: Syringomyelia and the Chiari Malformations. Park Ridge, Ill: AANS; 1997.

[52] Stevenson KL. Chiari Type II malformation: past, present, and future. Neurosurg Focus 2004;16(2):E5.

[53] Marlin AE. Management of hydrocephalus in the patient with myelomeningocele: an argument against third ventriculostomy. Neurosurg Focus 2004;16(2):E4.

[54] Piggott H. The natural history of scoliosis in myelodysplasia. J Bone Joint Surg Br 1980;62–B(1):54–8.

[55] Tubbs RS, et al. Chiari II malformation and occult spinal dysraphism. Case reports and a review of the literature. Pediatr Neurosurg 2003;39(2):104–7.

[56] Pollack IF, Kinnunen D, Albright AL. The effect of early craniocervical decompression on functional outcome in neonates and young infants with myelodysplasia and symptomatic Chiari II malformations: results from a prospective series. Neurosurgery 1996;38(4):703–10; discussion 710.

[57] Pollack IF, et al. Outcome following hindbrain decompression of symptomatic Chiari malformations in children previously treated with myelomeningocele closure and shunts. J Neurosurg 1992;77(6):881–8.

[58] Teo C, et al. The Chiari II malformation: a surgical series. Pediatr Neurosurg 1997;27(5):223–9.

[59] Vandertop WP, et al. Surgical decompression for symptomatic Chiari II malformation in neonates with myelomeningocele. J Neurosurg 1992;77(4):541–4.

[60] Park TS, et al. Experience with surgical decompression of the Arnold-Chiari malformation in young infants with myelomeningocele. J Neurosurgery 1983;13(2):147–52.

[61] Worley G, Schuster JM, Oakes WJ. Survival at 5 years of a cohort of newborn infants with myelomeningocele. Dev Med Child Neurol 1996;38(9):816–22.

[62] Tubbs RS, Oakes WJ. Treatment and management of the Chiari II malformation: an evidence-based review of the literature. Childs Nerv Syst 2004;20(6):375–81.

[63] Narayan P, et al. Clinical significance of cervicomedullary deformity in Chiari II malformation. Pediatr Neurosurg 2001;35(3):140–4.

[64] Barnet AB, Weiss IP, Shaer C. Evoked potentials in infant brainstem syndrome associated with Arnold-Chiari malformation. Dev Med Child Neurol 1993;35(1):42–8.

[65] Caldarelli M, Di Rocco C. Diagnosis of Chiari I malformation and related syringomyelia: radiological and neurophysiological studies. Childs Nerv Syst 2004;20(5):332–5.

[66] Worley G, et al. BAEPs in infants with myelomeningocele and later development of Chiari II malformation-related brainstem dysfunction. Dev Med Child Neurol 1994;36(8):707–15.

[67] Caldarelli M, et al. Surgical treatment of late neurological deterioration in children with myelodysplasia. Acta Neurochir (Wien) 1995;137(3-4):199–206.

[68] Milhorat TH, et al. Surgical treatment of syringomyelia based on magnetic resonance imaging criteria. Neurosurgery 1992;31(2):231–44; discussion 244–5.

[69] Cinalli G, et al. Failure of third ventriculostomy in the treatment of aqueductal stenosis in children. J Neurosurg 1999;90(3):448–54.

[70] Teo C, Jones R. Management of hydrocephalus by endoscopic third ventriculostomy in patients with myelomeningocele. Pediatr Neurosurg 1996;25(2):57–63; discussion 63.

[71] Pollack IF, et al. Neurogenic dysphagia resulting from Chiari malformations. Neurosurgery 1992;30(5):709–19.

[72] Bell WO, et al. Symptomatic Arnold-Chiari malformation: review of experience with 22 cases. J Neurosurg 1987;66(6):812–6.

[73] James HE, Brant A. Treatment of the Chiari malformation with bone decompression without durotomy in children and young adults. Childs Nerv Syst 2002;18(5):202–6.

[74] McLaughlin MR, Wahlig JB, Pollack IF. Incidence of postlaminectomy kyphosis after Chiari decompression. Spine 1997;22(6):613–7.

[75] Gardner WJ, Goodall RJ. The surgical treatment of Arnold-Chiari malformation in adults; an explanation of its mechanism and importance of encephalography in diagnosis. J Neurosurg 1950;7(3):199–206.

[76] Williams B. The distending force in the production of "communicating syringomyelia". Lancet 1969;2(7613):189–93.

[77] Ball MJ, Dayan AD. Pathogenesis of syringomyelia. Lancet 1972;2(7781):799–801.

[78] Milhorat TH, et al. Anatomical basis of syringomyelia occurring with hindbrain lesions. Neurosurgery 1993;32(5):748–54; discussion 754.

[79] Heiss JD, et al. Elucidating the pathophysiology of syringomyelia. J Neurosurg 1999;91(4):553–62.

[80] Greitz D, et al. Pulsatile brain movement and associated hydrodynamics studied by magnetic resonance phase imaging. The Monro-Kellie doctrine revisited. Neuroradiology 1992;34(5):370–80.

[81] Stoodley MA, Gutschmidt B, Jones NR. Cerebrospinal fluid flow in an animal model of noncommunicating syringomyelia. Neurosurgery 1999;44(5):1065–75; discussion 1075–6.

[82] Stovner LJ, Rinck P. Syringomyelia in Chiari malformation: relation to extent of cerebellar tissue herniation. Neurosurgery 1992;31(5):913–7; discussion 917.

[83] Hida K, et al. Pediatric syringomyelia with chiari malformation: its clinical characteristics and surgical outcomes. Surg Neurol 1999;51(4):383–90; discussion 390–1.

[84] Eule JM, et al. Chiari I malformation associated with syringomyelia and scoliosis: a twenty-year review of surgical and nonsurgical treatment in a pediatric population. Spine 2002;27(13):1451–5.

[85] Isu T, et al. Hydrosyringomyelia associated with a Chiari I malformation in children and adolescents. Neurosurgery 1990;26(4):591–6; discussion 596–7.

[86] Feldstein NA, Choudhri TF. Management of Chiari I malformations with holocord syringohydromyelia. Pediatr Neurosurg 1999;31(3):143–9.

[87] Sakamoto H, et al. Expansive suboccipital cranioplasty for the treatment of syringomyelia associated with Chiari malformation. Acta Neurochir (Wien) 1999;141(9):949–60; discussion 960–1.

[88] McIlroy WJ, Richardson JC. Syringomyelia: a clinical review of 75 cases. Can Med Assoc J 1965;93(14):731–4.

[89] Woods WW, Pimenta AM. Intramedullary lesions of the spinal cord: study of sixty-eight consecutive cases. Arch Neurol Psych 1944;52:383–99.

[90] Phillips WA, Hensinger RN, Kling TF Jr. Management of scoliosis due to syringomyelia in childhood and adolescence. J Pediatr Orthop 1990;10(3):351–4.

[91] Huebert HT, MacKinnon WB. Syringomyelia and scoliosis. J Bone Joint Surg Br 1969;51(2):338–43.

[92] Isu T, et al. Scoliosis associated with syringomyelia presenting in children. Childs Nerv Syst 1992;8(2):97–100.

[93] Mejia EA, et al. A prospective evaluation of idiopathic left thoracic scoliosis with magnetic resonance imaging. J Pediatr Orthop 1996;16(3):354–8.

[94] Williams B. Orthopaedic features in the presentation of syringomyelia. J Bone Joint Surg Br 1979; 61–B(3):314–23.

[95] Williams B. Syringomyelia. Neurosurg Clin N Am 1990;1(3):653–85.

[96] Kontio K, Davidson D, Letts M. Management of scoliosis and syringomyelia in children. J Pediatr Orthop 2002;22(6):771–9.

[97] Spiegel DA, et al. Scoliotic curve patterns in patients with Chiari I malformation and/or syringomyelia. Spine 2003;28(18):2139–46.

[98] Tomlinson RJ Jr, et al. Syringomyelia and developmental scoliosis. J Pediatr Orthop 1994;14(5): 580–5.

[99] Arai S, et al. Scoliosis associated with syringomyelia. Spine 1993;18(12):1591–2.

[100] Schwend RM, et al. Childhood scoliosis: clinical indications for magnetic resonance imaging. J Bone Joint Surg Am 1995;77(1):46–53.

[101] Zadeh HG, et al. Absent superficial abdominal reflexes in children with scoliosis. An early indicator of syringomyelia. J Bone Joint Surg Br 1995;77(5): 762–7.

[102] Evans SC, et al. MRI of 'idiopathic' juvenile scoliosis. A prospective study. J Bone Joint Surg Br 1996;78(2):314–7.

[103] Lewonowski K, King JD, Nelson MD. Routine use of magnetic resonance imaging in idiopathic scoliosis patients less than eleven years of age. Spine 1992; 17(6 Suppl):S109–16.

[104] Loder RT, Stasikelis P, Farley FA. Sagittal profiles of the spine in scoliosis associated with an Arnold-Chiari malformation with or without syringomyelia. J Pediatr Orthop 2002;22(4):483–91.

[105] Inoue M, et al. Preoperative MRI analysis of patients with idiopathic scoliosis: a prospective study. Spine 2005;30(1):108–14.

[106] Samuelsson L, Lindell D. Scoliosis as the first sign of a cystic spinal cord lesion. Eur Spine J 1995;4(5): 284–90.

[107] Ouellet JA, et al. Sagittal plane deformity in the thoracic spine: a clue to the presence of syringomyelia as a cause of scoliosis. Spine 2003;28(18): 2147–51.

[108] Barnes PD, et al. Atypical idiopathic scoliosis: MR imaging evaluation. Radiology 1993;186(1): 247–53.

[109] Winter RB, et al. Magnetic resonance imaging evaluation of the adolescent patient with idiopathic scoliosis before spinal instrumentation and fusion. A prospective, double-blinded study of 140 patients. Spine 1997;22(8):855–8.

[110] Maiocco B, et al. Adolescent idiopathic scoliosis and the presence of spinal cord abnormalities. Preoperative magnetic resonance imaging analysis. Spine 1997;22(21):2537–41.

[111] Whitaker C, Schoenecker PL, Lenke LG. Hyperkyphosis as an indicator of syringomyelia in idiopathic scoliosis: a case report. Spine 2003;28(1): E16–20.

[112] Ozerdemoglu RA, Denis F, Transfeldt EE. Scoliosis associated with syringomyelia: clinical and radiologic correlation. Spine 2003;28(13):1410–7.

[113] Ozerdemoglu RA, Transfeldt EE, Denis F. Value of treating primary causes of syrinx in scoliosis associated with syringomyelia. Spine 2003;28(8): 806–14.

[114] Tokunaga M, et al. Natural history of scoliosis in children with syringomyelia. J Bone Joint Surg Br 2001;83(3):371–6.

[115] Tubbs RS, et al. Scoliosis in a child with Chiari I malformation and the absence of syringomyelia: case report and a review of the literature. Childs Nerv Syst 2006.

[116] Brockmeyer D, Gollogly S, Smith JT. Scoliosis associated with Chiari 1 malformations: the effect of suboccipital decompression on scoliosis curve progression: a preliminary study. Spine 2003;28(22): 2505–9.

[117] Muhonen MG, et al. Scoliosis in pediatric Chiari malformations without myelodysplasia. J Neurosurg 1992;77(1):69–77.

[118] Farley FA, et al. Syringomyelia and scoliosis in children. J Pediatr Orthop 1995;15(2):187–92.

[119] Flynn JM, et al. Predictors of progression of scoliosis after decompression of an Arnold Chiari I malformation. Spine 2004;29(3):286–92.

[120] Mollano AV, Weinstein SL, Menezes AH. Significant scoliosis regression following syringomyelia decompression: case report. Iowa Orthop J 2005; 25:57–9.

[121] Charry O, et al. Syringomyelia and scoliosis: a review of twenty-five pediatric patients. J Pediatr Orthop 1994;14(3):309–17.

[122] Asch L. [Rheumatologic aspects of syringomyelia]. Rhumatologie 1972;24(6):207–11.

[123] Ghanem IB, et al. Chiari I malformation associated with syringomyelia and scoliosis. Spine 1997; 22(12):1313–7; discussion 1318.

[124] Sengupta DK, Dorgan J, Findlay GF. Can hindbrain decompression for syringomyelia lead to regression of scoliosis? Eur Spine J 2000;9(3): 198–201.

[125] Farley FA, et al. Curve progression in scoliosis associated with Chiari I malformation following suboccipital decompression. J Spinal Disord Tech 2002;15(5):410–4.

ELSEVIER
SAUNDERS

Neurosurg Clin N Am 18 (2007) 569–574

NEUROSURGERY
CLINICS
OF NORTH AMERICA

Index

Note: Page numbers of article titles are in **boldface** type.

1042-3680/07/$ - see front matter © 2007 Elsevier Inc. All rights reserved.
doi:10.1016/S1042-3680(07)00068-X

Moving?

Make sure your subscription moves with you!

To notify us of your new address, find your **Clinics Account Number** (located on your mailing label above your name), and contact customer service at:

E-mail: elspcs@elsevier.com

800-654-2452 (subscribers in the U.S. & Canada)
407-345-4000 (subscribers outside of the U.S. & Canada)

Fax number: 407-363-9661

Elsevier Periodicals Customer Service
6277 Sea Harbor Drive
Orlando, FL 32887-4800

*To ensure uninterrupted delivery of your subscription, please notify us at least 4 weeks in advance of move.

ELSEVIER